Human Rights and Social Justice

Human Rights and Social Justice: Key Issues and Vulnerable Populations is a comprehensive text that focuses on central issues of human rights and justice and links them directly with social work competencies and practice. Drawing attention to oppression and multiple forms of disadvantage and discrimination based on a person's identity and social location, this volume develops an integrated framework to advance human rights and social, economic, and environmental justice with vulnerable populations and communities across all three levels of practice.

Each chapter, written by leading scholars in their respective fields, is designed to enhance students' awareness, knowledge, and understanding of key theories and issues related to diversity, human rights, and equity. Broken into sections providing theory, practice, and case study illustrations, the chapters will first explain and argue that each person, regardless of their position in society, has basic human rights. Students will then see how these knowledges translate into practice through clear and engaging cases that reinforce skills and behaviors that social workers may use to advocate for human rights and ensure that they are distributed equitably and without prejudice.

Providing a broad overview of social justice and rights-based challenges and connecting theory to the profession's core competencies, this book is an excellent companion for social work students and faculty engaged in foundation and advanced courses in practice with individuals, groups, and communities and diversity and oppression.

Carole Cox is Professor at the Graduate School of Social Service at Fordham University. She is a Fellow of the Gerontological Society of America and the author of more than 75 journal articles and chapters focusing on various aspects of aging and caregiving, as well as nine books.

Tina Maschi is Associate Professor at the Graduate School of Social Service at Fordham University, with clinical and research experience in juvenile and criminal justice settings and community health settings.

Human Rights and Social Justice

Key Issues and Vulnerable Populations

Edited by Carole Cox and Tina Maschi

Routledge
Taylor & Francis Group
NEW YORK AND LONDON

Cover image: Shutterstock/Lars Poyansky

First published 2023
by Routledge
605 Third Avenue, New York, NY 10158

and by Routledge
4 Park Square, Milton Park, Abingdon, Oxon, OX14 4RN

Routledge is an imprint of the Taylor & Francis Group, an informa business

Library of Congress Cataloging-in-Publication Data
Names: Cox, Carole B., editor. | Maschi, Tina, editor.
Title: Human rights and social justice : key issues and vulnerable populations / edited by Carole Cox and Tina Maschi.
Description: New York, NY : Routledge Books, 2023. | Includes bibliographical references and index.
Identifiers: LCCN 2022015301 (print) | LCCN 2022015302 (ebook) | ISBN 9780367628819 (hardback) | ISBN 9780367628796 (paperback) | ISBN 9781003111269 (ebook)
Subjects: LCSH: Social work with minorities. | Social work with people with disabilities. | Social service. | Human rights. | Social justice. | Marginality, Social.
Classification: LCC HV3176 .H846 2022 (print) | LCC HV3176 (ebook) | DDC 362.84—dc23/eng/20220716
LC record available at https://lccn.loc.gov/2022015301
LC ebook record available at https://lccn.loc.gov/2022015302

ISBN: 978-0-367-62881-9 (hbk)
ISBN: 978-0-367-62879-6 (pbk)
ISBN: 978-1-003-11126-9 (ebk)

DOI: 10.4324/9781003111269

Typeset in Bembo
by Apex CoVantage, LLC

Contents

Contributors

Dean Adams, LMSW, is a recent graduate from Fordham University with interests in social justice, feminism, equity, and intersectionality. Dean is an aspiring LCSW, with goals of utilizing direct practice as a way to assist and empower the queer community through micro, macro, and research-oriented practices.

Keith Adamson is a social worker and Assistant Professor with the Factor-Inwentash Faculty of Social Work at the University of Toronto, where he is involved with the program's Teaching Stream. He has held positions in clinical, management, and professional practice roles for more than 20 years.

Wasif Ali is a postdoctoral associate in the Faculty of Social Work at the University of Calgary. Dr. Ali's research interests include green social work, environmental justice, and sustainable development. His practice experience has focused on water and environmental sustainability through community and stakeholder engagements.

Rachelle Ashcroft is a social worker and Assistant Professor with the Factor-Inwentash Faculty of Social Work at the University of Toronto. She has over 14 years of experience as a social worker in community health and tertiary care settings.

Rosemary A. Barbera is a social worker who has been working in human rights since the 1980s in the United States and Latin America, including roles helping immigrants fleeing war and the violence of poverty from Latin America and Africa. She lived in Bolivia and Chile and was a human rights worker in both countries, and she continues her work with survivors of human rights abuses in Chile as well as with the family members of the disappeared there.

Padma Christie is an MSW candidate, educator, and Research Assistant at Fordham University. Her interest areas include school social work, clinical practice, and LGBT+ research. Padma is an aspiring LCSW and looks forward to supporting children, adults, and families through group and direct practice.

Monique Constance-Huggins is Associate Professor and Undergraduate Program Director in the Department of Social Work at Winthrop University. She received her PhD, MSW, and MPIA from the University of Pittsburgh. She is a critical race social work scholar, who researches topics on race such as racial disparities, oppression, and ideologies.

Carole Cox is Professor in the Graduate School of Social Service at Fordham University. She is a Fellow of the Gerontological Society of America and a Fulbright Scholar. She also serves as a representative of the International Association of Gerontology and Geriatrics (IAGG) to the United Nations.

Smita Ekka Dewan, PhD, LMSW, is Assistant Professor in the Human Services department at New York City College of Technology, CUNY. Her teaching and scholarly interests include social work practice with immigrants and refugees, violence against women, international social work, human rights and social justice, and program evaluation.

Julie L. Drolet is Professor in the Faculty of Social Work at the University of Calgary and also Project Director of the Transforming the Field Education Landscape partnership. Dr. Drolet leads an international social work research program to advance knowledge in the fields of social work and social development.

Richard Enns, PhD RSW, is Associate Professor in the Faculty of Social Work at the University of Calgary. Dr. Enns has a background in forensic mental health and residential treatment of adolescents. His research interests include services for youth in transition and colonial and historical continuities between Canada's industrial and residential school systems for Indigenous students and current child welfare systems and practices.

Susan Gallagher, MSW RSW, is a clinical social worker who lives, teaches, and practices in Waterloo, Ontario. She views the world through a trauma-informed lens and embraces ongoing opportunities for integrating theory and practice.

Rina Goldstein, LSW, LMSW, is a recent clinical social work graduate whose interests lie in individual and group psychotherapy, clinical research, and holistic therapeutic interventions. Rina plans to contribute to mental health and substance use research and to apply innovative findings in her practice.

Jesse Henton is a research assistant and an MSW Foundation student in his second year at the University of Calgary. He holds an MA in Political Science.

Adriana Maya Kaye, LMSW, is a second-year doctoral student at Tulane University in Louisiana, a psychotherapist, and an emerging research and scholar.

Caroline Lee is Senior Lecturer in Social Work at Birmingham City University, UK. Prior to working in social work education, she worked with adults with a learning disability and complex needs, including work in forensic settings. Caroline's particular areas of interest and expertise are adult safeguarding and disability hate crime.

Sarah Malis is an MSW candidate and Research Assistant at Fordham University. Her research areas include clinical practice, qualitative research, and social justice. Sarah is an aspiring LCSW and has future goals of supporting others through direct practice.

Tina Maschi, PhD, LCSW, and ACSW, is a professor, researcher, scholar, professional musician, and an artist. She has more than 150 publications in peer-reviewed journals and five books, including her most recent co-authored book with Keith Morgen, *Aging Behind Prison Walls: Studies of Trauma and Resilience* (2020).

Anne Marie McLaughlin, PhD RSW, is Associate Professor on the faculty of Social Work at the University of Calgary. Dr. McLaughlin has a practice background in community mental health and child welfare. Her research interests are in the areas of professional social work practice, practice regulation, and the translation of professional values into practice.

Keith Morgen, PhD, LPC, ACS, is Associate Professor of Counseling and Director of the Graduate Counseling Programs at Centenary University in New Jersey. Dr. Morgen is the author of over 35 scholarly articles, the book *Substance Use Disorders and Addictions* (Sage 2016), and co-author of the book *Aging Behind Prison Walls: Studies in Trauma and Resilience* (Columbia University Press 2020).

Manoj Pardasani, PhD, LCSW, is Dean and Professor in the School of Social Work at Adelphi University. Previously, he served as Associate Provost (Graduate and Professional Schools) and Professor of Social Work at Hunter College in New York, Faculty Research Scholar at the Ravazzin Center for Social Work Research in Aging, and Senior Associate Dean at the Fordham University Graduate School of Social Service.

Stacey A. Shaw, PhD, MSW, is Assistant Professor in the School of Social Work at Brigham Young University, where she has worked since 2016. Her research examines refugee experiences and services in the United States and in Malaysia. Prior to obtaining a PhD in Social Work from Columbia University, she worked as a social worker in refugee resettlement services for the International Rescue Committee.

Peter Simcock, PhD, is Senior Lecturer in Social Work at Birmingham City University, UK. Prior to working in social work education, he was a specialist social worker with d/Deaf and deafblind people. His doctoral studies focused on the lived experience of vulnerability among adults ageing with deafblindness. Peter is the co-author of the Polity book *Social Work and Disability*.

Cassandra E. Simon is Associate Professor at the University of Alabama. Prior to her appointment there, she was on faculty at the University of Texas at Arlington. She has worked in higher education for over 30 years, focusing her work on justice, anti-oppression, and the promotion of an equitable world.

Sandra G. Turner, PhD, LCSW, is Associate Professor in the Graduate School of Social Service at Fordham University. Her research, scholarly, and clinical interests include sexual abuse, feminism, empowerment, depression among women, and substance abuse.

Nicola C. Williams is Assistant Lecturer in the Department of Sociology, Psychology, and Social Work at the University of the West Indies in Jamaica. As Community Organization and Policy Social Work Practitioner, her interests include human rights, environmental justice, sustainable development, and international social work.

Joseph Wronka is Professor in the School of Social Work and Behavioral Sciences at Springfield College in Massachusetts. In addition to his faculty position, Dr. Wronka is also Representative to the United Nations in New York for the International Association of Schools of Social Work (IASSW).

Foreword

Only chosen values endure. The continuing dearth of protections for workers, pregnant mothers and their children, the older adults, and other oppressed groups; humanity's almost suicidal path to environmental destruction; continuing structural racism, classism, xenophobia, disableism, religious intolerance, ageism, mass shootings, and violence in general; the ever-present pandemic of COVID-19 with the threat of other scourges on the horizon; and the threat of nuclear annihilation are just a few of a plethora of reasons for a global need for a human rights culture. From the Latin *cultura* meaning "the cultivation or tilling of the land to prepare the growth of plants or crops," such a culture can be defined as a "lived awareness" of human rights principles in our minds and hearts, and integrated into our everyday lives. Such principles like human dignity, non-discrimination, and solidarity are not values that can just be memorized, "spit back" to the instructor on a multiple-choice exam in courses on social justice or human rights. They are values that need to be learned, not merely in a cognitive sense but in ways that encompass an individual's "being-in-the-world," to borrow a term from the existential-phenomenologists, thus having repercussions for society as a whole. Let us recall that the word "education" comes from the Latin *educare* meaning "to grow, nourish, and strengthen." That is what human rights can and should do. Its principles can serve as guiding lights to lead us out of a cauldron of atrocities to a socially just world, constructed from the pillars of human rights. This compendium of works edited by Drs. Cox and Maschi provides a good and solid blueprint to move toward a socially just world, eradicating those and other social malaises and promoting well-being for every person, everywhere.

The key I think is to integrate. From the Latin *integrare* meaning "to make whole" the journey from the mind to heart to body, if you will, is a long one, but a voyage, while unknown and perilous at times, can nevertheless be filled with adventure and satisfaction. Like the famed refugee of the Trojan War, Odysseus, seeking to reunite with his beloved Penelope on his voyage to Ithaca, tying himself to a mast so as not to be tempted by the beautiful voices of the Sirens and steering perilously between the monsters Scylla and Charybdis, so too we must hold steadfast to our principles, keeping our eyes on our goals, in this instance to create a human rights culture. Yet, despite his best efforts, Odysseus's ship sank. But he did not give up. On the verge of drowning, he saw a twig on the shore, swam to it, grabbed it, pulled himself out of the waters, and continued to Ithaca. Similarly, we must not give up and have what can be called a "pathological belief in the impossible." There is always a twig somewhere, somewhat a forest of opportunity if we will only look for it and not give up. This inspiring text can serve as an impetus with its theoretic explanations and practical implications so as to persist in the struggles for social justice.

To emphasize, human rights, the pillars of social justice, thus are not some abstract cognitive concept, nor are they "emotional botch" to borrow a phrase from Rev. Dr. Martin Luther King. They are a way of life. I invite readers to partake on this journey in this compilation of works here on the cutting edge of the field, which ultimately should expand readers' consciousness about ways that this powerful social construct "human rights," which emerged from the ashes of World War II, can serve through direct non-violent social policies and actions to carve out a socially just world, not only locally, regionally, or nationally but throughout the global community.

Perhaps the words of the internationalist Antoine de St. Exupery, author of the famed *The Little Prince* have relevance here: "If you want to build a ship, don't drum up people to collect wood and don't assign them tasks and work, but rather teach them to long for the endless immensity of the sea." Thus, if you are looking for a cookbook approach to human rights and social justice *Integrating Human Rights and Social Justice into Social Work Practice*, go elsewhere. But if you want inspiration, constructed from sound scholarship and research, as you "long for" a socially just world, this is that book. Imagine then a world where we all have our human rights fulfilled and live with human dignity and in a world at peace. Who would have thought that with the invention of gunpowder centuries ago that the world would now have enough firepower to destroy itself almost literally in a flash within hours? Such a nightmare has become an ever-present reality. But can we not dream of a socially just world, where every person/everywhere has his/her human rights? Let us recall also the words of the late Senator Robert Kennedy: "Some men [or women] see things as they are, and say why. I dream of things that never were, and say why not?" Should not that vision of a socially just world be enough to move us to action? Are we so socialized by the media, our history textbooks, and the like to view violence and war as the only antidote to our contemporary problems? What was it that Gandhi said about violence? "When it appears to do good, the good is only temporary. The evil it does is permanent." And a strong devotee of Gandhi, Martin Luther King, echoing that sentiment said, "What we learn from history is that we do not learn from history." As an alternative, what has become known as "soft power," in this case social justice, thus human rights principles, if chosen freely and without coercion, can serve to have a world where humans can develop alone, yet in community with others and in harmony with the natural world.

Human rights principles, thus, discussed throughout this tome, an extremely timely work, can serve metaphorically speaking as the "seeds" for society's growth, actually the entire global community, our interconnectedness made more starkly apparent, given the COVID-19 pandemic. The maldistribution of vaccines throughout the world, favoring the rich at the expense of the poor countries will ultimately affect all of us. As the philosopher/social activist Eric Fromm and author of *The Art of Loving* stated: "unlived life leads to destruction." Whereas certainly Black, Indigenous, Asian, Latinx, "Third World," and other lives matter, the debates must be how we can move toward a society, or rather in the words of Martin Luther King a "Beloved Community" a perilous, yet challenging voyage perhaps metaphorically akin to the journey of Odysseus in search of his beloved. Thus, we must not neglect the self-determination of these and other populations discussed throughout this work but must be concerned about a socially just world, where every person, everywhere matters. Recall that Martin Luther King's March on Washington was a March for Jobs and Freedoms for *All* (emphasis added). Indeed, a lot of our work then as non-violent social justice/human rights activists is often about paradox, ambiguity, and struggle, which, while difficult to do, must be embraced wholeheartedly. Thus, while we must work to improve the situation of Black lives, somewhere we need also to combat hatred of our Asian brothers and sisters, for one. The answer is not simple and will perhaps always be a struggle, fraught with ambiguities and dangers along the way. Perhaps it is more a matter of priorities where a person in his/her meditative life has decided to expend his/her energies, which is an entirely personal decision. The answer then, paradoxically, is in the questioning together.

Yet, whereas it is easy to give into a labyrinth of despair, we ought to recall a recurring archetype in humanity's history evidenced, for example, by all the evils hurled into the world by the insolent Pandora, who in defiance of Zeus opened up a mysterious box. But buried somewhere at the bottom of Pandora's Box as it became known was "hope," which to this day remains a clarion call, a call to consciousness to battle those wanton acts of violence mentioned at the beginning of this Foreword. After World War II, there was an estimated 92 million killed in battles, atomic bombings, and policies of mass starvation among other things, and let us not forget the 10 million killed in concentration camps, primarily Jews, but also Jehovah's Witnesses, one-fourth of Poland, Roma, and those inimical to the Third Reich. But humanity could have said, "We will always have war"; "Humans are basically selfish;" or "There is a genetic propensity to do evil in the world." In effect, "a socially just world with human rights at its core is utopian idealism, so why bother?"

But humanity did not give in. In 1945 it chose to create a United Nations. Certainly, there was a reluctance to include human rights in its Charter.

Nevertheless, those founding nations, upon pressure from NGOs brought in largely by the United States to the San Francisco Conference, where the U.N. was founded set up a drafting committee headed by an American Eleanor Roosevelt to come up with a human rights document that ultimately all nations of the world should adhere to. So, in 1948 they came up with the Universal Declaration of Human Rights, a "milestone in the long and difficult struggle of the human race" as Saint John Paul II put it and now increasingly referred to as *customary international law*, which all nations must abide. But, the U.N. did not stop there. With a hopeful attitude and pulling the world out of the murky waters of despair, holding on to that "twig," much like Odysseus never gave up hope, that international voluntary organization developed other documents like the Convention on the Rights of Children (CRC), the Convention to Eliminate Racial Discrimination (CERD), and the Convention on the Elimination of Discrimination Against Women (CEDAW) that further defined the principles of the Universal Declaration of Human Rights, as well as, implementation measures, like World Conferences, the Universal Periodic Review, and special rapporteurs. Collectively, all these initiatives have been referred to as The Human Rights Triptych, substantive to the major themes of this book. In short, while the journey has not been easy and today continues to pose many challenges, humanity like Odysseus on his way to Ithaca had decided to move forward on the way to a socially just world, a Beloved Community.

"There is one thing stronger than all the armies in the world, and that is an Idea whose time has come," wrote Viktor Hugo author of the famed *Les Misérables*, a story about an unjust sentencing of a man condemned to many years in prison for having stolen bread to feed his family. Human rights, which ought to be at the basis of social justice, is that idea. Now, more than 80 years after the Conference of Evian (1938) called by the United States to stop the abuses of the Third Reich, no country would dare say it is against human rights. But, at that time, the conference ended in failure because bringing attention to Hitler's atrocities would also put a spotlight on other countries' abuses. There were public lynchings of African Americans, genocide against Indigenous Peoples, and sprawling urban ghettos in the United States; Russia's own concentration camps; and other European countries' policies of torture and bloodshed in Africa. But, after that war, the world having born witness to all its hideousness, things changed. Continuing up to today in 2022, whatever a country does to its citizens is within the purview of the entire global community.

To be sure, this idea has relevance beyond simply governments' obligations to implement human rights. Many of the helping and health professions, for instance, have endorsed such principles in their practices and ethics codes. The International Federation of Social Work (IFSW) has stated: "From its inception social work has been a human rights profession." Building upon these principles, IFSW came up with The Charter of Rights for Social Workers which includes healthy and safe workplaces free from abuse, empowers service users, speaks out and engages in social action, develops a professional relationship with service users, provides career progression routes which maintain practice, offers clear guides of accountability and delegated authority, ensures reasonable caseloads and protection from burnout, works critically effectively and reflectively, advocates and lobbies for service users, advices and makes representation, takes reasonable risks, belongs to a professional association, advocates good working conditions and reasonable wages, contributes to policy development, and ensures respect for professional ethics. And both IFSW and the International Association of Schools of Social Work (IASSW) in 2020 came up with a Global Standards for Social Work Education, stating that schools of social work should aspire to develop curricula based on human rights principles.

Finally, it is common for the helping and health professions, social work in particular, to develop strategies to promote well-being, thus eradicating social and individual malaises using multipronged approaches. Very briefly, these strategies, which will be further explained in this book, have become known as meta-macro, global; macro, whole population; mezzo, at-risk; micro, clinical; and meta-micro, everyday life approaches. In each of those approaches, human rights principles have relevance. Thus, in brief, we have to help the homeless, build homeless shelters, treat them with dignity and provide meaningful and gainful employment, more or less micro interventions, but we must also develop proactive strategies, roughly macro interventions by adding a right to shelter on the US federal constitution, if not states' constitutions, which in the words of former Supreme Court Justice Louis Brandeis ought to act as "laboratories of democracy."

The compendium of works here is broad, yet each article is moving in its own way. Taken altogether they can have a synergistic effect, undoubtedly stirring the reader to action. The articles include, but are not limited to, discussions on the interdependency and indivisibility or rights, governments' *a la carte* approach to human rights, integrated (a.k.a. advanced generalist) practice, oppression and diversity, Indigenous issues, economic inequality, environmental justice, health and mental health, children and families, the elderly, persons with disabilities, criminal justice, sexual orientation and identity, refugees, and socially just actions to move toward the creation of a socially just world, constructed upon the foundation of human rights principles. I ask readers to read them with a hopeful spirit, yet, critical attitude. Only then can they come to their own conclusions, to choose their own values. Only then can such values last. The challenges are there. It is up to us to live and implement them.

Joseph Wronka
Amherst, MA
February 2, 2022

Part 1

Setting the Foundation

The many chapters in this book focus on two issues that are central not only to social work but also to the well-being of both individuals and societies in which they live—human rights and social justice. Human rights pertain to every person, regardless of who they are or where they live. They are basic to the enjoyment of full humanity and participation in society. Simply being human means that you are assured of dignity and the freedom to live a fulfilled life. Social justice pertains to the opportunities and distribution of resources within a society that support human rights and thus permit all people to thrive and develop equally. The first two chapters in this section provide a historical overview of human rights, along with the key international instruments that clarify and support their foundation, and a framework for integrating human rights and social justice into social work practice.

The recognition and implementation of human rights and social justice continue to evolve as the specific concerns of populations and groups are acknowledged and addressed. Consequently, the acknowledgement of new awareness and understanding is often manifested in new terms and definitions. As an example, terms related to race, ethnicity, and gender continue to change in efforts to promote broader acceptance and equality. Most likely, these terms will continue to change, but these changes must not take away from the fundamental concerns that they describe.

DOI: 10.4324/9781003111269-1

1 Conceptualizing Human Rights and Social Justice in Social Work

Carole Cox and Tina Maschi

Social work is a profession that focuses on change, with change ranging from the individual to society. Critical to the profession is that this change aims to improve lives and reduce disparities and inequalities for individuals, families, groups, and communities. This book focuses on groups that unduly experience disparities and inequalities, associated with group characteristics that are related to social exclusion, marginalization, and, frequently, oppression. Accordingly, the United Nations refers to these groups as vulnerable populations (UNDP, 2021). We are using the same term in this book. Without always being conscious of it, human rights and social justice are the goals that practitioners seek. At the micro-level, this may assume the purpose of assuring that clients are eligible for specific services and that their concerns are recognized. At the mezzo-level, service accessibility is important, while at the macro-level, this goal may involve significant policy changes. All of these actions reflect human rights and frequently demand reforms to assure social justice (Wronka, 2017).

Social work based on human rights and social justice affirms each person's dignity and autonomy, independence, and freedom to make their own choices, putting humans at the center of social work (Androff, 2015). These rights are linked with social justice as it is in a just society, built on non-discrimination and participation, and in recognition of each person's worth and their ability to develop and reach their full humanity (Wronka, 2017).

L1 Human Rights

The idea of human rights has been discussed and reinterpreted for centuries. The Code of Hammurabi (1795–1750 BC) was composed of laws that outlined the ethical conduct to be expected of people in their relationships and obligations to each other with strict punishments for violators. The Judaic system in the Old Testament and compiled in the Ten Commandments dictates obligations and duties that support individuals and the society in which they live. The Hindu Vedas, the Quran, and the Analects of Confucius further dictate duties, rights, and responsibilities that people are expected to uphold in their lives and social interactions. However, it is Cyrus the Great

DOI: 10.4324/9781003111269-2

(539 BC), the first king of Persia, who freed the slaves, declared all people had the right to choose their religion, and established racial equality, who is believed to have written the first real charter on human rights, with the decrees written on a clay cylinder.

The Universal Declaration of Human Rights (UDHR), approved by the General Assembly of the United Nations in 1948, embodies the principles that all nations are expected to follow to promote human rights. The rights apply to all human beings, regardless of nationality, residence, sex, religion, or another status. The UDHR is considered the foundation for international human rights law as it presents specific obligations for governments to promote rights. Under international law, human rights violations and abuses subject a country to an investigation by the United Nations. However, these investigations must be agreed to by the specific country. The intention is that by working with the country, the issue may be resolved. If not, the UN has the authority to pass a resolution condemning the country for specific human rights abuses.

The fundamental belief underlying the rights is human dignity, inherent for all people, and which serves as the foundation for the rights for freedom, justice, and world peace. The Declaration comprises 30 Articles that articulate the standards that nations are expected to meet to secure this dignity. Critical to the framework is the universality of human rights. They apply to all people and their indivisibility; no one right is more important than another and violating one right impacts other rights. By signing the Declaration, the member states of the United Nations agreed to strive to promote the rights and freedoms they entail (Wronka, 2017)

The UDHR rests upon five core notions: the importance of human dignity; non-discrimination; civil and political rights; economic, social, and cultural rights; and rights to solidarity (Wronka, 2017). Together these rights contribute to societies where all people have the same opportunities, protections, and supports. These rights, as they affirm the value and worth of the person, their autonomy, and their right to make their own choices form the basis of a rights-based approach to social work practice (Androff, 2015. The UDHR is also used to inform empowerment-based assessment and social work interventions with vulnerable populations (Wronka, 2017).

The Human Rights Council within the United Nations is responsible for promoting human rights and addressing violations. Each country is reviewed every five years under The Universal Periodic Review (UPR). The review's results are compiled into a report with recommendations for improvements to be implemented before the next review. However, implementing changes can be difficult, mainly if recommendations depend on the support of many stakeholders (Although countries must express their responses to recommendations, they are not mandated to make the changes. The Council can pass resolutions regarding the outcomes, but it does not have the power to impose sanctions or provide a mandate to intervene.

Subsequent Human Rights Documents

Subsequent to the UDHR, nine binding conventions were developed to further elucidate, operationalize, and monitor the implementation of the 30 fundamental human rights of the UDHR. These are (1) The International Covenant on Economic, Social and Cultural Rights (ICESCR); (2) The International Covenant on Civil and Political Rights (ICCPR); (3) The International Convention on the Elimination of All Forms of Racial Discrimination (ICERD); (4) The Convention against Torture, and Other Cruel, Inhuman, or Degrading Treatment or Punishment (CAT); (5) The Convention on the Rights of the Child (CRC); (6) The Convention on the Rights of Persons with Disabilities; (7) The Convention on the Elimination of Discrimination Against Women (CEDAW); (8) The International Convention for the Protection of All Persons from Enforced Disappearance (CPED); and (9) The International Convention on the Protection of the Rights of All Migrant Workers and Members of Their Families (ICRMW).

In contrast to the UDHR, these conventions are binding to all parties ratifying them. The United States has ratified three of the Conventions: The International Covenant on Civil and Political Rights, The Convention on the Elimination of Racial Discrimination, and The Convention Against Torture. Each of the conventions has a committee that monitors their adherence to the treaties. States ratifying a treaty must submit periodic reports and respond to complainant comments regarding the implementation of the rights in the treaty. The reluctance to sign treaties has been attributed to a need for Senate ratification, isolationist attitudes, and a belief that such documents are not needed as they are protected by domestic legislation (Global Justice Center, 2017).

The Sustainable Development Goals (SDGs) to Transform Our World

The Sustainable Development Goals (SDGs) developed by the United Nations in 2015 have as their underlying theme the pledge that no one will be left behind (UN, 2015). The SDGs address global poverty, inequality, climate change, the environment, peace, and justice and closely reflect human rights principles. They are intended to be global benchmarks that all societies should reach by 2030 to ensure wellbeing and prosperity. Additionally, they aim to protect and promote human rights and freedoms, where all persons can live with dignity and security in societies free of violence and discrimination based on the foundation of universal human rights.

The 17 goals and their 169 targets cover a range of social and economic development issues from poverty and gender inequality to climate change and sustainable cities. Rooted in human rights principles, these goals are interrelated and indivisible, with each equally crucial for individual and social wellbeing. Thus, achieving gender equality is essential in eradicating poverty, while improved health is fundamental to increased personal productivity and economic growth. The 17 goals are as follows:

1) No poverty
2) No hunger
3) Good health and wellbeing
4) Quality education
5) Gender equality
6) Clean water and sanitation
7) Affordable and clean energy
8) Decent work and economic growth
9) Industry, innovation, and infrastructure
10) Reduced inequality
11) Sustainable cities and communities
12) Responsible consumption and production
13) Climate action
14) Life below water
15) Life on land
16) Peace and justice as strong institutions
17) Partnerships to achieve the goals

The 17 goals emphasize human rights and the responsibility of nations to address them. They also reflect the mission of social work to bring about change that benefits all members of society, recognize the most vulnerable, and provide social justice and security for all. The SDGs allow social workers to examine the policies in their own countries and, when necessary, to advocate for changes that target inequality and threaten security and wellbeing. With the goals significantly interconnected and global, applying to all nations, social work involvement at the state level can have a universal impact.

Rights and Needs

Human rights are frequently confused with needs, although the two are clearly distinguishable. Tangible needs exist as phenomena that can be objectively identified and measured, such as needs for food, housing, support, or income (Ife, 2012). However, needs can also be subjective, wherein society decides whether they actually exist. In contrast to human rights, which are constant, social values and perspectives influence needs. Social workers often determine needs by measuring them through methods such as needs assessments, which decide whether supports or services are warranted and how they may or should be met. Such needs are then often filtered through the prism of competing resources, where one vulnerable group may benefit at the expense of another dependent upon the values and viewpoints of policymakers and providers (Wronka, 2017).

In contrast to needs, the universality of human rights and their indivisibility means that they are substantiated in themselves and are not dependent on social values or perspectives. Moreover, human rights provide the mandate to fulfill human needs, with social policy acting as the means for attaining them. Consequently, social workers can play significant roles in assuring that, through policy and practice, needs are reframed and treated as fundamental human rights to which each individual is entitled. Doing so actually empowers clients, as they learn that expecting and demanding health care, or a decent income, is not an individual need but a universal human right to which they are entitled.

Human Rights and Social Work Practice

The International Federation of Social Work (IFSW) defines social work as a human rights profession, a definition found in many countries' codes of ethics. However, this relationship is notably absent in the code of ethics of the National Association of Social Work (NASW) in the United States. This code, revised in 2017, updated ethical issues such as those associated with technology but did not mention human rights (Mapp et al., 2019). The code highlights each person's dignity and worth, along with fundamental social work values and principles, yet with no reference to human rights. As shown in the work of pioneers such as Jane Addams, Edith Abbott, Jeannette Rankin, and Edward Devine, advocacy for human rights was an initial social work activity that has been superseded by a focus on needs.

Accordingly, the Preamble to the Code of Ethics states

> The primary mission of the social work profession is to enhance human wellbeing and help meet the basic human needs of all people, with particular attention to the needs and empowerment of people who are oppressed, and living in poverty.
>
> (NASW, 2017)

The continual emphasis on needs rather than rights undermines the work of a profession whose initial and enduring focus is social change. The Council on Social Work Education (CSWE), the accreditation body for schools of social work in the United States, has for many years been committed to the instruction of international human rights. Among its list of competencies expected of all graduating students is their ability to advance human rights and social, economic, and environmental justice, through knowledge, values, and skills that integrate these perspectives into practice. At the same time, the recent protests demanding racial equality in the United States have been a catalyst for NASW to affirm the necessity for real change at all levels by working for racial equity and justice through education, advocacy, and training. This new emphasis on rights rather than needs, as well as the urgency of structural social change, will, hopefully, now be incorporated into practice.

Applying the Human Rights Framework to Practice

A human rights framework is an overarching perspective that can inform social work interventions and the pathways to empower individuals, families, and communities at the local and global levels. It has underlying values and principles (UN, 2015), such as respect for all persons, the intrinsic value, dignity, and worth of each person, and the duty of governments (i.e., duty bearers) to their citizens (rights holders) and duty bearing citizens to other rights-holding citizens (UN, 1948).

The six major principles of a human rights framework are (1) universality, (2) non-discrimination, (3) the indivisibility and interdependence of rights (political, civil, social, economic, and cultural), (4) participation, (5) accountability, and (6) transparency, and are described later (Ife, 2012; UN, 2015). When applying this framework, these major principles inform social work interventions practice.

1) The principle of *universality* states that human rights belong to everyone, and there are no exceptions for any individual. The mere fact of being human entitles every human to have political, civil, social, economic, and cultural rights.
2) The principle of *non-discrimination* assures access to rights for everyone. In an ideal world, there should be no intentional or unintentional discrimination of national and international laws, policies, or practices.
3) The principle of *indivisibility and interdependence* guides governments to ensure political, civil, social, economic, and cultural rights to everyone. For example, suppose a government does not recognize a social right, such as the right to health and wellbeing. In that case, it challenges citizens' access to achieving other rights, such as the right to education and safety and protection from violence and discrimination.
4) The principle of *participation* refers to everyone's rights, especially those most affected, to participate in decisions that may infringe upon the protection of their rights. In the ideal situation, governments should engage, support, and provide a platform for the participation of civil society on political, civil, social, economic, and cultural issues.
5) The principle of *accountability* suggests that governments are responsible for creating a mechanism of accountability for the enforcement of equal rights, including monitoring and evaluating the implementation of laws and policies that protect rights.
6) The principle of *transparency* means that governments should communicate to civil society all information and decision-making processes affecting human rights. Society's members should be educated on becoming informed decision-makers and actively participating in making significant decisions that affect their rights. Such major decisions are at the national and international levels and at institutional levels such as social services and other institutions needed to protect such rights, including the right to social equality and education (UN, 2015).

A rights-based approach to social work practice means that practice must be consistent with human rights, related to human rights norms, affirming the whole person, their dignity, autonomy, and freedom to make their own choices (Androff, 2015). Rights-based practice reframes needs into human rights to which each individual is entitled. It focuses on the ways in which individual problems and concerns often result from social forces and structures rather than personal deficits. Consequently, interventions are often necessary for change to occur at all levels of practice, from the individual to society. The key to the helping process is that the individual is a true partner in the therapeutic relationship with the practitioner (Wronka, 2017).

At the micro-level, needs are reframed as rights. Therefore, social workers respect individuals' experiences and learn from them rather than act as an expert. The underlying premise is that the individual is the expert in their own life. Such practice necessitates understanding cultures and how they may impact the individual, their experiences, and affect one's own biases (Wronka, 2017).

The mezzo level of practice involves attention to the systems and structures with which individuals interact and their responsiveness. With human dignity at the core, services must be nondiscriminatory and accountable. Sensitive to cultural diversity and how lifetimes of experiences may influence individual responses and the people they serve are critical for service effectiveness. Interventions at this level may include education and advocacy for changes in practice that increase their relevancy to the people they serve (Wronka, 2017).

The macro-level focuses on policies and how governments and institutions support or violate human rights, thus impairing large population segments' quality of life. Macro-level interventions include advocacy and social action to bring about necessary systemic change. The recent focus on police brutality in the United States, particularly toward the Black community, is an example of macro interventions through social action in the form of protests focusing on changing governmental policies and procedures. In fact, as it represents the voices and participation of the people themselves, it represents a powerful type of advocacy.

Central Concepts: Human Rights, Social Justice, Wellbeing, and Cultural Relativism

The third aspect of understanding and applying a human rights lens involves being familiar with central concepts such as human rights, social justice, wellbeing, and cultural relativism. *Human rights* have been conceptualized as a necessary condition for achieving *social justice* and the *wellbeing* of all individuals, families, and communities. In theory, this suggests human rights are a mechanism to promote social justice and individual, family, and community wellbeing and are consistent with the mission of social work (Wronka, 2017).

Social Justice History and Meaning in Social Work

Social justice has been a term nearly consonant with social work. In social work, the realization of social justice meant that the quest for fairness, equality, and justice for all individuals had been achieved. Understanding how social justice values and thoughts have evolved in society and social work is a critical initial step toward incorporating it as a set of principles and approaches to guide practice with individuals, families, and communities.

The Pursuit of Social Justice

The pursuit of social justice has been a common thread throughout the history of social work. Although definitions of social justice vary, there are common themes that can be drawn from these definitions. Notions of social justice commonly embrace:

- values of fairness in the assignment of fundamental rights and duties,
- economic opportunities and social conditions,
- the equal worth of all citizens and their equal right to basic needs, and
- the importance of spreading opportunity and life chances to as many people as possible (Reisch, 2012).

Using a social justice lens helps reframe issues generally viewed as individual in origin to include broader social, political, economic, and cultural understandings. These open possibilities for new solutions for individuals, families, groups, organizations, and communities. It also focuses on social change efforts that extend from a solely national to a global or international perspective (Maschi, 2016; Maschi & Leibowitz, 2017).

Social Justice Balancing Act

An important aspect of social justice is the requirement to reduce and eliminate unjustified inequalities wherever possible. However, as easy as it sounds, it is a delicate balancing act. In remedying inequality, careful attention also must be paid to balancing the collective good without infringing upon basic individual freedoms (Finn & Jacobson, 2008).

History of Social Justice in Social Work

The history of social justice in social work has many religious and political roots that fueled social workers' activities. In the United States, social justice in social work has deep roots in Judeo-Christian religious tradition, 19th- and 20th-century Western philosophy (as early as Plato and Aristotle), and political theory (such as John Rawls). Throughout history, social justice notions that have emanated from religious thought have commonly been viewed as an abstract ideal that intersects with values related to what is good, desirable, and moral (Reisch, 2012). Social work also has been influenced by the ongoing social justice discourse that has been engaged in by many, including political theorists, philosophers, religious traditions, and social workers.

However, an ongoing critique among many social workers is that social justice definitions are extensive and also ambiguous, thus making it challenging to translate social justice into concrete practices (Reisch, 2012; Maschi & Leibowitz, 2017). Some theorists have argued that social justice reflects a concept of fairness in the assignment of fundamental rights and duties, economic opportunities, and social conditions. Others frame the concept into three components: legal justice, commutative, and distributive justice. Legal justice is concerned with what others owe society; commutative justice, which addresses what people owe each other; and distributive justice or what society owes the person (Wakefield, 1988, p. 193; Reisch, 2012). In social work, distributive justice is commonly referenced. Social justice entails approaches to societal choices regarding the distribution of goods and resources and the consideration of societal institutions' structure to guarantee human rights and dignity and ensure opportunities for free and meaningful social participation. Marion Iris Young (1990) also argued that social justice addressed the distribution of resources or institutional structures and the social processes and practices in which unfair treatment and oppression are transmitted.

Historically, social justice has been an organizing value of social work. However, particularly in America, the profession has been critiqued for not clearly defining it in the NASW code of ethics and putting it into practice. The following aspects of social work history, although not perfect, provide evidence throughout time of social workers attempting to achieve a social justice ideal by combating oppression. Social justice's origins in social work have commonly been traced to the early settlement house movement (Young, 1990).

In the early 20th century, social workers practiced in settlement houses, mostly in urban and impoverished communities, to provide a range of services to community members. The movement focused on addressing social-environmental conditions that impacted those living in poverty and substandard living conditions, especially immigrants. Resident workers sought social reform and followed what was referred to as "social gospel," or speaking about social justice issues, such as poverty, poor working conditions, and war and peace (Finn & Jacobson, 2008). Social work leaders, such as Jane Addams and Florence Kelly, are remembered for their advocacy efforts that led to systemic reforms in juvenile justice reform, workers' rights, and world peace. According to Finn and Jacobson (2008), these leaders represented social justice in practice because

> that called for them to see the viewpoint of those less powerful in society, to invite the participation of the affected in the understanding

> and resolution of social problems, to construct new forms of social life grounded in belonging, respect, and participation, and hold to a vision of a just world.
>
> (Finn & Jacobson, 2008, p. 8)

In the 1930s, the rank-and-file movement in the social work profession grew during the great depression as a reaction to unfair labor practices and oppressive conditions at that time. Group work was a standard vehicle for social justice during that time. Group work theory and practice were grounded in humanitarian and collective principles. Group work was used to harness collective energy to help achieve social justice aims in the broader society. Bertha Capen Reynolds, a rank-and-file movement leader, helped form unions and used principles of belonging, mutuality, power-sharing, and coalitions with clients, communities, groups, and professionals to help advance social justice (Finn & Jacobson, 2008).

In the 1940s and 1950s, group work and the rank-and-file movement declined with the rise of McCarthyism. In the 1960s, the civil rights movement and the struggle for equity gave rise to collective movements, group work, and social activism. During the 1960s, the profession began to reexamine how well it met its social justice aims. A growing anti-oppressive practice strand talked about developing critical consciousness, which is to move beyond individual pathology (such as Freudian theory) to sociopolitical structures for the underlying causes of inequality (such as feminist theory). In the late 20th century, the discourse on human rights and oppression as a social justice issue and empowerment theory and practice to achieve a socially just world. (Wakefield, 1988; Finn & Jacobson, 2008)

Since the 1970s, the philosopher John Rawls' theory (1971) strongly influenced social work practice. In his groundbreaking book, *Justice as Fairness: A Restatement*, Rawls described two fundamental justice principles: justice as fairness and just arrangements. Justice as fairness refers to that each person has an equal right to the most extensive essential liberty compatible with a similar liberty for others. Just arrangements are when social and economic inequalities are arranged so that they are both the most significant benefits of the least advantaged and attached to offices and positions open to all conditions of fair and equal opportunity. Rawls' concept of "redress" suggests social work redresses inequalities and shifts the balance of contingencies in the direction of equality (Wakefield, 1988; Reisch, 2012; Finn & Jacobson, 2008).

Rawls' view of social justice is an ideal theory of justice. It has an ideal set of distributive principles by which existing social orders must be judged according to the distribution of primary social goods. These social goods include liberties, opportunities, income, and wealth. This theory is grounded in an egalitarian view. Rawls asks, "[W]hat would be the characteristics of a just society in which basic needs are met, unnecessary stress is reduced, the competence of each person is maximized, and threats to wellbeing are minimized" (Rawls, 1971, p. 44). For Rawls, distributive justice refers to material goods and services, and social goods, such as opportunity and power (Wakefield, 1988).

In today's world of globalization, social workers are often called upon to assume a global outlook that envisions issues beyond borders. According to Finn and Jacobson (2008), a global approach views the world as a system made up of interdependent parts, that external structures shape human interactions and challenge cultural bound assumptions, for example, independence and self versus collectivism and interdependence of self. Social work has the potential to help facilitate global change and development. Central to this global view and social work practice in a global context is to incorporate human rights, multiculturalism, social exclusion/inclusion, security, and sustainability (Healey, 2001).

Visualizing Social Justice: The Glass Half Full or Empty?

Historically, social work has grappled with how social justice is defined and thus realized. There are many definitions and descriptions of social justice in social work. According to *The Social Work Dictionary*, social justice represents an "ideal" in the form of "an ideal condition in which all members of society have the same rights, protections, opportunities, obligations, and social benefits. Implicit in this concept is the notion that historical inequalities should be acknowledged and remedied through specific measures" (Barker, 2014, p. 405). A detailed examination of social work literature reveals that social justice is described in the literature in two ways: a positive ideal or value that envisions a just society and fair treatment for all (Maschi & Leibowitz, 2017).

Using a social justice lens necessitates that society perceives an ideal world in which equity and fairness are achieved for all. However, at the same time, social workers must also be fully aware of discrimination, oppression, and institutional inequities so that they are positioned to combat it. Similarly, in social justice practice, social workers must be prepared to look at all angles of an issue and willing to look beyond the glass for a global perspective (Maschi & Leibowitz, 2017).

According to Dewees (2006), social justice focuses on "institutional arrangements and systemic inequities that further the interests of some groups at the expense of others in the distribution of material goods, social benefits, rights, protections, and opportunities" (Dewees, 2006). Similarly, Wronka (2017) described social justice as a struggle to work toward a socially just world as well as to the adherence to the principles of the Universal Declaration of Human Rights (UN, 1948) in theory and in practice (p. 294).

For social work, social justice serves both a future goal-oriented and a present and past reality-oriented purpose:

(1) Using a present and future orientation, social justice can be conceived as a goal for an equitable and sustainable society. Using this orientation, social workers can develop interventions that help achieve this goal for individuals, families, groups, and communities (Barkers, 2014, p. 405).
(2) Using a past orientation, the stark reality of discrimination, oppression, and structural inequalities can be identified for assessment purposes to inform intervention planning. Using this orientation, social justice is a perspective through which social workers recognize and address the connection between personal struggles and society's structural arrangements. In this light, social justice entails the use of advocacy and other strategies to confront discrimination, oppression, and institutional inequities (Barker, 2014, p. 405).

Theorizing Social Justice for Action

Social justice is often premised on the notion of distributive justice, how these resources are "distributed," and how society is accountable to the individual and collective (Reisch, 2012).

Social workers have been influenced by the different philosophical approaches developed in the past two centuries about social justice. These theories have been used to inform how societal decisions are made and actions related to the distribution of resources, including psychological, economic, social, legal, material, work, civil, cultural, and political resources. Some of these theories are more consistent with social work ethics and values, while others are not. According to some scholars, social justice is premised on distributive justice. That is, how these resources are "distributed," how society is accountable to the individual and collective, and what principles guide the distribution of goods and resources (Reisch, 2012).

Van Soest and Garcia (2003) describe five perspectives of distributive justice: (1) libertarian, (2) utilitarian, (3) egalitarian, (4) racial contract, and (5) human rights envision what a socially just world should be.

1) Libertarian theories assume an individual focus and a fair playing field for all. This perspective argues that individuals are entitled to any resources they legally required, and there should be no societal obligation that resources should be distributed equally. Using this view, individuals, and not collective, are the focus and what an individual has obtained is fair and square. It justifies personal hardship for some (Van Soest & Garcia, 2003).
2) Utilitarian theories assume an individual and collective view. This perspective argues that the socially just world is achieved when seeking the greatest benefit and the least harm for the most significant number

of people. Infringing upon individual rights is acceptable if it results in meeting the needs and interests of the majority. Overall, it justifies personal hardship for some as long as people are treated fairly (Van Soest & Garcia, 2003).

3) Egalitarian theories view equity for the collective. Egalitarian theories argue that every member of society should be guaranteed the same rights, opportunities, and access to goods and resources. Using this view, the redressing or redistribution of resources should be to the advantage of society's most vulnerable members (Van Soest & Garcia, 2003; Rawls, 1971).
4) The racial contract perspective offers a sober view of the current situation of societal inequities, the unequal system of privilege, racism, sexism, etc. According to this view advanced by Black and women scholars, the stark reality is that the social contract of equality has not extended beyond white people. For other racial groups to be treated as equal recipients of social justice, the white privilege must be dismantled. In the case of women and other marginalized groups, multiple intersectional identities such as gender, class and cultural identity, sexual orientation, immigration, incarceration, and disability status must also be addressed (Crenshaw, 1991; Jordan, 2010).
5) The human rights perspective visualizes all individuals as having the right to equitable distribution of resources instead of it being a need. Every human is expected to be treated with dignity and respect, and institutions and governments should be structured in a way to foster full human development. Some argue that a human right perspective provides a global and political language for social justice with international support across nations and a comprehensive and defined set of guidelines that can be easily implemented (Reichert, 2011)

Social work also has been influenced by two opposing theoretical viewpoints: the order and change perspectives. These perspectives inform social justice-based practice on the origins of social problems and human behavior. As its name suggests, the order perspective views society as stable, ordered, and harmonious, in which all people are united and in consensus as part of a shared culture. In contrast, the conflict perspective views groups in society in a conflict in which dominant groups have power and subordinate or oppressed groups do not. There is differential control of resources, and political power organizes society, and the motivation of oppressed groups it to remedy societal injustices. Although these perspectives differ in their underlying assumptions, explanations, and solutions for social problems, they have been used interchangeably by social workers (Reichert, 2011).

The order perspective views the relationship between people and society in which members conform to the mutually agreed upon societal norms. Problems are conceptualized as an individual defect and their inability to conform to group expectations. It rises to be social problems when large groups of individuals with similar issues deviate from the norm. When using an order perspective, interventions target individual behavior change and resocialization. Social reform efforts are minor in scope to not tinker with the nature of the existing system. Social work traditionally has embraced order perspectives that target the individual level (Reichert, 2011). Examples are psychodynamic, behavioral perspectives, or perspectives that recalibrate a system to return to harmony (e.g., the systems, ecological, problem-solving, strengths perspective).

In contrast, the conflict perspectives see society's nature as based on structural inequality and group conflict. Dominant groups maintain power through control and coercion over subordinate groups that are expected to conform. Social problems are reviewed due to oppressive conditions transmitted through a dominant ideology, social processes, practices, and institutions. Therefore, issues target large-scale social change. Using strategies such as behavioral change of individuals is viewed as "blaming the victim" and is not a recommended strategy (Other views of social justice include the capabilities framework. Based on the work of Amartya Sen, the capabilities perspective focuses on the fair distribution of "capabilities." That is the resources and power to exercise self-determination and to achieve wellbeing (Morris, 2002). It goes beyond the importance of securing primary social goods and sees these as an essential part of achieving social justice but not the goal. "Capability is based on what a person wants to achieve and what power he or she has to convert primary goods to reach her or his desired goals" (p. 368). In contrast to the Rawlsian perspective uses societal level principles, the capabilities perspective begins at the individual level and imagines what a person can do and become (Nussbaum, 2004).

The capabilities approach is also referred to as the human development approach. In this approach, materials and resources create and facilitate the development of human capabilities. Rights are viewed as entitlements to capabilities. The contemporary philosopher, Martha Nussbaum (2004), developed a list of capabilities that provides a quality-of-life assessment and for political planning (Nussbaum, 2004). This list of central human capabilities represents the benchmarks for a minimally decent life. These capabilities are as follows:

1. Life
2. Bodily health
3. Bodily integrity
4. Senses, imagnation, and thought
5. Emotions
6. Practical reason
7. Affiliation
8. Other species
9. Play
10. Control over one's environment

This capabilities approach recognizes that there is a socially unjust world and expands upon distributive justice, commonly referred to in social work and which includes other central social work values, such as self-determination, human dignity, and wellbeing. McGrath Morris (2002) notes the congruence between the capabilities perspective and social work's dominant theories that focus on strengths, person-in-environment, and empowerment. Nussbaum's work has been used to guide advocacy work when societal circumstances are "outside of one's control and do not permit some people, especially women and persons of color, to develop their capabilities" (p. 53).

The Social Worker's Path to Transformation of Self and Society

Social justice commonly refers to the vision of a society comprised of fairness, equality, and justice for all individuals juxtaposed against the reality of unfairness, inequality, and injustice. How social justice is realized continues to generate a creative tension and lively debate within the profession of social work. Understanding how social justice values and thoughts have evolved in society and social work is a critical initial step toward incorporating it as an overarching theme into one's practice paradigm (Maschi, 2016; Nussbaum, 2004).

How do social workers put social justice into action? Jane Addams once said, "*Action is indeed the sole medium of expression for ethics*." One possible interpretation is that it is the commitment to social justice values and the ethic of service to others that can act as a springboard. This next section outlines strategies to move from social justice values to action. Empowerment and transformation action strategies have been used by social workers to promote social justice, including personal transformation for social justice work. Empowerment and anti-oppressive theory and practice seek transformation and liberation as the goals. Transformation is expected to occur from inside one's self (i.e., to the individual), between one's self and others (i.e., to the relationship), and at the political level (i.e., collective political liberation). Therefore, social work interventions must focus on individual and sociopolitical levels to increase the chances of lasting individual and social change.

As health, social, cultural, and political systems disarray, it becomes even more evident how oppression (e.g., racism, sexism, ageism, classism) is a complex interplay of psychological, sociopolitical, economic, interpersonal, and institutional processes. The Black Lives Matter Movement's responses are unifying diverse constituencies and beckon us to be kinder and gentler humanity instead of what is being perpetuated. Oppressive thought and practices are weaved throughout the fabric of society through dominant perspectives. It is also transmitted through private and public attitudes that advance power over and control hierarchical approaches, fear tactics, divisive social norms and practices, laws and policies, pitting social and cultural practices, and social media messaging.

According to intersectionality theory and models, the Levels of Oppression Framework consists of four levels: structural, cultural, individual (personal/interpersonal), and internalized. **Structural oppression** refers to the oppression that is transmitted via institutions (e.g., economic and social institutions), organizations (e.g., mental health, aging, and criminal justice service providers), structures (e.g., local, state, and federal governments), laws, and policies. Structural oppression can be found when the society disproportionately allocates good jobs, health care, and housing to the dominant group (Mullaly & West, 2018).

Cultural oppression consists mainly of overall societal attitudes and judgments. In cultural oppression, there is a dominant cultural messaging that promotes, universalizes, and imposes on everyone, while oppressing, suppressing, and repressing other cultures (Mullaly & West, 2018). **Individual oppression (or personal/interpersonal oppression)** consists of every experience with individuals in one's immediate micro-level network. This contact can be with family members, neighbors, strangers, and professionals. Individual oppression is characterized by the transmission of thoughts, attitudes, and behaviors that depict subordinate groups' negative prejudgments, usually based on stereotypes. It occurs overtly or covertly and may or may not be intentional. It may manifest in the form of conscious acts of microaggressions, overt aggression, and hatred, including violence. It also may manifest as unconscious acts of aversion and avoidance (Mullaly, 2010; Mullaly & West, 2018).

The Relationship of Social Justice to Oppression

The year 2020 has created a historical turning point in which we, as a society, have found ourselves in global "lockdown" due to the spread of COVID-19 and the concomitant rise in deaths. It behooves us to continue to reflect individually and collectively on its meaning, especially as we also strive to achieve equality and justice, especially for Black, Indigenous, and people of color in America and disparities and inequalities impacting older adults (Maschi & Morgen, 2020, Cox, 2020).

Historically, social work was birthed in the early 20th century by concerned citizens who were fueled by compassion as an act of "doing good" and assisting others by alleviating their suffering. Many communities were grappling with social problems such as mass industrialization, immigration, racism, and ethnocentrism. The remnants of the enslavement of African Americans as part of America's history morphed into different forms of post-emancipation, including being excluded from the early settlement house movement (Maschi & Morgen, 2020). The continued prevalence of flawed and oppressive dominant beliefs influenced the narrative that racial, ethnic, and other minorities, such as women and LGBTQIA+ people, were less than the "dominant norm," represented by the white Anglo Saxon, wealthy, Protestant, able-bodied, and heterosexual male. All the while, globally, ageism and negative stereotypes of older adults continue to impact their health and wellbeing (Stuart, 2013, WHO, 2018).

The UN's Sustainable Developmental Goals (SDGs, UN, 2015 and the National Association of Social Worker's (NASW, 2017 social justice priorities are used to illustrate the ongoing social problems of the social structural determinants of health and justice and apply to the health and wellbeing of the wider world. These NASW priorities include the intersectional social concerns of economic justice (e.g., poverty), criminal justice and juvenile justice (e.g., policing, mass incarceration, institutional and community trauma and abuse), environmental justice (e.g., pollution), immigration, health and social wellbeing (e.g., health disparities, access to services and rights), and the political, governmental system (e.g., participation, voter rights).

Oppression at all these levels must be addressed, especially the psychological and emotional internalization of the dominant group's collective and cultural narratives (e.g., racism, ageism, sexism, homophobia), which leads to a fear- or problem-based forms of thinking. Such ways of thinking are characterized by survival mode with outcomes marked by a mental contraction in which individuals tend to see each other as "separate" (Mullaly & West, 2018).

Conclusion

Human rights and social justice are intrinsically connected to the mission of social work. Integrating both into practice is critical for attaining the goals of assuring human dignity in a responsive and supportive society that respects diversity and seeks equality for all. At the same time, it is important to recognize that while human rights are unalterable, pertaining to all people in all societies, there are varying perspectives of social justice.

In the following chapters, authors share their expertise on specific vulnerable groups and issues and the ways that rights-based practice and a social justice focus relate to them. As found in society itself, the subjects that are discussed are not static; they shift with interrelated events and factors that influence social change. Even while these changes occur, the principles that underly social work practice, when based upon the human rights approach that recognizes the worth of each person, will offer a blueprint for pursuing a just society in which human dignity is recognized and fulfilled.

References

Androff, D. (2015). *Practicing Rights: Human rights-based approaches to social work practice.* Practicing Rights: Human Rights-Based Approaches to Social Work Practice. New York: Routledge.

Barker, R. L. (2014). *The social work dictionary* (6th ed.). Washington, DC: National Association of Social Workers Press.

Cox, C. (2020). Older adults and COVID-19; social justice, disparities, and social work practice. *Journal of Gerontological Social Work, 6*, 611–624.

Crenshaw, K. (1991). Mapping the margins: Intersectionality, identity politics, and violence against women of color. *Stanford Law Review, 43*, pp. 1241–1299.

Dewees, M. (2006). *Contemporary social work practice*. Boston, MA: McGraw-Hill.

Finn, J., & Jacobson, M. (2008). *Just practice: A social justice approach to social work* (2nd ed.). Peosta, IA: Eddie Bowers Publishing, Inc.

Global Justice Center Blog. (2017). U.S. Aversion to International Human Rights Treaties. Retrieved from https://globaljusticecenter.net/blog/773-u-s-aversion-to-international-human-rights-treaties

Healey, L. (2001). *International social work: Professional action in an interdependent world*. New York, NY: Oxford University Press.

Ife, J. (2012). *Human rights and social work: Towards rights-based practice*. New York: Cambridge University Press.

Jordan, J. (2010). *Relational cultural therapy*. Washington, DC: American Psychological Association.

Mapp, S., McPherson, J., Androff, D., & Gabel, S. (2019). Social work is a human rights profession. *Social Work, 64*, 259–269.

Maschi, T. (2016). *Applying a human rights approach to social work research and evaluation: A rights research manifesto*. New York, NY: Springer Publishing.

Maschi, T., & Leibowitz, G. (2017). *Forensic social work: Psychosocial and legal issues across diverse populations and settings* (2nd ed.). New York, NY: Springer.

Maschi, T., & Morgen, K. (2020). *Aging behind prison walls: Studies of Trauma and Resilience*. New York, NY: Columbia University Press.

Morris, P. (2002). The capabilities perspective: A framework for social justice. *Families in Society, 83*(4), 365–373.

Mullaly, B. (2010). *Challenging oppression and confronting privilege* (2nd ed.). New York, NY: Columbia University Press.

Mullaly, R., & West, J. (2018). *Challenging oppression and confronting privilege*. Oxford: Oxford University Press.

National Association of Social Workers (NASW) (2017). *Code of ethics* (Rev. ed.). Washington, DC: Author.

Nussbaum, M. C. (2004). Beyond the social contract: Capabilities and global justice. *Oxford Development Studies, 32*(1), 1–17.

Rawls, J. (1971, 1999). *A theory of justice*. Cambridge, MA: Harvard University Press.

Reichert, E. (2011). *Social work and human rights: A foundation for policy and practice*. (2nd ed). New York, NY: Columbia University Press.

Reisch, M. (2012). Defining social justice in a socially unjust world. *Families in Society: The Journal of Contemporary Social Services, 83*(4), 343–354. Doi: 10.1606/1044-3894.17

Smith, P., & Max-Neef, M. (2011). *Economics unmasked; From power and greed o compassion and the common good*. Devon: Green Books.

Stuart, P. (2013). Social work profession: History. *Encyclopedia of Social Work*. Doi: 10.1093/acrefore/9780199975839.013.623

United Nations (1948). *Universal declaration of human rights*. Retrieved from https://www.un.org/en/ universal-declaration-human-rights/index.html

United Nations (2015). *The Sustainable Development Goals*. Retrieved from https://www.undp.org/sustainable-development-goals

United Nations Development Programme (UNDP) (2021). *Vulnerable and key populations*. Retrieved from www.undp-capacitydevelopment-health.org/en/legal-and-policy/key-populations/

Van Soest, D., & Garcia, B. (2003). *Diversity education for social justice: Mastering teaching skills*. Alexandria, VA: Council on Social Work Education. www.undp-capacitydevelopment-health.org/en/legal-and-policy/key-populations/

Wakefield, J. C. (1988). Psychotherapy, distributive justice, and social work—Part 1: Distributive justice as a conceptual framework for social work. *Social Service Review*, *62*(2), 187–210.

World Health Organization (WHO) (2018). *Global campaign to combat ageism*. Retrieved from www.who.int/ageing/ageism/campaign/en/

Wronka, J. (2017). *Human rights and social justice: Social action and service for the helping and health professions* (2nd ed.). Thousand Oaks, CA: Sage Publications.

Young, I. (1990). *Justice and the politics of difference*. Princeton, NJ: Princeton University Press.

2 A Human Rights Framework for Integrated Practice

Joseph Wronka

At the outset of the COVID-19 Pandemic, Antonio Gutteres, secretary general of the United Nations, said:

> The COVID-19 pandemic is a . . . human crisis that is fast becoming a human rights crisis. . . . In February I launched a Call to Action to put human dignity and the promise of the Universal Declaration of Human Rights at the core of our work. . . . Human rights cannot be an afterthought in times of crisis-and we now face the biggest international crisis in generations.
>
> (Gutteres, 2020)

Those words concerning the pandemic illustrate the importance of adhering to fundamental human rights principles to promote well-being and eradicate social and individual malaises, goals that are fundamental not only to the profession of social work but also to the helping and health professions in general. However, for the purposes of the fundamental focus of this work, as well as, brevity, this chapter, without minimizing the importance of a human rights framework to the helping and health professions in general, will emphasize social work, albeit a particular "kind" of social work that of "integrated practice," sometimes referred to alternately as advanced generalist practice.

Whereas this article emphasizes relevance to social work, which according to the International Federation of Social Work has stated that "from its inception social work has been a human rights profession," and, indeed, has a long history in that profession (Healy, 2008, 2020) many of the helping and health professions also emphasize the need for human rights in their professions. The American Nurses Association (2007) asserts, for instance, "a fundamental principle that underlies all nursing practice is respect for the inherent work, dignity, and human rights of every individual" (p. 3). Regarding quarantining note that the 2019 Code of Ethics for the American Public Health Association asserts: "[I]f public health subjects individuals to compulsory quarantine or social distancing measures, it is the ethical

DOI: 10.4324/9781003111269-3

responsibility of public health and other officials and agencies to provide appropriate medical assistance, housing conditions, nutrition, access to outside communication, and other *human rights protections* (italics added) throughout the course of their isolation." Human rights thus can often provide a common language among the helping and health professions, thus enabling interdisciplinary cooperation, so necessary in these days of pandemics, particularly COVID-19, which has brought to fore the inadequacy of these and perhaps other professions to work in solos and the stark reality, yet utmost importance of our global and professional interconnectedness.

The word "integrate" is from the Latin *integrare* meaning "to make whole" (online Etymology, 2020a); the word "practice" is from the Latin *praxis* meaning "practice, exercise, action" (Etymon on line, 2021). Integrated practice, therefore, from an etymological standpoint means, to have a holistic (the "w" often dropped in academic parlance) view of things, very briefly, to look at the big picture and to put this view into action. Such a holistic view as this essay argues is for the social worker in tandem with other helping and health professions to have a repertoire of actions that are both proactive to prevent social and individual malaises in the first place, yet reactive to curtail, if not eradicate those malaises if they have occurred.

A human rights framework, which ought to be seen as the theoretic foundation of social justice, for socially just policies and actions advocated in this essay can best be defined by the Human Rights Triptych. (see Wronka, 2017; unless otherwise noted, references here are from that work). Indeed, the etymology of social justice is from the Latin *socius* meaning "friend, ally, partner" and *justia* meaning "equal treatment." Thus, literally, it is important to treat our friends equally, thus in socially just ways. But social justice can often be seen as too broad in scope without definitional parameters, that can further concretize this notion, thus providing a framework to engage in socially just actions. This Human Rights Triptych thus can elucidate and concretize this framework, hence, giving the foundation for effective interventions for integrated social work practice. Readers may also wish to note how powerful this idea of "human rights" is, which can move us to action. To say, for example, that health care is a human right, seems more formidable than to say that it is socially just to have health care.

Readers should note also that this article emphasizes "a" not "the" human rights framework. This is a framework advocated here by this author, who encourages readers to develop their own notions of what a human rights framework is or ought to be, thus, seeing the relevance of this powerful "social construct," which arose from the ashes of World War II, as unique to their own practice situations. This article therefore consists of four sections: (1) an explanation of the meaning of the Human Rights Triptych; (2) select implications of the Human Rights Triptych for practice; (3) elaborating upon integrated practice; and (4) general suggestions for future directions for integrated a.k.a. advanced generalist practice.

Preliminary Comments

Before going into depth into those sections, it is sufficient to say at this point and roughly by way of example that housing, which is a human right, can be provided by multi-pronged interventions consistent with integrated practice. Looking at the big picture, thus it would be important to prevent homelessness in the first place by having an amendment to the US Constitution that asserts that housing is a human right, echoing the Universal Declaration of Human Rights (UDHR). But, despite such an amendment, or lack thereof, if homelessness exists it would be important to set up shelters. Legislation, decrees, declarations, and the like are no guarantee that they will promote well-being and eradicate a social problem. More importantly, it is the values that have crystallized into such edicts that play the most important role. Only the values that "work" are the ones that society has chosen and have come about through open and honest debate, if you will, a "free market" of ideas.

One often hears that social justice with human rights at its core is struggle. To work proactively and reactively at the same time is an almost infinite struggle. This is possible, nevertheless, if one is willing to dive into the ambiguities and complexities involved. Metaphorically speaking, this struggle can be akin to the actions of the Greek mythological character Sisyphus who, because of his antics by putting Death in handcuffs and hiding the key from him, was condemned by Zeus to push a boulder up a hill, only to watch it fall again. Such a struggle, a seemingly arduous task, would need to be repeated over and over again. But, as the existentialist Albert Camus (1991, p. 123) stated, "We must imagine Sisyphus happy." That is, he found joy in struggle. Indeed, that literary metaphor speaks to the struggle of intervening both proactively and reactively, thus being a social worker who engages in integrated practice, thus realizing the importance and necessity of multi-pronged levels of intervention, which often overlap.

It ought to be emphasized that the Council on Social Work's (CSWE, 2015) Educational Policies and Accreditation Standards (EPAS) states explicitly the importance of human rights in the profession's curricula. Indeed, EPAS asserts *inter alia*: "the purpose of social work is actualized through its quest for social and economic justice, the prevention of conditions that limit human rights, the elimination of poverty, and the enhancement of the quality of life for all persons, locally and globally." More emphatically Competency three asserts that social work curricula must: "Advance Human Rights and Social, Economic, and Environmental Justice," further elucidating that competency by asserting, "Social workers understand that every person regardless of position in society has fundamental human rights. . . . Social workers understand strategies designed to eliminate oppressive structural barriers to ensure that social goods, rights, and responsibilities are distributed equitably and that civil, political, environmental, economic, social, and cultural human rights are protected [and] . . . apply their understanding of social, economic, and environmental justice to advocate for human rights at the individual and system levels; and engage in practices that advance social, economic, and environmental justice." Despite CSWE's emphasis on competency 3, however, it ought to be acknowledged that, whereas the National Association of Schools of Social Work (NASW) Code of Ethics mentions social justice in its Code of Ethics seven times, there is no mention of human rights. This lack indicates that much more work is necessary to go beyond and concretize traditional notions of social justice in social work and to acknowledge human rights as social justice's theoretic practice underpinnings, thus providing an adequate framework for integrated practice. Indeed, NASW's "effectiveness in the 21st century will depend on the extension of its social justice values within the context of global human rights" (NASW, 2021, p. 196).

Furthermore, the Global Standards of Social Work Education (GSSWE, 2020), a joint project of the International Federation of Social Work (IFSW) and the International Association of Schools of Social Work (IASSW), emphasizes human rights. When speaking about the profession of social work, it states in Principle 4:

> Social, Economic and Environmental Justice are fundamental pillars underpinning social work theory, policy and practice. All schools must: Prepare students to be able to apply human rights principles to frame their understanding of how current social issues affect social, economic and environmental justice . . . [and] Ensure that their students understand the importance of social, economic, political, cultural, and environmental justice and develop relevant intervention knowledge and skills.

Given this emphasis then of human rights in GSSWE and in CSWE's accreditation standards, as well as, other allied professions, this powerful social construct, "human rights," can serve as a thread to weave theory with integrated practice, thus a framework, much like a scaffolding to build a home for constructing a socially just world. Note that the aim of such a framework is to construct a "home," not necessarily a "house." People want to have not only a home, with adequate structural integrity certainly, but also a place that is inviting to others and can feel literally "at home," in a caring environment with loved ones. Human rights can serve as that framework for the entire world.

It is indeed a powerful idea whose time has come. As the author Viktor Hugo (2020, p. 1) stated rather eloquently: "Nothing is as powerful as an idea whose time has come. There is one thing stronger than all the armies in the world and that is an idea whose time has come." Human rights is that idea.

The Human Rights Triptych

The question becomes what precisely are human rights. Or, as some would say what "is" human rights, given they are interdependent and indivisible, thus plural in form but singular in meaning. These rights can be best grasped by understanding what has become known as The Human Rights Triptych as displayed in Table 2.1. It consists of the UDHR at the center panel; the guiding principles, declarations, and conventions on the right panel; and implementation measures on the left.

But to elaborate, the UDHR, a progeny of the U.N. Charter, is a historical-philosophical-religious compromise. It consists of five crucial notions: (1)

Table 2.1 The Human Rights Triptych

Implementation	*The Authoritative Definition of Human Rights Standards*	*Documents Following the Universal Declaration*
1. Thematic and Country-Based Reports for Charter-Based Concerns 2. Dialogue with the Human Rights Monitoring Committees of Major Human Rights Conventions consisting of: a. the filing of reports; b. the response of the human rights monitoring committee; and c. the informing of the appropriate governmental bodies of the positive aspects and concerns of the committee. 3. World Conferences and Action Plans 4. The Universal Periodic Review	1. The United Nations Charter, which has the status of Treaty 2. The Universal Declaration of Human Rights (UDHR)—the Authoritative Definition of Human Rights Standards, increasingly referred to as Customary International Law and consisting of five crucial notions: a. human dignity b. nondiscrimination c. civil and political rights d. economic, social, and cultural rights e. solidarity rights	1. Nine Major Human Rights Conventions having the status of Treaty a. The International Covenant on Civil and Political Rights (ICCPR) b. The International Covenant on Economic, Social and Cultural Rights (ICESCR) c. The Convention on the Rights of the Child (CRC) d. The Convention on the Elimination of Discrimination Against Women (CEDAW) e. The Convention Against Torture (CAT) f. The International Convention on the Elimination of All Forms of Racial Discrimination (CERD) g. The Convention on Migrant Workers and Their Families (CMW) h. International Convention on the Rights of Persons with Disabilities (CRPD) i. International Convention on Enforced Disappearances (CED) Other human rights protocols and documents, like the Genocide Convention and the Draft Declaration on the Rights of Indigenous Peoples

Adapted from Wronka, J. (2017). Human rights and social justice: Social action and service for the helping and health professions (Los Angeles, Sage. P. 59) human dignity in Article 1, reflecting substantively the Judeo-Christian-Islamic tradition; (2) non-discrimination in Article 2 on the basis of such characteristics as race, gender, national origin, or political opinion integral also to those traditions; (3) civil and political rights in articles 2–21, such as freedoms of speech, the press, worship, and peaceful assembly reminiscent of the Age of Enlightenment, which some authors have argued rests heavily upon Indigenous knowledge (Graeber & Wengrow, 2021); (4) economic, social, and cultural rights, in articles 22–27 as rights to meaningful and gainful employment, rest and leisure, medical care, including thus mental health care, security in old age, social protections for the family as the fundamental unit of society, special protections for motherhood and children, education teaching tolerance and friendship, and participation in cultural life, evoking the Age of Industrialization; and (5) solidarity rights, reflecting the failure of domestic sovereignty to solve global problems, in articles 28–30 calling for a "just social and international order," intergovernmental cooperation, duties, and limitations of rights. Those final articles have given sustenance to rights to peace, a clean environment, humanitarian disaster relief, development, self-determination, global distributive justice, the preservation of the common and cultural heritages of humanity, like the oceans, space, and cultural and religious landmarks, and the promotion of world citizenship (Davis, 2010). Note, moreover, that when we speak of a "just social and international order," it is important to be cognizant of unjust social and economic arrangements that can lead to human rights violations in the first place as Pope Francis stated when addressing the joint session of the US Congress back in 2015. Such an unjust social arrangement can be defined as a capitalist order, which prioritizes capital from capital, that is, money from money. Such a notion is antithetical to employment, which ought to be socially useful, contributing to the development of the human personality and with reasonable wages as a human right, as asserted by the US delegation to the drafting committee for the Universal Declaration of Human Rights (Wronka, 1992). It may well be that "Capitalism" is indeed the "dung of the devil," as Pope Francis also asserted. That human rights are interdependent and indivisible is integral to human rights discourse. What, after all, is freedom of speech and the press (civil and political rights) to a person who is homeless, lacking access to health care (economic and social rights), and lives in a world at war and environmentally devastated (solidarity rights)?

On the right panel, there are nine major international conventions, which largely elaborate upon rights in the UDHR. While called conventions or covenants, they are also considered international treaties: Civil and Political Rights (ICCPR); Economic, Social, and Cultural Rights (ICESCR); the Elimination of Discrimination Against Women (CEDAW); the Elimination of All Forms of Racial Discrimination (CERD); the Rights of the Child (CRC); the Protection of the Rights of All Migrant Workers and Members of Their Families (CMW); the Rights of Persons with Disabilities (CRPD); The Convention Against Torture (CAT); and the

International Convention for the Protection of All Persons from Enforced Disappearances (CED). Thus, the UDHR urges "special care and assistance" for motherhood and children (Article 25). CEDAW elaborates that such protections "should be accorded to mothers during a reasonable period before and after childbirth . . . wherein working mothers should be accorded paid leave or leave with adequate social security benefits" (Article 10). The United States, which is a primary focus of this article, has ratified ICCPR, CAT, and CERD, which, according to the Supremacy Clause of the US Constitution, Article VI, must, because they have the status of international treaty, become "law of the land . . . and the judges bound thereby" (Weissbrodt et al., 2009). It is important to note that the late Ramsey Clarke at a side event sponsored by the U.N. Human Rights Council spoke about the "failure of the legal system" to implement that Supremacy Clause.

Select other documents, are in brief, the Principles for the Protection of Persons with Mental Illness (PPMI), Principles of Medical Ethics (PME), the Declaration of Human Rights Defenders (DHRD), Guiding Principles on Extreme Poverty and Human Rights GPEP), Universal Declaration on the Eradication of Hunger and Malnutrition (DEHM), The Declaration on the Rights of Indigenous Peoples (DRIP), Declaration on the Rights of Peasants (DRP), and the Genocide Convention (GC). Very roughly, these documents on the right panel first come about after global sentiment, which is a measure of evolving values in the global sphere, arises as mirrored in meetings of the UN Human Rights Council which meets periodically in Geneva, three times a year on average, barring emergency sessions. There is thus generally first a guiding principles document, followed by a declaration, and then covenant or convention, the latter, in actuality being treaties. This right panel can ultimately inform the debates concerning how the core notions of the Universal Declaration can be further elucidated, rather than relying on a kind of intuition alone.

The left panel on implementation consists briefly of world conferences, the periodic filing of reports by countries roughly every five years on progress toward compliance with ratified documents; taking part in the Universal Periodic Review (UPR), where every U.N. member country's human rights practices, which can be defined not only by conventions but also by declarations and guiding principles, coming before the Human Rights Council every four years; the appointing of special rapporteurs who report on select themes, such as on cultural rights and public spaces (2019), human rights defenders (2018), eradication of extreme poverty (2017), privacy (2015), contemporary forms of slavery (2014), and democracy and a just equitable order (2012); world conferences, such as on Climate Change (2017), Indigenous Peoples (2014), and Water (2013) generally with follow-ups every five years; and select countries' situations, such as by special rapporteur on extreme poverty Philip Alston (2017) on extreme poverty in the

United States It is noteworthy, that regarding mental health, a major area of social work practice, Philip Alston stated, *inter alia*:

> Poverty, unemployment, social exclusion and loss of cultural identity also have significant mental health ramifications and often lead to a higher prevalence of sub-stance abuse, domestic violence and alarmingly high suicide rates in indigenous communities, particularly among young people. Suicide is the second leading cause of death among American Indians and Alaska Natives aged between 10 and 34.
>
> (2017, pp. 16–17)

The point of these implementation measures, ultimately, is a creative dialogue with member states, relevant U.N. bodies, including countries and supranational organizations like the World Trade Organization (WTO), World Bank (WB), and the International Monetary Fund (IMF) and non-governmental organizations (NGOs) and civil society in general. Consequently, positive aspects and select concerns are discussed openly with countries at least, and hopefully, in a spirit of humility and dignified compromise, as the social activist Mahatma Gandhi advocated should we desire a socially just world (Guha, 2018) constructed from the pillars of human rights.

Select Implications of the Human Rights Triptych for Practice

Professional settings ought to first encourage the creation of a human rights culture, which is a "lived awareness" of human rights principles in one's mind and spirit and integrated into one's everyday life (humanrightsculture.org, 2020). Ultimately, however, it must be recognized that one does not just "do" human rights in professional situations. Rather, what is tantamount is the importance of human rights as a way of life in one's everyday life. Thus, when speaking about social work (or the helping and health professions in general), it is not "really" the profession we are talking about but rather it is life as the profession. Thus, we must learn to treat others with human dignity and non-discriminatory ways, seeing others as possibilities for tremendous growth, rather than as "actualities," finite persons viewed within the confines of our own narrow viewpoints, if not prejudices. Indeed, the UDHR must be "lived in letter and in spirit," as Saint John Paul II had asserted.

Given that the UDHR is a set of guiding principles and values that ought to be woven into socially just policies, a major guiding principle can be found in Article 28, which asserts the necessity of a just "social and international order" in which rights can be realized. Practice settings, therefore, *inter alia* ought to serve as a setting where social workers can help facilitate changing the social order, so rights can be realized. Thus, if a free market economy that emphasizes profit, rather than the fulfillment of human needs, thus human rights, which can be described as the legal mandate to do so, has resulted in such things as exorbitantly high medical costs, lack of adequate respirators, and hoarding of vaccines by predominantly the Global North at the expense of the Global South during the COVID-19 outbreak, and exorbitant tuition in higher education, practitioners who espouse an integrated practice model, must work toward ways to move toward a human needs, thus a human rights-based society. Ultimately, this can be defined as a democratic-socialist commonwealth which can, in part, be constructed by the practitioner joining political action committees and finding ways to have civil society, in this case, the voices of the poor and marginalized and groups representing them, such as done by the ATD [All Together in Dignity] Fourth World Movement to provide input into the policy debates. Taking article 28 even further, with its emphasis upon a socially just "international order," the intern can declare him or herself a world citizen, apply for a world passport, and work toward a world government. Whereas one may not see the results immediately, the fact that just 2% of money spent by countries on armaments, just to keep their boundaries intact, could feed and educate every man, woman, and child on the earth (IASSW, 2013), the need to declare oneself a world citizen is especially poignant.

The UDHR also speaks of other sets of rights, such as civil, political, economic, social, and cultural. As a general rule, people, at least in the United States tend to equate human rights with civil and political rights, such as freedoms of speech, the press, and religion, as embedded largely in the US Constitution's Bill of Rights. They are important certainly, but it is important to relay to the general populace that other rights, such as economic, social, and cultural ones like employment, food, education, adequate sanitation, health care, security in old age, and shelter, are important. This relaying of information can be done in a variety of ways, such as commemorating international days, like World Water Day (March 22), International Day of Older Persons (October 1), World Food Day (October 16), and World Toilet Day (November 19). The social worker can also work trying to add a constitutional amendment to have a right to employment, shelter, and/or security in old age. As mentioned, while having such an amendment is no guarantee that the right would be implemented, the point is to expand the debates concerning what human rights really are in ways that they make sense to the general populace, so that public sentiment, thus laws and policies, will eventually mirror human rights values. Only chosen values endure. Whereas it might take a relatively long time to expand the debates largely through international, the point is that society in part through the institutions that serve others must have such robust debates, so indeed a human rights culture can flower. Changes in society might even take generations, but, considering in contemporary times an almost suicidal path of humanity evidenced in part by environmental destruction and increasing proliferation of nuclear arms, we must join in solidarity with those who are coming after us, which appears largely an Indigenous value (Weaver, 2019).

The social work practitioner can also play a role in participating in some of the implementation measures as enunciated earlier. She or he can take part in participating at world conferences and provide input into human rights reports and the Universal Periodic Review. They can also work with executives, legislators, and appropriate committees that ought to serve as conduits to ratify human rights documents, such as the US Senate Foreign Relations Committee. Social workers can also show human rights reports to elected officials to get their opinions, which they can then distribute to their constituents, if not write shadow reports, that is alternative reports, such as the Indigenous Peoples and Nations Coalition Shadow Report (2006), speaking of the right to resist colonialization in response to a US human rights report. They can also look at what is often a "litany" of recommendations to a state party to implement socially just policies and choose which ones the intern feels might be most useful. The Report of the Special Rapporteur on trafficking in persons (2017) in the United States, for instance, has roughly 50 recommendations for the state party ranging from the ratification of CEDAW and the CRC to strengthening

> the coordination between government officials and the private sector, particularly in the tourism industry, on the Internet and in the field of telecommunications [and] encourage service providers, banks, trade unions and the media to identify cases of trafficking in persons, disseminate information and share best practices.
>
> (p. 22)

The possibilities actually are limitless as one must be creative and persistent until there is an acceptance of human rights principles but one that is not just "lip service" but actually results in implementation.

Elaborating Upon Integrated (Advanced Generalist) Practice

Integrated practice, strongly aligned with the public health model of intervention, can be defined as a multi-pronged approach that is both proactive and reactive to promote societal and individual well-being, thus eradicating social and individual malaises. This approach can first be further defined as the "meta-macro," which, while recognizing the global interconnectedness of things, made especially apparent during the Coronavirus, calls for interventions that are international in scope, reminiscent of the words of Martin Luther King in his 1963 Letter from a Birmingham Jail that "[i]njustice anywhere is a threat to justice everywhere." (2020, p. 1).

More recently, as the scholar/social activist Angela Davis asserted in regard to police brutality:

> The struggles that we have engaged in against institutionalized police violence are very much related to what is happening in Europe, and Australia, and Latin America, and Africa, and Asia, and the Middle East. . . . We have to learn how to value those who have expressed solidarity for our struggles in the U.S.—We need to not think of ourselves as so ensconced in domestic struggles that we fail to recognize how important international solidarity is.
>
> (Chicago Defender, 2021)

Indeed, an increased sensitivity to our global connectedness can also be found in the words of Philonius Floyd responding to the guilty verdict for Derek Chauvin who murdered his brother. He said:

> I get calls from Brazil, Ghana, Germany, everybody, London, Italy [and they said] 'we won't be able to breathe until you are able to breathe'. . . . I am going to put up a fight . . . not just fighting for George anymore, but for everyone around the world.
>
> (Democracy Now, April 21, 2021)

Indeed, writing about his death, and other African Americans, such as Breonna Taylor, and Jacob Blake, the global COVID pandemic and within the context of Asian American solidarity, Liu (2021) writes: "[T]he pandemic requires us to engage in the racial justice and antinativist struggles in our different localities as well as hold one another's movements accountable to an *internationalist vision* (emphasis added) of collective survival" (p. 4). Certainly, thinking of Sisyphus again, social justice is struggle. Thus, we must stop Asian hate, as well as such irrational fears against Muslims and foreigners referred often to as Islamophobia and Xenophobia, respectively. The debates ultimately must be for human rights for every person, everywhere.

Thus, in the global arena, working with the United Nations and regional organizations, such as the African Union, the European Union, and the Organization of American States, and the ratification and implementation of all human rights documents are examples of such interventions, which ought to be part of the social worker's repertoire for integrated practice thus to play a role in their ratification and implementation, which can have far-reaching effects. As discussed, ratifying CEDAW thus may lead to paid maternity leave and even government-sponsored quality daycare for parents desiring to work in the formal sector. But, whereas ratifying those documents is no guarantee of implementation, the point is that framing, for example, parental leave with pay, a major aspect of President Biden's Build Back Better Act, in human rights terms could give further impetus to the debates, which can help create public sentiment to support such principles.

It cannot be overemphasized that only chosen values endure and having robust debates about such principles could lead to a "lived awareness" of human rights principles in our minds and hearts and integrated into our everyday lives, called a "human rights culture," a major "key" to socially just policies. The social worker thus can play a role in fostering those debates by commemorating international days, creating awareness of human rights documents, and distributing findings of human rights reports, as discussed earlier. Actually, there is a plethora of things social workers can do on the meta-macro level. However, it is necessary to acknowledge that results may not be seen immediately, which is why it is important to understand that implementing human rights is a struggle and the importance of taking on the toga of "Sisyphus" to find joy in struggle.

The "macro level" can be defined as a whole population approach, which attempts to prevent problems before occurring. An example is substance abuse prevention, which is integral to such curricula as Families First or Here's Looking at You. Very briefly, they might teach children and adolescents other ways, than abusing substances to deal with stress or rejection in social situations, such as speaking with the school social worker or a trusted friend, taking up sports like skiing, swimming, or jogging and/or cognitive-behavioral approaches in brief to "evaluate the source." The theory is if at an early age a person can find positive ways of coping, rather than ones that can have deleterious consequences, such as addiction, such consequences could be prevented. Regarding human rights, more specifically, human rights education has been shown to prevent bullying (Rights Sites News, 2020), a global surge to be sure as the 21st century builds up steam, due perhaps to violence in the media, a culture of every person for him or herself, and a culture of profit versus the fulfillment of human needs. But, schools, for example, that have instituted human rights education, in brief, to teach and "live" human rights principles, have been shown to have significantly lessened the impact of bullying. It doesn't take much to realize that if students are taught to treat others with human dignity (Article 1 of the Universal Declaration) and in non-discriminatory ways (Article 2), eventually, such principles will sink into their consciousness and they will act accordingly.

The "mezzo level" can be defined as an at-risk approach that attempts to work with populations that have not reacted successfully to whole populations approaches. Thus, while having attended classes to prevent substance abuse or human rights education, the individual may come home to a dysfunctional family with possibly a violent alcoholic parent or be the member of a community gang that focuses on intimidation and bullying. In both instances, social workers as part of their responsibilities ought to engage in the founding and implementation of such groups. Another case in point is the child who is quiet and shy but may be at risk for mental illness and ultimately suicide. Generally, it can be said that such children are not referred for treatment, which often includes medication, as opposed to more aggressive and acting out ones, who are generally the most referred. It is here where the social worker needs an understanding of human rights documents, which can serve as guiding principles for socially just policies, in this instance The Principles for the Protection of Persons with Mental Illness and the Improvement of Mental Health Care (PPPMI), which is Article 10, asserts: Medication shall never be administered as punishment or for the convenience of others.

The "micro" level often referred to as a clinical approach necessitates interventions when symptoms are fully blown, previous levels of interventions just not working. It is here where individual and group counseling, often the domain of internships, an important one certainly, but one that is only part of the equation. Whereas these skills need to be learned, certainly documents like the PPMI can serve as a framework for the clinician's skills set as it emphasizes *inter alia* that treatment should take place in the least restricted environment, non-exploitation of the labor of the patient, appropriate disclosure of treatment in language understood by the patient, and the right to treatment suited to the person's cultural background. Other documents, such as the CRPD, can also serve as a set of substantive guiding principles for treatment for those having a disability (actually a differing ability), which speaks of the cultural and evolving nature of disability, calling for their full and effective participation and inclusion and the right of opportunity to earn a living. These documents, among others, in brief, set out the goals that social workers must move toward if integrated practice with human rights at its core is to be taken seriously.

The "meta-micro" level often referred to as the realm of the everyday life emphasizes the importance of non-professional interventions, which emphasize in part strengths in a person's environment, such as trusted friends, relatives, and colleagues, but also the many "anonymouses" that exist, such as Alcoholics, Narcotics, Food Addicts, Emotions, and Depressions Anonymous. There are also now many groups on the Internet, such as on Facebook and Twitter, where people may find, solace, comfort, and advice. Noteworthy here is that CEDAW, noting the significant roles that women in rural areas play in the economic survival of their families, including non-monetized work, has expressed the need for self-help groups (Articl14(e)), particularly among women in rural areas, which mirrors the need for this level of intervention. The professional thus ought to be sensitive to this level, facilitating the setting up of such groups, making note also of other connections on the Internet, often as an adjunct to professional levels of intervention.

Research, both quantitative and qualitative, provides a dynamic interplay among these levels of intervention, providing input as necessary, examining the efficacy of best practices and looking at practices that have failed, suggesting corrective measures. A major research approach is to determine the extent that policies and practices compare with fundamental human rights principles. On the state level, a case in point was Massachusetts House Bill

706, which this author worked in tandem with the Massachusetts chapter of Women's International League for Peace and Freedom (WILPF), a legacy of Jane Addams, aimed to assess how Massachusetts laws and policies measure up to human rights standards. Certainly, social workers can propose to legislators similar bills, which would require extensive research. Social workers can also examine how agency policies measure up to human rights principles, but in ways that produce a creative dialogue among supervisors, administrators, and boards. Whereas it may be interpreted that by doing so, social workers may be whistleblowing, that is, calling the agency to the floor of human rights violations, thus needing protection as outlined by the United Nations Declaration on Human Rights Defenders (DHRD), such an assertion appears too strong. Social workers need to learn ways to work positively to resolve conflict with a number of individuals and parts of an organization, in a spirit of humility and compassion.

To be sure, these levels, while distinct, tend at times to overlap, and have their own concerns and struggles. The meta-macro, for example, if advocating for peace and world citizenship will face tremendous pushback after years of socialization from a culture that may believe that war is inevitable as humans are basically selfish and believe in the priority of the nation state. The macro will require approval of human rights education curricula ultimately by school boards that may have ties to elitist institutions and corporations (Gil, 1992) that might feel threatened by such principles in human rights education like rights to health care, to form unions, to employment and to rest and leisure. It also may be difficult to get funding for such an approach as results may not be seen immediately, often a requirement to receive continued funding. The mezzo has its own problems as when one "targets" a group as at-risk, those at risk for substance abuse if having "alcoholic" parents, it may unwittingly create a self-fulfilling prophecy. The micro level generally services a small number of people creating a kind of band-aid approach to social problems. Thus, while it is important to have homeless shelters and counsel the homeless, an unjust social order will continue to result in the homeless to keep on coming. The meta-micro may be seen as negating professionalism, possibly not getting support from professionals and professional organizations. Given these concerns, however, the professional needs to jump into the fray, acknowledge these concerns, and learn to deal with ambiguity, doing research to examine which interventions work effectively and to act accordingly.

General Suggestions for Future Directions

The need to have human rights as the basis of social work's mission and practices in the future can perhaps be summed up by this statement in the *Routledge Handbook of Social Work Ethics and Values* (2020):

We encourage social workers to (1) infuse the specific term "human rights" into their daily practice; (2) critically evaluate how the use of alternative language can impact social workers' responsibility to clients, the profession, and society; and (3) reference and refer to the UDHR, in addition to their country-specific formalized codes of ethics. We call upon *all* social workers to recognize that in addition to their professional roles (e.g., brokers, educators, facilitators), they should consider themselves first and foremost as *human rights advocates* (Keeney et al., p. 13).

Indeed, this powerful idea has tremendous implications during the COVID pandemic, which can continue, in post-COVID times, having tremendous relevance to what social workers do (Quzack et al., 2021). Based on the foregoing discussion of human rights and integrated practice, therefore, here are some general suggestions, with their rationales, that the profession ought to move in the future.[1]

1) First and perhaps most importantly, there ought to be mass social movements in one's country and through the world, as channeled perhaps by CSWE (at least in the USA), IFSW, and IASSW to add provisions to job descriptions, that say something to the effect in regard to the specific population served: "the professional must engage in both proactive and reactive measures to promote well-being"; "the social worker must engage in social justice and social change activities, constructed from the pillars of human rights, to move toward a culture of human rights in society and the world"; and/or "the social worker must engage in multi-faceted approaches (aka integrated practice) with human rights at its core to alleviate social and individual malaise and promote well-being, thus able to tolerate ambiguity."

The rationale for those provisions is really rather simple. As a general rule, there is a conservative tendency to leave things the way they are, to not get out of one's comfort zone, and to deal with only symptoms of an unjust social order. A case in point is that domestic violence and child abuse are functions of unemployment (Gil, 2013) and recall that employment is a human right. There are, for instance, numerous domestic violence shelters staffed by social workers, who provide a number of practical and therapeutic services for their populations. Certainly, these services are important and must be provided. Yet, should we have an integrated practice approach, with human rights providing the framework for action, there would need to be an acknowledgment at least of a "meta-macro" intervention such as implementing the United Nations Charter, which states that nations should commit themselves to full employment, which is antithetical to a capitalist order. Social workers must ultimately as part of their job descriptions work for social justice and human rights, thus requiring finding alternatives to capitalism, such as having a democratic-socialist commonwealth. Also, not very well known is that the US delegation to the committee that drafted the UDHR asserted that employment meant work that was socially useful, contributed to the development of the human personality, and increased purchasing power (Wronka, 1992).

It is important to acknowledge that in regard to funding agencies, it is their money and, as a general rule, want to see the results of interventions within a reasonable amount of time. Professionals, however, can perhaps point out the importance of funding of integrated practice interventions that are multi-pronged, thus being both proactive and reactive. The plethora of jobs in the helping and health professions generally emphasize clinical practice, a micro level of intervention, which deals with symptoms of an unjust order and mirrors a general conservative tendency of the human condition (Gil, 2013). While important, micro practice will not necessarily get at the roots of the causes of societal malaises. Having a human rights culture should get at these roots. There is nothing wrong certainly with having such job descriptions as "doing intakes," "participating in utilization reviews and case conferences," "giving diagnoses," "doing treatment," and the like. But the social worker must also grapple with causes of such social and individual malaises, whether such causes are the lack of a helping ethic in society, a blind adherence to a supposed "free market," and/or lack of human rights education in the schools. Social workers thus need employment where they can support themselves and families becomingly. If they are to do social work right and change "the social and international order" (as asserted in Article 28 of the UDHR) in socially just ways, they should be able to make a living doing that in order to have long-lasting social change.

2) In addition to including, or at least linking to, ethics codes for domestic, if not international social work organizations, such as the National Association of Schools of Social Work (NASW), even the International Federation of Social Workers (IFSW), or the International Association of Schools of Social Work (IASSW), there ought to be included in-field or personnel manuals in places of employment, a copy of at least the UDHR. There also ought to be some discussion in manuals of select salient articles of the Universal Declaration, such as Articles 1 and 2, which assert respectively and inter alia that "[a]ll human beings are . . . equal in dignity and rights and should act towards one another in a spirit of brotherhood [or sisterhood as Eleanor Roosevelt initially wanted]" and that with all these human rights there should no "distinction of any kind, such as race, color, sex, language, religion, political or other opinion, national or social origin, birth or other status." Certainly, such articles can serve as a framework for integrated practice, thus fostering professional growth, for things like supervisory sessions, case conferences, and utilization reviews.

But such discussions must be done with tact and concern certainly for the human dignity of the supervisee and other members of the helping team. It is very easy to get defensive with even the slightest hint that clients are not treated with dignity and are not acting with others in a "spirit of brotherhood" [or sisterhood] or in discriminatory ways, as asserted in the UDHR. To rectify the situation it is probably best, therefore, to merely have a discussion of those and other issues in practice settings, frankly stating with humility that adhering to human rights principles is not simple and "automatic." It is always a challenge. In fact, it will be a lifelong challenge to implement them in one's everyday life and in the professional situation. The point, however, is not that the UDHR and other documents ought to be memorized, understood only in a cognitive way but rather that they are lived in the sense that clients and colleagues are treated with human dignity and in non-discriminatory ways. Certainly, treating others in such a way need not be limited only to the field setting, and the population served. Rather, and to emphasize, every person, everywhere must be treated with dignity and policies reflective of treating others with dignity. Indeed, if one "does" social work correctly, then ultimately we are speaking about the fact that "life" is the profession to treat others with dignity, rather than finding a profession in life.

3) Pendant upon the practicum setting, copies of other human rights documents, the progeny of the UDHR ought to be included in field and agency manuals that work with specific populations. Thus, if the setting concerns itself with domestic violence, then copies of CEDAW ought to be included in the manuals. Whereas it is true that men are also abused, articles from CEDAW can be extrapolated as they relate to men, as well as, have a discussion of how a human rights document on the rights of men might look. In that regard, with contemporary discussions of gender and sexual identity being more fluid nowadays, CEDAW can perhaps serve as a "springboard" for the need to treat LGBTQIA+ populations with human dignity and respect for their diversity. Whereas a fully fledged human rights document on the rights of that latter group has not yet been developed, other guiding principles documents, such as the Yogyakarta Principles Plus 10 (2017) a precursor to such a fully fledged human rights document, can also be displayed as appropriate in field and agency manuals. Other examples are if the agency deals with children, then the Convention on the Rights of Children (CRC) ought to be integrated; if it deals with people with disabilities then the Convention on the Rights of People with Disabilities (CRPD); and if it deals with Indigenous People, which the UN has referred to as having a "special situation," then the Declaration on the Rights of Indigenous People (UNDRIP) ought to be integrated and so on. A problem is that whereas Eleanor Roosevelt wanted human rights documents "not for the doctorate in jurisprudence . . . but for the educated layperson," many such documents, nevertheless, tend to border on "legalize," if

not elitist language and salient points need to be written for the educated layperson. Such an activity can also be grist for the professional to have such documents be understood without pretense for the population served, even if the population includes children for discussion and debate with the possibility of presenting workshops and doing community outreach on a particular human rights document.

It is perhaps necessary here to further discuss UNDRIP, which may have led to CSWE's Statement of Accountability and Reconciliation for Harms Done to Indigenous and Tribal Peoples (Weaver et al., 2021), as well as, the American Psychological Association's Apology (2021) to People of Color for APA's Role in Promoting, Perpetuating, and Failing to Challenge Racism, Racial Discrimination, and Human Hierarchy in the United States. That document speaks, *inter alia*, of full guarantees against genocide, including, but not limited to, the prohibition of the removal of Indigenous children under pretext, the right to be educated in one's own language in a manner appropriate to cultural methods of teaching and learning, but with access to non-Indigenous cultural diversity, and to be treated in ways that are culturally relevant. If working with an Indigenous population, the social worker can thus compare agency policies with that document attempting to implement the multipronged levels discussed, such as creating awareness of UNDRIP throughout the world (metamacro), informing the Department of State about some of its provisions (macro); working with the media, which might be at risk of not paying sufficient attention to Indigenous issues (mezzo); counseling children in ways urging an appreciation of traditional cultural values, such as the avoidance of conflict and respect, for elders (micro); and culturally appropriate ways of peer support, in regard to addiction to alcohol, such as the Native American Church (Prue, 2013; Canda et al., 2019), as an alternative to Alcoholics Anonymous. It appears that this group is often forgotten in governmental, if not public, discourse, an unfortunate occurrence, given that they consist of 6.2% of the world's population, are roughly four times more likely on average to live in poverty, and are guardians of the most varied and nearly extinct languages on this planet, exacerbated most recently by COVID-19. The urgency of informing others of UNDRIP and using it as a set of important guiding principles for integrated practice is noteworthy for as stated by Martin Luther King:

Our nation was born in genocide when it embraced the doctrine that the original American, the Indian, was an inferior race. Even before there were large numbers of Negroes on our shores, the scar of racial hatred had already disfigured colonial society. From the 16th century forward, blood flowed in battles over racial supremacy. We are perhaps the only nation that tried as a matter of national policy to wipe out its Indigenous population. Moreover, we elevated that tragic experience into a noble crusade. Indeed, even today we have not permitted ourselves to reject or to feel remorse for this shameful episode. Our literature, our films, our drama, our folklore all exalt it (cited in De Zayas, 2020).

4) In addition to documents that deal with specific populations, there are various other documents that have relevance that cut across populations. Examples are The Principles for the Protection of Persons with Mental Illness and the Improvement of Mental Health Care (PPMI), The Principles of Medical Ethics Relevant to the Role of Health Personnel, Particularly Physicians in the Protection of Prisoners and Detainees Against Torture, and Other Cruel, Inhuman, or Degrading Treatment or Punishment (PME), the Universal Declaration on the Eradication of Hunger and Malnutrition (DEHM) and The Declaration on the Right and Responsibility of Individuals, Groups, and Organs of Society to Promote and Protect Universally Recognized Human Rights and Fundamental Freedoms (DHRD) and the U.N. Declaration on the Rights of Indigenous Peoples (UNDRIP). These documents, which may need to be "paired down," so they are understood by the educated layperson, can be included in field manuals and agency settings as necessary goals that the setting can work toward. This is not to say that one should immediately "whistleblow," which can be synonymous with defending human rights (Wronka, 2020), that is to call out the setting for failures to meet the principles of those documents but rather to participate in productive sessions with the supervisor, staff, administration, and clients in ways that can progressively move toward implementing those principles. However, history has been replete with whistleblowers, aka human rights defenders being ostracized for calling attention to an organization's violation of human rights principles. A case in point is Albert Woodfox (2019), an African American who was in solitary confinement for 44 years for allegedly killing a prison guard, which he denied. Rather, he felt he was punished extensively for forming a chapter of the Black Panthers in the prison. He went thus against the status quo in the prison culture. Whatever the reasons for Woodfox's punishment, 44 years in solitary violates the "cruel and unusual punishment" clauses of the UDHR and CAT, and he makes a strong plea for society to heed and practice human rights principles. Human rights documents in this case, CAT, can thus serve as guiding principles for social action on the part of the social worker. The social worker, therefore, needs to be aware of such infringements of human rights, take appropriate action as necessary, and needs protections in ways as elucidated in the DHRD. Regarding those documents, the social worker ought to compare those principles with the policies of the agency at which she/he works and suggest constructive and positive ways that the agency can be improved through an integrated practice lens.
5) Before concluding, it must be said that social work and the helping and health professions do not have a "monopoly on human rights."

Thus, while human rights are substantive to the social work profession, as discussed, CEOs, presidents of organizations, administrators, and all those at every level of the organizational structure that ultimately deal with the levels mentioned earlier can and should implement human rights principles. First and foremost, recall that human rights is a way of life for us all. And certainly, human rights documents, as discussed, tend to mirror fundamental spiritual principles, such as human dignity, non-discrimination, direct non-violence, duties to our neighbor, and treating others as we would like to be treated, aka, The Golden Rule. Thus, an easy argument could be made that living and furthering such spiritual principles in our everyday lives and our work is most important. This can be done, perhaps without an in-depth knowledge of the workings of the UN and regional systems and human rights principles, which, ultimately, have as their foundation a profound spirituality.

6) Settings ought to encourage among its employees a tolerance for ambiguity and ultimately a concern for intergenerational solidarity. It is here where taking on the toga of Sisyphus as discussed earlier is especially relevant. But this is generally only possible of course if funding sources are aware of the importance, if not paradox, of tolerating ambiguity and acknowledging that results of certain advanced generalist interventions will not be readily apparent, but may ultimately have long-lasting effects for later generations. Yet, whatever funding agencies do, the practicum site must never lose the vision that human rights entail and the courage necessary to implement them, the "vision and courage of the eagle," as the great spiritual leader of the Sioux, Crazy Horse, advocated. Indeed, what has become known as the Spirit of Crazy Horse, which is "peace, humility, and everlasting love," ought to be at the basis of everything that social workers and certainly others in the helping and health professions do. Thus, human rights, which ought to serve as the pillars of social justice, can provide a stalwart framework for creating the world as a home, if not the thread to tie together, thus integrating, and making whole the multipronged interventions as advocated by integrated practice.

Note

1 Vignettes of these suggested directions, as well as other practice illustrations, can be found in Wronka, J. *Human rights and social justice: Social action and service for the helping professions* (2017; Forthcoming).

References

Alston, P. (2017). Rep*ort on poverty in the United States of America*. Retrieved from www.ohchr.org/EN/NewsEvents/Pages/DisplayNews.aspx?NewsID=22533

American Nurses Association Center for Ethics and Human Rights (2007). *Code of ethics for nurses with interpretive statements*. Retrieved from www.nursingworld.org

American Psychological Association (2021). *Apology to people of color for APA's role in promoting, perpetuating, and failing to challenge racism, racial discrimination, and human hierarchy in U.S.* Washington, DC: APA Press. Retrieved from www.apa.org/about/policy/racism-apology.

Camus, A. (1991). *The myth of Sisyphus and other essays.* (J. O'Brien, Trans.). New York: Random House.

Canda, E., Furman, L., & Canda, H. (2019). *Spiritual diversity in social work practice: The heart of h^el^ping.* (3rd ed.). New York, NY: Oxford University Press.

Chicago Defender (2021). *Angela Davis speech encourages international solidarity.* Retrieved from https://chicagodefender.com/angela-davis-speech-encourages-international-solidarity/

Council on Social Work Education (2015). *Educational policy and accreditation standards.* Retrieved from www.cswe.org/getattachment/Accreditation/Accreditation-Process/2015-EPAS/2015EPAS_Web_FINAL.pdf.aspx

Davis, G. (2010). *My country is the world.* Scotts Valley, CA: Create Space Independent Publishing.

De Zayas, A. (2020). *Reflections on the "discovery" of America.* Retrieved from https://mail.google.com/mail/u/0/#search/alfreddezayas%40gmail.com/CllgCHrg-DRxZQwNhPdTDPcMPZNrWTDzXLzkHcdjxCvnlGNsNqzSfNdDZlLftHmhvQZCJXlXzGlq?projector=1&messagePartId=0.1

Gil, D. (1992). *Unraveling social policy.* Rochester, VT: Schenkman.

Gil, D. (2013). *Confronting injustice and oppression. Concepts and strategies for social workers.* New York, NY: Columbia University Press.

Global Standards of Social Work Education (GSSWE). (2020). Retrie ved from: https://www.iassw-aiets.org/wp-content/uploads/2020/11/IASSW-Global_Standards_Final.pdf

Graeber, D., & Wengrow, D. (2021). *The dawn of everything: A new history of humanity.* New York, NY: Farrer, Straus and Giroux.

Guha, R. (2018). *How Gandhi gave India a sense of dignity and national purpose.* Retrieved from https://qz.com/india/1409887/gandhis-methods-gave-india-dignity-and-purpose-says-ramachandra-guha/

Gutteres, A. (2020). *We are all in this together: Human rights and COVID-19 response and recovery.* Retrieved from www.un.org/en/un-coronavirus-communications-team/we-are-all-together-human-rights-and-covid-19-response-and

Healy, L. (2008). Exploring the history of social work as a human rights profession. *Journal of International Social Work, 51*(6), 735–748.

Healy, L. (2020). *International social work: Professional action in an interdependent ^w^orld.* (3rd ed.). New York, NY: Oxford University Press.

Hugo, V. (2020). *Wikiquote.* Retrieved from www.google.com/search?q=nothing+more+powerful+than+an+idea&oq=nothing+more+powerful&aqs=chrome.0.0j69i57j0l6.5943j0j4&sourceid=chrome&ie=UTF-8

Humanrightsculture.org (2020). *Website for Dr. Joseph Wronka.* Retrieved from www.humanrightsculture.org

Indigenous Peoples and Nations Coalition Shadow Report (2006). Retrieved from https://tbinternet.ohchr.org/Treaties/CCPR/Shared%20Documents/USA/INT_CCPR_CSS_USA_16635_E.pdf

King, M.L. (2020). *Brainyquote: Letter from a Birmingham Jail.* Retrieved from www.goodreads.com/quotes/631479-injustice-anywhere-is-a-threat-to-justice-everywhere-we-are

Liu, W. (2021). *Internationalism beyond the "Yellow Peril"; On the possibility of transnational, Asian-American solidarity*. Retrieved from https://escholarship.org/content/qt3n6934zz/qt3n6934zz_noSplash_3b922bc760a0e91e8b497c31c09bd840.pdf?t=qliv2a

NASW. (2021). International policy on human rights. In *Social Work Speaks: NASW policy statements 2021–2023*. (12th ed.), 193–198.

Online Etymology Dictionary. (2020a). Retrieved from www.etymonline.com/search?q=integrate

Online Etymology Dictionary. (2020b). Retrieved from www.etymonline.com/search?q=core

Prue, R. (2013). Indigenous supports for recovery from alcoholism and drug abuse: The Native American Church. *Journal of Ethnic and Cultural Diversity in Social Work, 22*(3–4), 271–287.

Quzack, L., Picard, G., Metz, S., & Chiarelli-Helminiak, C. (2021). A social work education grounded in human rights. *Journal of Human Rights and Social Work, 6*, 32–40. Doi: https://doi.org/10.1007/s41134-020-00159-5

Rights Sites News. (2020). *Bullying and human rights*. Retrieved from www.theadvocatesforhumanrights.org/uploads/rights_sites_bullying.pdf

Weaver, H. (2019). *Trauma and resilience in the lives of contemporary Native Americans: Reckoning our balance, restoring our well-being*. New York, NY: Routledge.

Weaver, H., Sloan. L., Barkduli, C., & Lee, P. (2021). *Statement of accountability and reconciliation for harms done to Indigenous and Tribal Peoples*. Alexandria, VA: CSWE Press. Retrieved from https://cswe.org/getattachment/Education-Resources/Indigenous-and-Tribal-Content/CSWE-Statement-of-Accountability-and-Reconciliation-for-Harms-Done-to-Indigenous-and-Tribal-Peoples.pdf.aspx.

Weissbrodt, D., Ni Aolain, F., Fitzpatrick, J., & Newman, F. (2009). *International human rights: Law, policy and practice*. (4th ed.). New York: Lexis/Nexis.

Woodfox, A. (2019). *Solitary: Unbroken by four decades in solitary confinement*. New York: Grove.

Wronka, J. (1992). *Human rights and social policy in the 21st century: A history of the idea of human rights and comparison of the United States federal and state constitutions with the United Nations Universal Declaration of Human Rights*. Lanham, MD: University Press of America.

Wronka, J. (2017). *Human rights and social justice: Social action and service for the helping and health professions* (2nd ed.). Los Angeles: Sage.

Wronka, J. (2020). *Whistleblowing, human rights, mental health/well-being: Implications for advanced generalist practice*. Retrieved from www.researchgate.net/publication/339131451_Whistleblowing_Human_Rights_and_Mental_HealthWell-being_Implications_for_Advanced_Generalist_Practice.

Yogyakarta Principles Plus 10. (2017). Retrieved from http://yogyakartaprinciples.org/wp-content/uploads/2017/11/A5_yogyakartaWEB-2.pdf

Additional Readings

Androff, D. (2015). *Practicing rights: Human rights-based approaches to social work practice*. New York, NY: Routledge.

Berthold, S. (2014). *Human rights based approaches to clinical social work*. New York, NY: Springer.

Davis, A. (2022). *Angela Davis: An Autobiography*. Boston, MA: Haymarket.

De Zayas, A. (2022). *The human rights industry*. Atlanta: Clarity.

De Zayas, A. (2021). *Building a just world order*. Atlanta: Clarity.

Edward Clown Family. (2016). *Crazy Horse: The Lakota warrior's life and legacy*. Kaysville, UT: Gibbs Smith.

Gatenio-Gabel, S. (2015). *A rights-based approach to social policy analysis*. New York, NY: Springer.

Ife, J. (2012). *Human rights and social work: Towards rights based practice*, (3rd. ed.). London: Cambridge University Press.

Libal, K., Berthold, S., Thomas, R., & Healy, L. (2014). *Advancing human rights in social work education*. Alexandria, VA: Council of Social Work Education.

Mapp, S. (2020). *Human rights and social justice in a global perspective: An introduction to International Social Work* (3rd ed.). London: Oxford University Press.

Reichert, E. (2011). *Social work and human rights. A foundation for policy and practice* (2nd ed.). New York, NY: Columbia University Press.

Sikkink, K. (2017). *Evidence for hope: Making human rights work in the 21st century*. Princeton, NJ: Princeton University Press.

Van Wormer, K., & Link, R. (2018). *Social work and social welfare: A human rights foundation*. New York, NY: Oxford University Press.

Part 2

Key Issues

The chapters in this section explore key human rights issues that impact large populations of people and the societies in which they live. Oppression based on race, ethnicity, culture, and religion remains a powerful factor in denying the rights of people across the globe. Those in power set the standards that enable the full participation and development of significant populations in society. Group membership in any specific group can be a key factor in integration and success or a basis for discrimination, marginalization, and oppression.

At the social level, economic inequality, health equity, and the environment are critical to assuring that people live in societies that facilitate their well-being and security. Justice in each of these spheres is essential to both individuals and the interests of the societies in which they live.

DOI: 10.4324/9781003111269-4

3 Oppression and Diversity

Race and Social Justice

Cassandra E. Simon and Monique Constance-Huggins

Introduction

Social work's focus on social betterment with an emphasis on social justice makes it mandatory that race be a central part of social work's knowledge base. Understanding the place of race in society, both historically and contemporarily, is necessary to engage in race-centric approaches to social work practice that acknowledge, consider, and apply the significant role of race in many life conditions. Without examining policies, practices, and research within the context of race, the profession overlooks a major life determinant and does much of humanity a disservice. This chapter provides a historical overview of race in U.S. society and current-day racial conditions while presenting Critical Race Theory (CRT) as a valid approach to engaging in social work practice. This will be done through an overview of CRT and its application to social work practice with case studies at different levels of practice.

History of Race in the United States

Race. It has no absolute meaning. Yet, it affects absolutely everything for so many, if not all. How is it that something that does not really exist influences life and life outcomes with such power and veracity? The earliest of civilizations have separated themselves into different groupings, beginning with things like living conditions and developing into distinctions made on things like religion, language, and status. Early interactions between Native Americans and English colonists did not place great meaning on the physical differences between them as status was of significant importance in determining one's place in society. Early colonial days placed more emphasis on economic status than physical differences, with indentured servants of European descent and enslaved Africans being friends and developing intimate relationships (Harvey, 2016). It was not until the popularization of slavery, in what is now the United States, with the moral, political, and social crises that accompanied it did the term "race" emerge.

DOI: 10.4324/9781003111269-5

Although preceded by focused efforts to separate poor, indentured servants from enslaved Africans to dismantle a growing economic connection between them, the critical use of race as a major divider among humans became a major force in the later days of the colonies and subsequently the United States. Given an opportunity to fold into others who physically resembled them, poor "immigrant" Whites were given an opportunity to uplift their status and separate themselves from their darker complexioned counterparts. Indentured servitude decreased and enslavement of Africans increased. Africans began to be noted as an ideal labor force with a major reason being their inability to blend in with tribes and others due to their physical differences. The enslavement of Africans and their descendants soon began to be written into laws and Whites began to separate themselves even more, identifying more with the already wealthy Whites. As the moral crises presented by slavery grew, those in power who benefitted greatly by the free labor provided by enslaved persons began to develop ways of thinking to justify slavery. This justification was intricately connected to skin color, equating Blackness with justified enslavement. This idea of anti-Blackness continues today, permeating different cultural groups effecting everything from daily experiences, to job opportunities and healthcare. One of the most comprehensive examinations of race, its origins and its implications for where we as a society today is Race: The Power of an Illusion. The author strongly suggests viewing it for a comprehensive biological, social, economic and political fact-based foundation of race its development and influence.

Thus, a number of rationalizations were given in defense of slavery, from religious to biological. Many explained away the cruel ownership of other human beings by presenting how uncivilized the enslaved were, lacking an ability to care for themselves. Colonization, along with slavery, became reframed as noble. Other explanations and attempted justifications for slavery, along with the genocide of Native Americans, were unsubstantiated theories of inherent superiority of those of European descent. This all laid the foundation for what we know as race.

Race is a relatively modern concept that is closely associated with physical traits and characteristics, especially skin color. Numerous efforts have been made to find a biological basis for race and the differences we see between those grouped together racially. Yet, the most sophisticated of modern-day technology confirms that there is more genetic variability between those in one "racial group" than between individuals in different "racial groups". The physical commonalities of one so-called race have more to do with ancestry, social groupings, and ethnicity than some biological differences between them. The scientific community acknowledges this and the National Cancer Institute has acknowledged that race is not a good identifier, suggesting it is a proxy for ethnicity. Race is so greatly embedded in our infrastructure and society that to move away from race would require a major paradigmatic shift (Simon, 2006). In fact, the way race is defined in one country can vary.

Brazil is one country often given as an example regarding the complexities of defining race. With five racial categories that are primarily based on skin color and physical characteristics, nuclear family members often identify as belonging to different races. Recent data suggests a growing redefinition of race in Brazil, with many more identifying as Black than ever before (McCoy & Traiano, 2020). So, race as most people perceive it does not exist. It is a concept constructed by man to obtain and perpetuate dominance of some. It has no real biological meaning but significantly affects the life experiences of all.

Racial Groups

Race has greatly contributed to quality-of-life differences seen between Whites and others. And while racial categories have changed over time, White is generally used today to refer to those individuals of European, Middle Eastern, or Northern African ancestry. "Others" are further racially categorized and collectively known as first minorities and more recently as people of color (POC). Other terms like "marginalized," "under-represented," and "at-risk" have been used to refer to these "otherized" people but have been criticized for having negative connotations to the populations to whom they refer. Others put forth the term "minoritized populations" to emphasize what is being done to these populations that limit protection of rights, safety, equality, and equal opportunity, as emphasizing the situation or process. These terms continue to be used among people who are not of primary European ancestry. Currently in the United States, there are five recognized racial categories. These are the major five used on the 2020 Census. In addition to White, there are Black or African American (a person having origins in any of the Black racial groups of Africa), American Indian or Alaskan Native (a person having origins in any of the original peoples of North and South America (including Central America) and who maintains tribal affiliation or community attachment), Asian (a person having origins in any of the original peoples of the Far East, Southeast Asia, or the Indian subcontinent), and Native Hawaiian or Other Pacific Islander (a person having origins in any of the original peoples of Hawaii, Guam, Samoa, or other Pacific Islands). Hispanic and non-Hispanic are provided as ethnicity (place of national origin) options and people who identify as such may be of any race. It is important to note that the five categories used by the U.S. Census Bureau are based on self-identified socio-cultural groups to which one belongs, and an individual may identify with more than one.

Ethnic groups' options provided by the U.S. government are Hispanic/Latino or non-Hispanic/Latino, although the general public loosely refers to ethnic groups when speaking of what is referred to as racial groups (U.S. Census Bureau, 2020). The previous discussion of race, its development, its fluidity in meaning, and the dominance of whiteness in defining others is important in understanding how race has maintained its power over time and continues to determine so much at so many levels in our society. These conditions have led to structural barriers to equality embedded at all levels of the U.S. society. This contributes greatly to negative health, employment, housing, social mobility, economic, education, and mental health outcomes of people of color.

Impact of Race on Well-Being

The impact of race on people of color cannot be denied. The dominance of Eurocentrism, along with notions of white superiority and supremacy, is predicated on laws, principles, and practices that throughout history have situated people of color in a state of oppressive conditions. Each group has its own unique history with this country; yet, they all share the inability to escape the penalization of not being White.

The legacy of genocide, displacement, stolen property, slavery, segregation, Jim Crow, mass incarceration, internment, voting restrictions, and anti-immigrant sentiments along with other factors have and continue to greatly shape the conditions in which POC must live in this society. The overall result has been increased social, political, and economic challenges that make it more difficult to meet life demands and improve the conditions in which they live. A comprehensive overview of each of these groups and their specific experiences in the United States is warranted but beyond the scope of this chapter. Yet, an examination of some of the indicators of quality of life conditions for these groups will illustrate the stark differences in what exist for people of color as compared to Whites.

Income and wealth inequality by race and ethnicity are starkly present in the United States today. Little progress has been made over time in closing race-based wealth gaps with Whites, on average, having eight times the wealth of Black families and five times that of Hispanic families. In addition, Whites have the highest mean and median incomes as Black Americans have the lowest of these. All other racial groups, including Asian, American Indian, Alaska Native, Native Hawaiian and Pacific Islander, and those identified as multi-racial had higher median and mean incomes than Blacks and Hispanics, but less than that of Whites (Bhutta, 2020).

Prior to the 2020–2021 COVID-19 pandemic, the overall U.S. poverty rate had been declining, hitting its lowest (10.5%) in 2019 since 1959, when it first began being reported. While Black (18.8%) and Hispanic Americans (15.7%) reached historic poverty rate lows, they both remained over-represented in poverty in the United States in proportion to their populations. Whites remain under-represented in poverty based on their population number, and Asian Americans have remained consistently below the poverty line over time (Creamer, 2020). It is important to remember that within these broad groupings of race, there are a number of differences among populations within them.

Health disparities by race in the United States are another factor where inequity persists. The past decade has seen an overall decline in health disparities for all racial groups with remaining significant negative outcomes for people of color compared to Whites. Overall Black Americans have poorer health outcomes than any other racial or ethnic group. Black Americans possess the highest mortality rates from cancer, cardiovascular disease, infant morbidity and mortality, and increased negative human immunodeficiency virus (HIV)-related outcomes. Black Americans have over a 30% chance of dying early from heart disease and are twice as likely as White people to die from strokes (Baciu, 2017). Other health problems experienced disproportionately by African Americans are diabetes and obesity.

Although these are conditions of concern in Hispanic communities, especially the Mexican American community, certain Hispanic populations have been known in some instances to have better health outcomes than Whites (Lara, 2005). This, however, seems to depend largely on the country of origin and length of time in the United States. With a 66% increased chance of developing diabetes and having poorer outcomes at a rate higher than Whites, diabetes remains a formidable challenge to this community (Fortman et al., 2019). As is the case for all racial groups, heart disease and cancer are the leading causes of death in Hispanic Americans. For those born in 2020, American Indian/Alaskan Natives have a life expectancy slightly lower than that of Whites, with high causes of death beyond cancer and heart disease being from diabetes, stroke, hepatitis, substance abuse, and suicide. The CDC highlights tuberculosis as a major health threat to American Indians/Alaska Natives with a 2019 incidence rate seven times higher than that of Whites (OMH, 2021).

Geography and poverty are significant obstacles to reducing health disparities for this population (IHS, 2019). Although Asian American and Pacific Islanders have mixed health care outcomes compared to Whites, in many instances they fare better than other racial groups. There are a number of historical, contextual, policy, and practice variables that have combined to put communities of color at increased risk for decreased health and higher morbidity and mortality rates. These disparities are currently being seen with the COVID-19 pandemic.

COVID-19

On March 11, 2020, the World Health Organization (WHO) declared a worldwide pandemic due to the coronavirus disease or what became known as COVID-19 (Cucinotta & Vanelli, 2020). What started out as an outbreak of pneumonia in Wuhan, China, was now considered a public health threat to the world. The economic, political, and social ramifications of this disease are devastating. Although there are challenges to getting exact numbers, recent estimates indicate that worldwide approximately 7 million persons have died from COVID-19, although some estimates are as low as

3.24 million, with over 900,000 deaths in the United States alone (IHME, 2021).

COVID-19 highlighted the racial health inequities discussed previously, demonstrating the ever-important role of race and related social determinants (access to health care, insurance, housing, income, racism, wealth, occupations, etc.) in determining life chances. Data regarding the impact of COVID-19 has shown an all too familiar pattern of increased risk of contracting, getting severely ill, and dying from COVID-19 if you are a person of color. Deaths from COVID-19 have consistently shown that more Whites have died from COVID-19, but persons of color are disproportionately represented in the death toll from the disease (Stokes et al., 2020; Killerby et al., 2020). At the time of writing, vaccines to guard against contraction and severity of COVID-19 indicate that racial disparities continue to exist in terms of the number of persons receiving the vaccine by race, as compared to their number in the population or number of deaths from the disease.

Beyond the health consequences, the reaction to the geographic origins of the virus resulted in a great deal of racial violence against persons of Asian descent across the world. Increased violence against persons of Asian descent has been reported across the United States, Canada, Europe, and England. The UK reported an increase of 300% in Asian hate crimes in 2020 as compared to 2018 and 2019 (Clements, 2020). Although the United States demonstrated an overall 7% decrease in overall hate crimes in 2020, it has an estimated 150% increase in hate crimes against Asian Americans (These crimes have been random, individualized physical attacks, verbal abuse, workplace discrimination, refusal of services, and even being spit or coughed on. These increases in hate crimes have largely been noted in large cities, but the mental health effects on the Asian community have been great causing anxiety and fear regardless of location. A mass shooting in Asian business districts in Atlanta, Georgia, in March of 2021 resulted in the death of eight persons, further amplifying Anti-Asian hate crimes in the United States. And while there were heightened concerns about the rise in anti-Asian sentiments since the pandemic began, the mass shooting led to public outcry and shortly after the Senate passed anti-Asian hate legislation. These conditions, combined with other societal events, have placed the United States at a renewed focus on race, racism, and racialized violence and how these influence all aspects of our lives.

Racial and ethnic violence has been a part of the North American story from the beginning of its formation. Yet, its relationship with Black Americans has been far more complicated and excessively horrific and shaming. On May 25, 2021, the world watched in horror as one Minneapolis police officer, Derek Chauvin, kneeled on the neck of 46-year-old George Floyd, an African American man who was being questioned about an alleged counterfeit 20-dollar bill. Chauvin kneeled on Floyd's neck for over 9 minutes and 29 seconds, cutting off his air supply as Floyd begged for his life and called for his mother who had died a few years before. Three other law enforcement officers stood by while Chauvin murdered Mr. Floyd and citizen bystanders pleaded for mercy and attempted to intervene. Video footage of the murder was shared on social media and viewed worldwide. Another Emmett Till (murdered in1955), another Rodney King (beaten in 1992), some might say Mr. Floyd's death initiated a second Civil Rights Movement of sorts or at least an awakening. This took place within a historical context of violence against enslaved Africans by slave traders and carried on through plantation overseers and runaway slave patrols to current day law enforcement. Contemporarily, this took place within the context of almost a decade of highly publicized shootings and deaths of Black men (Eric Garner, Michael Brown, etc.), women (Sandra Bland, Breonne Taylor, etc.), and children (Tamir Rice, Antwon Rose, etc.) by law enforcement.

In a decade characterized by protests, riots, and the Black Lives Matters (BLM) Movement, there is an acknowledgment by many now who never saw before that the experience of Black Americans is different than that of White Americans with restricted opportunities and access and a devaluation of lives. Subsequently, Derek Chauvin was convicted and sentenced for the murder of George Floyd.

Many remain surprised that he was actually convicted, as the 1992 Rodney King videotaped beating did not result in a conviction. Some of the raised social consciousness regarding race and racisms has resulted in some movement that indicates more ownership of the history, definition, and effects of race (Lemaire, 2020 June). For example, there is more legitimacy given to and in support of the Black Lives Matter movement and LM, a changed definition of racism in the Merriam-Webster dictionary to include the systemic nature of it. Other examples include capitalization of the letter b in Black in mainstream publications, new legislative actions, removal of confederate memorial statues, naming of governmental sites to honor African Americans in place of White persons who supported eugenics and racism and an increase in the number of diversity, equity, and inclusion initiatives and positions in the private and public industries. As encouraging as this sounds, there are also efforts to counter these measures to remove these negative impacts of race and improve race relations.

Racism and its related effects exist due to the combination of several historic, personal, societal, and governmental factors intertwined intergenerationally that have at the base race and the idea of inferiority that still operates today. And while race has no real meaning, other than the meaning we as a society give it, its impact on our lives is real. There are so many ways in which race intermingles with income, wealth, quality of life, increased death rates, life chances, illness, and other aspects of life, that it is impossible to deny its effects.

Hopefully, the complexity and impact of race are examined enough in this chapter to warrant closer examination of the role of race in the lives of the clients or client systems we serve. Each group discussed in this chapter warrants a complete study, exploration, examination of their experience in this country, and how to best work toward equitable treatment to improve their life conditions. This, however, goes beyond the scope of this chapter. What is hoped is that you have come to realize that assessment and intervention in many clients' or client systems' situations may require a closer examination of the role of race in how they experience the world. Critical Race Theory (CRT) is a lens that social workers can use to examine the role of race in lived experiences.

Discussion of Critical Race Theory

CRT draws attention to the centrality of race and racism in American society. Its initial contributors, Derrick Bell and Richard Delgado, postulated that the deep-rooted nature of race is the reason for the stalled progress for Blacks despite the efforts of the civil rights movements (Delgado & Stefanic, 2001). Several scholars have conceptualized different tenets of CRT (Constance-Huggins, 2012; Kolivoski et al., 2014; Ortiz & Jani, 2010). From these scholars, six (6) main tenets of CRT emerge—the endemic nature of racism, interest convergence, critique of liberalism, whiteness as privilege, intersectionality, and advancing the unique voice of those who are marginalized.

The endemic nature of racism emphasized that race is tightly woven into all aspects and dimensions of society. It manifests itself through social processes, institutions, and policies. Accordingly, race is not a marginal factor in the lives of racial minorities, but it is a central force that shapes their outcomes and experiences. Another tenet of CRT is the critique of liberalism. This tenet argues against the idea that policies are neutral and therefore calls for a critique of policies to examine the ways that they disadvantage racial minorities. The tenet suggests that society cannot reach a state of equality for all people through a neutral view of laws and policies.

The critique of liberalism also argues against colorblindness, which is one of the most popular racial ideologies in the United States since the 1960s. Color blindness is the idea that race should not matter and therefore does not matter (Neville et al., 2001). This ideology is characterized by three dimensions. The first dimension is the denial of White privilege. That is, it does not acknowledge that Whites, by virtue of their skin color, enjoy unearned benefits compared to racial minorities. Second, color blindness does not acknowledge the existence and role of institutional racism. Specifically, it overlooks the disadvantages that exist in policies and procedures that block opportunities for racial minorities. The third dimension of colorblindness is the denial that racial discrimination still exists. CRT argues that these dimensions of colorblindness should be challenged as they overlook the lived experiences of people of color. Further, they are destructive to the advancement of people of color.

Another tenet of CRT is interest convergence. This suggests that policies that are targeted to benefit racial minorities would be supported by the dominant culture only if they also stand to benefit from those policies. Further, it suggests that these policies would be supported as long as they do not represent fundamental disruptions to the way of life for most Whites. In sum, the tenet suggests that there is a lack of interest among the dominant culture to dismantle racism if doing so does not support and advance their positionality.

The CRT tenet of whiteness as property draws attention to the social and economic privileges that Whites enjoy as a result of skin color. This tenet intersects skin color with property value to demonstrate how it can be used to benefit those who are White. On the other hand, racial minorities suffer social and economic disadvantages as a result of their skin color. For example, people of color might be more likely to be followed in a store under suspicion of stealing compared to those who are White. Also, they are more likely to be seen as perpetrators of abuse compared to their White counterparts (Kolivoski et al., 2014). In other words, skin color conveys a positive reputation and elevated status to Whites simply because of skin color.

Another tenet of CRT is the intersectionality of identities and oppression. The idea of intersectionality was popularized by Kimberle Crenshaw (1991), who wanted to center the experiences of Black women. She argued that much of the conversation on women excluded the experiences of women who were Black. Further, conversations on Blacks tended to overlook Blacks who were women. In addition to looking at how identities intersect, the tenet looks at how different forms of oppression intersect. Specifically, it highlights how race intersects with other forms of oppression to compound people's lived experiences. Collins (2005) refers to this intersection of oppression as the matrix of domination.

Advancing the voice of those who are marginalized is another tenet of CRT. This acknowledges the legitimacy of the lived experiences of racial minorities and the stories they tell. By sharing stories of the oppression they face, racial minorities are able authentically shed light on their experiences. This highlights the need for counter storytelling to dispel the negative narratives about people of color that are constructed by the dominant culture.

These tenets represent a commitment to social justice as they draw attention to the disadvantages that people of color face through various mechanisms. The attention to vulnerable populations is an important aspect of social justice, and so by centering on race, CRT is advancing social justice. This is with the hopes of creating more equitable outcomes for people of color.

CRT is a vehicle for advancing human rights and its six major principles. In this section, we will demonstrate how the tenets of CRT are intrinsically linked to the principles of human rights (Table 3.1). The six guiding principles of a human rights framework are (1) universality, (2) non-discrimination, (3) the indivisibility and interdependence of rights (political, civil, social,

Table 3.1 Linking human rights principles and CRT tenets

Human Rights Principles	*CRT Tenets*
Principle of *universality*	Racism is endemic
Principle of *non-discrimination*	Critique of liberalism
Principle of *indivisibility and interdependence*	Intersectionality
Principle of *participation*	Advancing the voice of those who are marginalized
Principle of *accountability*	Critique of liberalism
Principle of *transparency*	Interest convergence

economic, and cultural), (4) participation, (5) accountability, and (6) transparency (United Nations Population Fund, 2005). Each of these principles is consistent with key tenets of CRT.

The principle of universality suggests that no individual or groups of individuals should be devoid of human rights. This can be linked to the general premise of CRT but more specifically to the endemic nature of race and racism. The connection to this tenet, which highlights how racism can manifest itself in every aspect of society, ensures that no area—including political, civil, social, economic, and cultural lives—is overlooked for anyone, including racial minorities.

The principle of non-discrimination can be linked to the CRT tenet of critique of liberalism. This principle ensures that no one faces discrimination whether through direct acts or through policies and practices. The critique of liberalism advances this right by arguing against a neutral view of laws and policies. It acknowledges that these policies and laws can indeed restrict the rights of individuals and that a neutral view of the law is ineffective in fighting racism. The critique of liberalism also challenges color blindness, a dimension of which is the denial of discrimination against Blacks. Drawing attention to the persistent discrimination that racial minorities face, even today, advances the principle of non-discrimination.

Another principle of human rights is that of indivisibility and interdependence. This is supported by the CRT tenet of intersectionality. This principle draws attention to the fact that when rights in one area, for example social rights, are ignored, it can impact rights in other areas. This highlights the intersection of different forms of oppression, such as oppression based on race and gender that a Black woman would experience.

The human rights principle of participation is supported by the CRT tenet of advancing the voice of the marginalized. This principle calls for full participation of everyone, especially those who are marginalized, in the decision-making process. CRT supports this by postulating that the experiences and voices of the marginalized must be heard as their experiences of oppression are valued as a legitimate source of information. As racial minorities share their stories, Whites gain a deeper understanding of their struggles.

The principle of accountability offers that governments should ensure that equal rights are enforced especially through the evaluation of laws and policies. This principle is supported by the critique of liberalism, especially with regard to the neutrality of the law. As part of the government's role to ensure that they are maintained through laws, they must provide a critical analysis of policies to ensure that they do not disadvantage racial minorities.

Lastly, the principle of transparency is advanced by the CRT tenet of interest convergence. This principle suggests that governments should be transparent about the decision-making process of policies that impact society. The CRT tenet of interest convergence can shed some light on the role of governments in ensuring that the decision-making process is fair and equitable, not that the policies to improve the well-being of racial minorities are inhibited by the dominant culture because they do not simultaneously stand to benefit.

Discussion of Critical Race Theory and Levels of Social Work Practice

Advancing human rights means paying attention to the role of race in restricting the rights of people of color, and social workers are called to do this. Social work is a human rights profession. Competence 3 of the 2015 CSWE EPAS states that social workers should "Advance Human Rights and Social, Economic, and Environmental Justice." It further states that,

> Social workers understand that every person regardless of position in society has fundamental human rights such as freedom, safety, privacy, an adequate standard of living, health care, and education. Social workers understand the global interconnections of oppression and human rights violations and are knowledgeable about theories of human need and social justice and strategies to promote social and economic justice and human rights. Social workers understand strategies designed to eliminate oppressive structural barriers to ensure that social goods, rights, and responsibilities are distributed equitably, and that civil, political, environmental, economic, social, and cultural human rights are protected.

As a human rights profession, social work must continue to explore the mechanisms through which the rights of people of color are violated at the micro, mezzo, and macro levels. When rights such as freedom, safety, privacy, an adequate standard of living, health care, and education are violated, it amounts to social injustice. Attention at each level is essential in order to arrive at sustainable and impactful change. Gill (2004) supports this multidimensional level approach to social justice. According to him, social justice can be seen at the levels of the individual or human relations, social institutions and values, and global human relations.

The individual or human relations level of social justice signals the way human beings should be treated. That is, they should be treated with worth and dignity as well as be afforded all human rights. This cautions against treating individuals as objects to be used. The second dimension of social justice draws attention to the policies and laws that restrict opportunities for individuals and communities, thereby not allowing them to reach their full potential. Gill (2004) adds a global dimension to social justice by focusing on the need to improve relations and policies that can impact global communities. The two cases next highlight how social injustice can manifest itself at the individual level as well as through a policy that appears race-neutral on the surface.

CRT Under Attack

Despite the importance of CRT in providing a framework to understand how race impacts the lived experiences of people of color, it has come under attack within the last year. Specifically, CRT has been dubbed a divisive tool, which aims to create instability in American society. Advocates also argue that teaching about race and racism is un-American and is in fact racist (Harmon, 2020). As such, there have been rallies, disruptions to school board meetings, and legislation introduced to remove content on race and racism from public schools. The latter is particularly unfortunate, given that public school is an opportunity for children to learn about the truth of our history and the reality of current lives. The curriculum, as it stands, is already Eurocentric, so removing content on race and racism from the classroom further denies all students the opportunity to learn about race and how it impacts people.

These attacks on CRT in essence are attempts to silence the voices of those who are marginalized and to render their everyday lived experiences illegitimate. It seeks to nullify the historical and contemporary representations of race and racism and their socio-economic backgrounds. It is for this same reason why the CRT tenet of advancing the voice of those who are marginalized is necessary. The attack on CRT is also used to instill fear in society about people of color increasingly taking positions of power and participating in the democratic process. According to Harmon (2020), such fear tactics are used by the far right to "influence political discussions in a way that furthers their ideological agenda (p. 276)."

However, scholars suggest that this attack on CRT is only the latest in the long history of attacks against an effort to accurately represent the manifestation of race in the United States. Attacks on the Civil Rights Movement and Black Lives Matter were all part of this agenda to delegitimize the experiences of people of color. All these attacks are clear reminder of the length and breadth to which individuals and groups would go to undermine advancing social justice in the United States, which is the core of CRT.

Conclusion

Race is a central element in the conversation on human rights and social injustice. People of color have historically and in contemporary times been marginalized and have faced discrimination. These acts represent social injustice and are antithesis to the principles of human rights—universality, non-discrimination, the indivisibility and interdependence of rights, participation, accountability, and transparency. Race is a central, not a marginal factor that impacts the lived experiences and outcomes of people of color. Consequently, it must be centered in our quest for social justice and human rights. CRT, through its tenets, has provided a framework to help us understand how race works and how it can be addressed. Should we remain committed about advancing social justice and human rights in our nation, race must be a central part of this conversation.

Hurricanes of Destruction—Micro, Mezzo, and Macro Practice Example

Rebecca, aged 40, has worked for the Bayou Community Center for the last 10 years in X town. The Community Center is situated in the economically depressed side of town, where the majority of residents are working-class Blacks. Bayou is situated in the northern portion of her adopted hometown. Rebecca relocated there after Hurricane Katrina devastated New Orleans in 2005. Bayou serves as a primary service provider for residents on the North end of town, providing basic medical and dental services, along with utility and food assistance. For the last week Rebecca has been working overtime, following up on her regular caseload to assess their safety and post-hurricane needs. Two weeks ago, the town was hit by a category 4 hurricane, destroying businesses and homes across the county. Residents were encouraged to evacuate the town and many did. Some residents did not evacuate and others returned as soon as they were allowed several days later. It was declared a national disaster. Essential businesses like stores, restaurants, gas stations, and banks were closed or destroyed. Electrical and gas lines were destroyed, along with the water treatment system. There was no water, gas, or electricity for days, and telecommunications were limited. Small progress was made in restoring the infrastructure of the town; people who evacuated began returning to their destroyed homes, many uninhabitable. Others who were evacuated were still out of town. Families were separated. Before significant progress could be made, 43 days later another hurricane hit the town, further devastating it. It was one week post the second hurricane, and as in the first Bayou became the command station and central location for hurricane relief in the northern part of town. This continued and Rebecca had been seeing clients continually. One, however, was Ms. Theresa, a 64-year-old Black woman who was overweight, insulin dependent with high blood pressure, had heart failure, and was stuck with COPD. She has four children and while not estranged from them, she has a strained relationship with all four. None of the children ensured Ms. Theresa was evacuated for either hurricane, although the three who live in Town X evacuated themselves and their families.

Despite the third-world living conditions brought on by the first hurricane, none of the children were willing to take Ms. Theresa with them to where they evacuated. Ms. Theresa came to the Center to get a hot meal since she could not cook at home, some water and other supplies being provided by volunteer agencies being dispersed from the Center. Ms. Theresa was really upset. She talked incessantly about her living conditions and how there was no electricity, no water, and no grocery stores opened. She talked about the racism in the town and how frustrating it was to see the other side of town that was predominately White and more affluent getting services restored and resources on their side of town since the first hurricane hit, while the north side of town lagged significantly behind. Rebecca knew this was true as grid surveys and assessments of resource restoration showed this was the case.

Although the city leadership had explanations for this, Ms. Theresa let Rebecca know that she was tired of the city legislators putting resources in the South part of town and not in the North part of town. Her immediate frustration though was there was no way for her to get her medicines as the only open pharmacy was on the other side of town and Ms. Theresa had no way to get there as gas was unavailable. Rebecca had heard the same frustrations since the first hurricane hit from her clients. She listened intently to Ms. Theresa, nodding, giving her eye contact, attempting to convey empathy, and let Ms. Theresa know her concerns were valid. She shared with Ms. Theresa some people might attempt to dismiss the race-based concerns she has, the response models showed that what she said was true. She briefly shared her experience and the experiences of other New Orleans residents post Katrina. She empathized with her fear and anger. Rebecca also reinforced that it was not fair and seemed to be connected to privilege, but that the Center had been discussing disaster-related disparities since the first hurricane. She also informed Ms. Theresa that the Center was able to build on the work done with the first hurricane and was able to have many of the services that were provided on the South side of town, offered now on the North side of town and at the Center with stations from the different service providers because they in the parking lot.

Rebecca was proud to tell Ms. Theresa that she and other staff had listened to concerns since the first hurricane hit and sought ways to address those concerns as best as they could when the second hurricane hit, given the relatively short interval between them. Based on that and the obvious disparities in recovery, the Center had discussed changing policies that prevented duplication of services for clients under any circumstances and having other agencies come to the Center to provide services. Previous to this, the policy was for no other service providers to be on site at the Center, although referrals could be given. For this reason, there was now the ability to get all services provided on the South side of town to those on the North side of town, including medication pick up? Ms. Theresa was pleased with the Center's advancements, and she left the Center feeling heard and somewhat vindicated. She also left with her medication in hand.

Case Review Questions

1 How did CRT play a part in the way Rebecca responded to Ms. Theresa?
2 Examine each tenet of CRT and which could be applied to this case example. How was CRT applied and how could it be applied at all three levels of social work practice?

The Radcliff Reemployment Center

The Radcliff Reemployment Center has a high sanctioning rate among welfare recipients, compared to other welfare-to-work agencies in the city and state. Almost 80% of the individuals who participate in the welfare-to-work program are Blacks, and they bear a disproportionate share of those who are sanctioned for non-compliance. That is, they lose portions and, in some cases, all of the welfare benefits because they are not able to meet their hours of work requirement each week.

James is the new manager at the Radcliff Reemployment Center. He has recently moved to the area and was hired for the position, which was vacant for about four months. As part of James' acclimation to the new position, he was to review the center's reports, including the monthly work participation report. He was also meeting with each of the supervisors to learn about their various duties and to hear about any concerns in the RRC. Alarmed by high sanctioning rates that he found in the reports, James decided to ask each of the supervisors whom he met with for their thoughts on the issue. Shelia, who was the longest-serving employee, said that, since she joined the company seven years ago, she noticed the issue but never really took it to be a big deal. Other staff with fewer years of service also said the same thing. In fact, most of them were all surprised that the new Director was magnifying the issue by bringing it up in the one-on-one meetings with them. They felt this is the way it had always been and that there was no need now to discuss that, especially when participants were simply not motivated to meet their hours. One staff member said they are basically following the state rules, which state that if a parent is unable to meet their 20 or 30 hours a week, then they lose their benefits. It's as simple as that, she said. James was, however, not satisfied and still considered this a problem. He kept thinking about how parents would be able to feed themselves and their children and keep a shelter over their heads if they are sanctioned. Were they being sanctioned for things outside their control? Was the sanction fair across the different participants?

These questions prompted James to take a closer look into the disparities and take action to help rectify the issue. One of the first things he decided to implement was a series of cultural competence training sessions for the staff. The training sessions highlighted things such as implicit biases and drew attention to structural barriers in society that can impact people of color. This was the first time the staff had any such training. James felt it was necessary for staff to be aware of their implicit biases as that could impact their decision on the frequency and the nature of sanctions given to welfare participants of color. He felt that they should not only be aware of their biases but also have an understanding of the real barriers to employment that participants, especially those of color, faced. James noted that many people may not be able to find work because of the high unemployment rate and the discrimination they may face because of their race. If this is our reality, he told the staff, then we cannot continue to heavily sanction people for things they cannot control. Although some of the staff members were reluctant to attend the training at first, they all found much value in it. They felt themselves become more culturally sensitive and began paying attention to contextual factors. At the same time, the welfare participants were more satisfied with the services at the agency. James also formed a task force to review and revise their internal sanctioning policies. After the first six months of the changes and two workshops, there was a significant reduction in the length and extent of the sanctions. James also noticed that the racial gap in sanctions was beginning to close. He was pleased with the trend and commended the staff for being flexible and responsive to change.

Case Review Questions

1 What are the social justice issues in this case?
2 What aspects of critical race theory are in this case? How did James use these in his approach?
3 In the same situation, would you have done anything differently than James? Why or why not?

References

Anti-Asian Prejudice March (2020). *Fact sheet—center for the study of hate & extremism center for hate and extremisms*. Retrieved from www.csusb.edu/sites/default/files/FACT%20 SHEET-%20Anti-Asian%20Hate%202020%203.2.21.pdf

Baciu, A., Negussie, Y., Geller, A., & Weinstein, J. (Eds.) (2017). *Communities in actions: Pathways to health action. National Academies of Sciences, Engineering, and Medicine; Health and Medicine Division; Board on Population Health and Public Health Practice; Committee on Community-Based Solutions to Promote Health Equity in the United States*. Washington, DC: National Academies Press.

Bhutta, N., Chang, A. C., Dettling, L. J., & Hsu, J. W. (2020). *Disparities in wealth by race and ethnicity in the 2019 survey of consumer finances, FEDS Notes.* Washington, DC: Board of Governors of the Federal Reserve System. Retrieved from https://doi.org/10.17016/2380-7172.2797

Clements, L. (2020). *COVID in Wales: Racist incidents take your breath away.* Retrieved from www.bbc.com/news/uk-wales-56323775

Collins, P. H. (2005). *Black sexual politics: African Americans, gender and new racism.* New York: Routledge

Constance-Huggins, M. (2012). Critical race theory in social work education: A framework for addressing racial disparities. *Critical Social Work, 13*(2), 1–16. Retrieved from http://www1.uwindsor.ca/criticalsocialwork/

Creamer, J. (2020). *Inequalities persist despite decline in poverty for all major race and Hispanic Origin Groups.* U.S. Census Bureau. Retrieved from www.census.gov/library/stories/2020/09/poverty-rates-for-blacks-and-hispanics-reached-historic-lows-in-2019.html.

Crenshaw, K. W. (1991). Mapping the margins: Intersectionality, identity politics, and violence against women of color. *Stanford Law Review*, 43(6), 1241–1299.

Cucinotta, D., & Vanelli, M. (2020). WHO declares COVID-19 a pandemic. *Acta Biomedical, 91*(1), 157–160. Doi: 10.23750/abm.v91i1.9397.

Delgado, R., & Stefanic, J. (2001). *Critical race theory: An introduction.* New York, NY: New York University Press.

Fortmann[1], A. L., Savin, K. L., Clark, T. L., & Philis-Tsimikas, A., Gallo, L. (2019). Innovative Diabetes Interventions in the U.S. Hispanic Population. *Diabetes Spectrum,* 32(4): 295–301.

Gill, D. G. (2004). Perspectives on Social Justice. *Reflections: Narratives of Professional Helping, 10*(4) 32–38.

Harmon, M. G. (2020). Policy distraction: Sentencing reform adoption as a diversion from rising social inequality. *Crime, Law and Social Change, 73*(3), 275–295.

Harvey, S. P. (2016). Ideas of race in early America. *American History.* https://doi.org/10.1093/acrefore/9780199329175.013.262

Indian Health Services. (2019). *The Federal Health Program for American Indians and Alaska Natives Disparities.* U.S. Department of Health and Human Services. Retrieved from www.ihs.gov/newsroom/factsheets/disparities/

Institute for Health Measurement and Evaluation (2021). *COVID-19 has caused 6.9 million deaths globally, more than double what official reports show.* Retrieved from www.healthdata.org/news-release/covid-19-has-caused-69-million-deaths-globally-more-double-what-official-reports-show

Killerby, M. E., Vet, M. B., Link-Gelles, R., Haight, S. C., Schrodt, C. Lucinda England, L., Gomes, D. J., Shamout, M., Pettrone, K., O'Laughlin, K., Kimball, A., Blau, E., Burnett, E., Ladva, C., Szablewski, C. M., Tobin-D'Angelo, M., Oosmanally, N. Drenzek, C., & Murphy, D. J. (2020). *CDC COVID-19 response clinical team characteristics associated with hospitalization among patients with COVID-19—metropolitan.* Atlanta, GA: MMWR Morbidity and Mortality Weekly Report. DOI: http://dx.doi.org/10.15585/mmwr.mm6925e1external *icon*

Kolivoski, K., Weaver, A., & Constance-Huggins, M. (2014). Critical race theory: Opportunities for application in social work practice and policy. *Families in Society: The Journal of Contemporary Social Services, 95*(4), 269–276. DOI: 10.1606/1044–3894.2014.95.36

Lara, M., Health R., & Rand C. (2005). *Acculturation and Latino health in the United States: A review of the literature and its sociopolitical context.* Santa Monica, CA:

RAND Corporation; 2005. Division of Minority Health. U. S. Department of Human Services Profile Native American/Alaskan Natives. Retrieved from ssshttps://minorityhealth.hhs.gov/omh/browse.aspx?lvl=3&lvlid=6

Lemaire, S. (2020, June 26). *How George Floyd's death has acted American life*. Race in America. Retrieved from www.voanews.com/usa/race-america/how-george-floyds-death-has-impacted-american-life.

McCoy, T., & Traiano, H. (2020, November 15). *He grew up White. Now he identifies as Black. Brazil grapples with racial redefinition*. Retrieved from www.washingtonpost.com/world/the_americas/brazil-racial-identity-black-white/2020/11/15/2b7d41d2-21cb-11eb-8672-c281c7a2c96e_story.htm

Neville, H. A., Worthington, R. L., & Spanierman, L. B. (2001). Race, power, and multicultural counseling psychology: Understanding White privilege and color-blind racial attitudes. In J. G. Ponterotto, J. M. Casas, L. A. Suzuki, and C. M. Alexander (Eds.), *Handbook of multicultural counseling* (pp. 257–288). Thousand Oaks, CA: Sage.

Office of Minority Health (OMH) (n.d.). *Profile: Asian Americans. U.S. Department of Health and Human Resources*. Retrieved from https://minorityhealth.hhs.gov/omh/browse.aspx?lvl=3&lvlid=63

Ortiz, L., & Jani, J. (2010). Critical race theory: A transformational model for teaching diversity. *Journal of Social Work Education, 46*(2), 175–193. doi:10.5175/JSWE.2010.26090007

Simon, C. E. (2006). Breast cancer screening: Cultural beliefs and diverse populations. *Health & Social Work, 31*(1), 36–43. https://doi.org/10.1093/hsw/31.1.36

Stokes, E. K., Zambrano, L. D., Anderson, K. N., Marder, M., Raz, K. M., Felix, S. E., Tie, Y., & Fullerton, K. (2020). Coronavirus disease 2019 case surveillance—United States, January 22—May 30, 2020. *Morbidity and Mortality Weekly Report*, 69, 759–765. DOI: http://dx.doi.org/10.15585/mmwr.mm6924e2external icon external icon

United Nations Population Fund (2005). *Human rights principles*. Retrieved from https://www.un.org/en/universal-declaration-human-rights/

U.S. Census Bureau. (2020). *About race*. Retrieved from www.census.gov/topics/population/race/about.html

4 Oppression and Diversity

Ethnicity, Culture, Religion

Carole Cox

Setting the Stage

Oppression is a threat to individuals and society as it serves to denigrate and divide. The oppressor or dominant group perceives others with specific characteristics as subordinates and is able to convey these beliefs through social, political, and economic assumptions and values that focus on differences depicting the subordinate group as unworthy or incompetent (Mullaly, 2010). The underlying intent of oppression is to maintain the power of the oppressing group through beliefs and ideologies, often institutionalized, that support the powerful and disadvantage others. Oppression is a violation of basic human rights and a perpetrator of social injustice as it focuses on marginalizing and subordinating groups while refuting their basic human dignity.

As discussed earlier in this book, oppression occurs at several levels: cultural, structural, and individual with each interacting with the other (Mullaly, 2010). Cultural oppression reflects social attitudes, beliefs, and stereotypes about a specific group. Structural oppression occurs when these beliefs are institutionalized in society through policies, institutions, and organizations. Individual oppression refers to the personal experiences of those targeted by these attitudes and stereotypes. Moreover, as these biases are internalized by those victimized, they can shape self-concepts and identity, thus affecting individual responses (McIntosh, 2012).

The key element in oppression is power, which is closely tied to positionality, one's place in society. Positionality influences access to resources and opportunities, contributes to identity formation, and recognizes that individuals have many interacting positions (Kesar, 2002, Sloan et al., 2018). Understanding one's own position and multiple identities is essential for practice with diverse persons and groups.

Challenge social injustice while promoting sensitivity to and knowledge about oppression and cultural and ethnic diversity are central tenets of social work practice (NASW Code of Ethics, 2017). The profession's ethical responsibilities call upon social workers to be culturally aware and understanding of diversity and oppression as it occurs in many forms, including

DOI: 10.4324/9781003111269-6

race, ethnicity, sex, sexual orientation, gender, status, ability, and religion. Cultural competency, the ability to understand the unique experiences of diverse groups with an awareness of one's own privilege and power is essential to combating oppression (NASW Standards of Cultural Competence, 2016).

The Council on Social Work Education (CSWE, 2018), the accreditation body for schools of social work in the United States, specifies ten competencies expected of graduating students. Among these competencies, Competency 4: Engage diversity and difference in practice and Competency 5: Advance Human Rights and Social, Economic, and Environmental Justice offer a foundation for anti-oppressive practice. Both competencies attest to the importance of social work's role in combating oppression and the role of social work education in addressing it.

Ethnicity

The term "ethnicity" connotes both psychological and social identity and has been defined as the shared values and beliefs of a group (Spenser, 2006). From a psychological perspective, ethnicity refers to the way in which the individual develops a sense of self. It is a complex term, in that it has multiple and varying definitions and interpretations. Gordon (1964) defines an ethnic group as individuals with a shared sense of peoplehood based on race, religion, or national origin. Shibutani and Kwan expand this definition by including the perception of the individual and others in the definition, "[A]n ethnic group consists of those who conceive of themselves as being alike by virtue of their common ancestry, real or fictitious, or are so regarded by others" (1965, p. 47). Cohen (1974) includes the role of interaction in his definition, "a collectivity of people who (a) share some patterns of normative behavior and (b) form a part of a larger population interacting with people from other collectivities within the framework of a social system" (1974, ix). As reflected in these many definitions, ethnicity is a complex term that continues to be operationalized in many ways, with little consensus as to how exactly it should be measured (Juby & Conception, 2005).

Race is not the same as ethnicity although the two terms are often used interchangeably. Ethnicity refers to shared social, cultural, and historical experiences stemming from common national or regional backgrounds (Smedley, 1998). Ethnic groups are subgroups of a population that share common historical experiences, beliefs, values, and behaviors and identify with belonging to the group (Smedley, 1998). Multiple ethnic groups can be subsumed within one racial group, each with their own experiences and traditions. In comparison, race is used to define groups that share distinctive physical traits such as skin color or hair texture although the term itself has no genetic basis (Blakemore, 2019). Physical characteristics, often in conjunction with language and traditions, connote ethnic ties.

Individuals belonging to an ethnic group are governed by the values and normative expectations adhered to by the group members. Such forces shape ethnic identity, which can give persons a sense of belonging and even pride and self-worth. At the same time, when ethnic groups are perceived as a threat to the majority, they may be the target of discrimination and oppression. In the extreme, this can lead to ethnic cleansing, with those in power besieging an entire group for removal or even annihilation. The Turkish massacre of the Armenians, the persecution of the Jews in Nazi Germany, the Khymer Rouge attacks on Chinese in Cambodia, and the oppression of the Rohingya in Myanmar are striking examples of ethnic cleansing.

However, it is essential to recognize that ethnicity is not a constant. Thus, among immigrants, ties to ethnic traditions and culture frequently wane among the generations. First-generation immigrants tend to adhere more strongly to values than subsequent generations who become acculturated to the new society.

Culture

Culture systematizes interactions as individuals learn what to expect from each other and how they themselves should behave and interact. Culture is both shared and inherited as it is passed to subsequent generations, influencing both life experiences and the roles that people play (Lum, 2000). However, as culture is a social definition, it is dynamic and constantly constructed in response to challenges and experiences that people have through their own interactions (Yan, 2008). Consequently, comparable to ethnicity, generalizations about culture and its influence on an individual must be made cautiously as interactions and experiences are unique. Culture may act as a foundation for understanding action but should not be treated as an immutable blueprint for characterization.

Cultural responsiveness is an ongoing process that requires self-awareness in order to understand others, the systems in which they interact, and the factors that influence them. Cultural humility, which seeks to see the world as others experience it, including the biases and oppression that have impacted them can increase sensitive responsiveness (Abe, 2020). Moreover, such humility can only be learned through direct interactions with clients that enable the practitioner to be immersed in the others' world and thus understand their reality (Abe, 2020). This humility validates the other's reality, distinguishing it from the power and privilege of the practitioner.

Religion

Among the rights that compose the UNDHR is Article 18, "everyone has the right to freedom of thought, conscience and religion." Religion differs from spirituality as it describes the institutionalized systems of beliefs, rituals, and behaviors related to a supreme being to which adherents submit

(Black & Stone, 2005). However, religious freedom is frequently challenged as religious oppression remains globally prevalent. Religious persecution, severe discrimination based on a person's faith, continues with religious minorities who lack access to political or cultural power and are frequently the targets of oppression (Hodge, 2006).

Religion is closely connected with ethnicity and culture as it gives identity, a sense of meaning, and traditions. Even though America is perceived as a pluralistic country, it is also a religious country with almost half of all Americans (47%) identifying themselves as Christian and with 55% of that group defining themselves as Evangelical, while among the non-Christian faiths, 1.9% identify as Jewish, and 0.9% as Muslim (Pew Research Center, 2015).

Religious institutions themselves tend to be segregated and support specific ethnic groups. Ethnic churches that serve predominantly one ethnic group with services in the group's language continue to exist along with multi-ethnic churches. These churches play important roles in assisting new immigrants to assimilate (Arkash, 2011). They act as comfort zones, where congregants can enjoy their own identity and culture, prayers, and communal life (Kim, 2011, Raphael, 2011).

Restrictions through laws and actions that target religious groups are widespread, reaching a global high in 2018 (Majumdar, 2020). These include laws that restrict beliefs and practices ranging from bans on clothing to acts of armed conflict. Most of such restrictions are on Christians and Muslims who compose the largest religious groups while Jews, who account for 0.2% of the world's religious population, are the third most-persecuted religious group.

Since its founding, the United States has been predominantly a Christian country. Despite its increasing diversity, those viewing it as a Christian nation have increased (Straughn, and Feld, 2010). Although liberty and tolerance are a part of the American credo, discrimination against Catholics, Jews, and Muslims is prevalent. Findings from a national survey found 82% of respondents stating Muslims suffer discrimination, 64% stating that Jews suffer discrimination, and 50% stating that Evangelical Christians are discriminated against (Masci, 2019).

Recently, white supremacy in the United States, frequently associated with Christianity, has been linked with racism, xenophobia, and Islamophobia and increases in anti-Muslim and anti-Semitic attacks (Perry et al., 2019, Scala, 2020). "Jews will not replace us" chanted at a demonstration in Charlottesville, Virginia, in 2017 by white supremacists as well as signs such as "Camp Auschwitz" displayed in the January 2021 attack on the US capital suggest the extent of racism, hate, and division in the country.

Religious intolerance has long been a part of American life and thus those in power are able to draw upon and encourage these sentiments as Muslims, immigrants, and Jews are described as threats to Christian society (Corrigan, 2020). Building upon these fears fuels intolerance and is particularly notable in the rise of anti-Semitism, as Jews are perceived as dangers to traditional American society (Dias, 2020; Vasques & Acosta, 2019).

Ethnicity and American Immigration

Over a period of decades, the diversity, often identified as "pluralism" or "multiculturalism," has been perceived both positively and negatively by American society. The growth and development of the nation were dependent upon the skills and manpower offered by succeeding waves of immigrants, while their acceptance and integration into society were and are often met with conflict.

Africans, the first large group of immigrants, were brought to America involuntarily and were followed by northern and then central and eastern Europeans. The first Africans arrived in Virginia in the early days of the colony, probably as indentured servants, a position shared with many of the whites in the colony (Takaki, 1993). This status changed in 1661 when the Virginia Assembly institutionalized slavery, eventually defining slaves as property. With this definition and concerns over discontent among white laborers, landowners and planters were instrumental in the development of a racially subordinated labor force (Takaki). Subsequently, new laws dictated the interactions between whites and Blacks, subordinating Blacks to a lower status, and establishing the framework for subsequent relationships between the races.

The following waves of immigrants came voluntarily to America, often seeking refuge from economic and religious persecution. In a country shifting from a primarily agricultural society to an increasingly urban one, these groups were essential to the new developing industries. These early immigrants were mainly English, (49%), German, and Scot and shared religion and culture with the Americans (Archdeacon, 1983). By the time of the Revolutionary War, there were more than 75,000 German residents in Pennsylvania (Glatfelter, 1990). Between 1820, the time of the first census, and 1890, nearly 15 million immigrants had settled in the United States (Archdeacon, 1983).

The influx of immigrants coincided with the urbanization and industrialization of the country. They provided a critical labor force but given their poor wages, they tended to concentrate in tenements and slums in urban areas where factors were established. Although needed for their labor, there were also fears that the new immigrants were taking jobs away from the native Americans. These fears coupled with the problems of urbanization, poor living conditions, overcrowding, and lack of sanitation, coupled with foreign languages and traditions, contributed to increasing contempt for immigrants and restrictive immigration policies (Young, 2017).

One of the earliest groups to experience mass anti-immigrant feelings was the Irish who composed nearly half of all immigrants in the 1840s (Ó Gráda, 1999). Given their large numbers, poverty, and poor education, they were seen as a menace to American society. This threat was magnified by their Catholicism, a glaring contrast to the predominantly Protestant middle class. In the 1850s, the anti-immigrant sentiments coalesced in the development of The Know-Nothings, a political party whose primary goal was to keep out all foreign influences and preserve traditional American values. Among its aims were the elimination of all foreigners and Roman Catholics from public office, the establishment of a 21-year naturalization period for all aliens, the deportation of foreign paupers and criminals, mandatory bible reading in public schools, and the preservation of Protestant domination in all areas of public life (Spann, 1981). Although the Party dissolved in the 1860s, it elected ten governors and hundreds of legislators and local politicians and was thus influential in American policy and society (Boissoneault, 2017).

From the late 19th Century through the first half of the 20th Century, diverse groups of immigrants entered America distinguished by religion, traditions, and language, coming primarily from Southern and Eastern Europe. As well as fears about losing jobs to the immigrants, traditional cultural prejudices contributed to resentment (Young, 2017). These included concerns that the Catholics would undermine society through their allegiance to the Pope while Jews were viewed through historical anti-Semitic stereotypes portraying them as greedy and untrustworthy (Schragm, 2010).

As their numbers grew in the 1850s, particularly in the Western states, resentment and discrimination against the Chinese also increased. Their labor was needed for building railroads and in mining, but this need was accompanied by resentment as they were viewed as competitors for jobs. Distinguished by their appearance, traditions, and behaviors, they were easily marginalized and victimized, identified as the "Yellow Peril." Such oppression resulted in The Chinese Exclusion Act of 1882, which suspended the immigration of Chinese laborers for ten years and mandated that the Chinese had to obtain certificates proving their eligibility to live and work in the United States. The Act stayed in effect until 1943.

Although sometimes called the "model minority," Asian Americans continue to encounter hatred and violence in the United States, particularly in urban areas (Yancy-Bragg, 2021). Such violence, fueled by rhetoric that often sees them as responsible for the COVID-19 pandemic, has led in recent years to a soaring rate of attacks on Asians, particularly on older adults in many urban areas (Yancy-Bragg, 2021). Such attacks are often accompanied with verbal harassment, being shunned, or being denied services (Asian American Commission, 2021).

Other groups continue to be marginalized and oppressed as they are perceived as threats to the stability of the country. Following the attacks on the World Trade Center in 2001, Muslims were viewed with suspicion and distrust and often considered unassimilable (Young, 2017). More recently, strict immigration laws have targeted Mexican immigrants, dissuading them from entering the country as they were described as dangers to American society (Israel & Tatalova, 2020). As these oppressive policies prevail, human rights are violated.

Social Work and Ethnicity

Social works involvement with ethnic groups can be traced to the settlement movement in the late 19th Century. From the 1880s American cities became the focus of large concentrations of immigrants eager to settle in the new country. These immigrants concentrated in major cities, such as New York, Philadelphia, Boston, and Chicago, dramatically increasing both the numbers and diversity of these cities' populations. Between the years 1866 and 1917, more than 200,000 Europeans entered the United States each year, with most settling in these cities. In 1910, in the eight largest cities of America, more than one-third of the population were foreign born (Trattner, 1994).

For the most part, these people were unskilled and poor, and unable to speak English. The most visible of these immigrants were those who concentrated in the centers of these cities, lived in the poorest housing, and lacked the basic amenities common to the majority of the American population. The settlement house movement sought to improve the conditions of these people and to institute social and economic changes, which would assist them in assimilating into American society. Thus, in contrast to earlier social work movements such as the charity organization societies, which focused on individuals and their needs for help, the settlements were concerned with the broader acculturation, action, and reform that were integrated into these groups and the communities.

Settlement houses legitimated ethnicity in several ways. The movement saw neighborhoods as basic social units for teaching skills necessary for social action and citizenship, and the vast majority of urban neighborhoods were organized and defined by ethnicity. Thus, ethnic identifications became a part of the settlement houses. Settlements helped neighborhoods to celebrate ethnic "national days," worked as forces for inter-ethnic tolerance, and promoted the concept that becoming American did not mean renouncing cultural heritage and traditions.

Even today, society plays a major part in the shaping and determination of ethnicity. Although individuals may seek to shed their ethnic identity and assimilate into the mainstream, society itself may act as a barrier. To the extent that persons are perceived as being ethnically different, they may be excluded or find themselves the target of oppression (Villa, 2020). Although they may no longer adhere to strict traditional values, their appearance often implies differences that separate people from the majority. Consequently, this exclusion may serve to strengthen ethnic ties, even for those seeking to acculturate.

Conspiracy Theory and Oppression

Particularly troubling is the recent emergence of conspiracy theories that fuel prejudice against specific ethnic and minority groups. Such theories act as a foundation for overt oppression and continue to be spread by powerful groups seeking to maintain control by threatening specific groups and praising those who adhere to their beliefs (Kruglanski et al., 2019). Research suggests many factors underlie persons' adherence to the theories, including feelings of uncertainty, a need for control and security, and a need to maintain a positive self or group image (Douglas et al., 2017).

The theory attempts to explain the causes of significant political and social circumstances, with claims that they are due to two or more powerful causes (Aaronovich, 2010). Widely circulated through white supremacists' groups and the media, these theories build on negative attitudes and stereotypes that depict racial and ethnic groups as threats to society. As an example, the terrorist attacks of 9/11 were blamed on the Bush administration, the Saudi government, corporations, financial industry, and the Jews. Conspiracy theories that the Chinese created global warming, immigrants plot to attack the British government, and that Jews are plotting to take over the world continue to fuel prejudicial attitudes, oppression, and violence (Jolley & Douglas, 2019).

A notorious example of conspiracy theory is *The Protocols of the Elders of Zion* that appeared in a Russian newspaper in 1903 and was adapted by Henry Ford into a newspaper series, *The International Jew*, in the 1920s, (Baldwin, 2002). The protocols describe the Jewish people as a cunning elite, whose goal is to dominate the world by destroying institutions, the church, and society. Although a fabrication based on ancient stereotypes and attitudes, the book continues to be sold across the world and to stir anti-Semitic acts and violence. Among the more recent claims are that Jews caused the COVID pandemic (Zipperstein, 2020) and claims that Jewish bankers are using lasers to start forest fires to finance railroads (Chaitt, 2021).

Conspiracy theories can be powerful tools for oppression as they are easily spread through social media. The violent attack on the US Capital in January 2021 is illustrative of the role that conspiracy theory and social media can play in encouraging and supporting violence. Beliefs in a fraudulent election, treachery forums, and right-wing websites that warned of minority groups taking over the country, spurred on by those in power, underscore the danger that such theories pose to social justice and society itself (Djupe & Dennon, 2021).

Social Work Practice With Diverse Groups

Critical social work is an important approach in working with diverse groups as it recognizes that large social processes including race, gender, and socioeconomics, are associated with power and status in society. It recognizes the social structures that impact life experiences of others (Payne, 2014). As such, it focuses on social injustice and the analysis of institutional contexts of practice as well as the social location of privilege and power (Dominelli, 1997). Structural inequalities and inequities are key elements of oppression and demand actions and discourse that deconstruct them and reveal their impact). Consequently, practice with clients must be a collaborative process that works to identify these elements as well as an empowering one that works toward change (Hick et al., 2005).

Critical thinking necessitates understanding the complexity of forces that affect different groups and affect their advantages and disadvantages in society (Hardiman et al., 2007). A vivid example of these disparities is found in the overrepresentation of racial and ethnic minority persons affected by the COVID-19 pandemic. Living situations, chronic health conditions, and types of employment increased exposure to the virus, a higher prevalence of the illness, greater mortality, and a lack of access to vaccination underscore the inequality in society and its impact on the lives of specific disadvantaged groups (Ellis & McPhillips, 2021).

At the same time, critical social work recognizes the roles that ethnic norms and traditions can have on the perception of problems, both physical and mental, and the decisions to seek professional help. Beliefs can influence the perception of help, the kind of problems that require professional assistance, and who should be included in the help-seeking process. Stigmas associated with problems and the help-seeking process can act as formidable barriers to care. As an example, research on help-seeking behavior of Asian Americans finds that they tend to delay care due to a focus on emotional self-control, factors that contribute to personal responsibility, social harmony, and saving face (Kim et al., 2016). These attributes also reflect the collectivist focus of the culture and the stigma associated with professional help seeking (Sue et al., 2012).

Anti-oppressive practice begins with understanding one's own biases and stereotypes. Reflecting on one's own beliefs and thoughts is essential for developing new ways of understanding and acting. Critical reflection helps to bring out unconscious thoughts and feelings, which contribute to oppression and injustice (Mattison, 2014). It increases awareness of cultural attitudes and beliefs that influence perceptions, which may then be institutionalized into varying social structures. This begins with practitioners' awareness of their own power, biases, and stereotypes that can impact their perspectives and interactions.

The Lens Model and Practice

The lens model (Cox & Ephross, 1998) refers to the lens through which we all see the world and attribute meanings to the experiences of both ourselves and others. It is a tool that is directly applicable to critical social work as it is based on the premises that meanings influence actions and that meanings are unique to experience.

The lens is influenced and shaped by one's own values, norms, stereotypes, and expectations. As with all lenses, accuracy is important, in that they must be transparent if they are to clearly show the meanings and intentions of others. An opaque lens suppresses and even negates true understanding of the individual's responses as it reflects the viewer's experience. Consequently, social workers must be knowledgeable about their own beliefs, biases, and stereotypes to work effectively with diverse clients (Nguyen et al., 2020).

Practice also demands that culturally aware social workers are knowledgeable about the values and norms of those with whom they are working. As an example, self-determination is a guiding principle of the profession. However, this emphasis on the "self" may be contradictory to the cultural values that stress the importance of the group over the individual. The emphasis on the individual reflects the Western notion of individualism, which may not apply to other groups where collectivism is emphasized with self-actualization and determination secondary to the well-being of the group.

As well as distortions caused by the viewer's own attitudes, it is essential that the social worker is knowledgeable of the individual's previous experiences with the formal system. As an example, previous negative experiences, such as long waits, indifferent or poor treatment, and insensitive providers, can act as barriers to care. Concomitantly, it is important to recognize that any one individual may be influenced by specific experiences, values, or traditions. Generalizing negates the individual's own unique history and responses and can be a deterrent to care.

Practice with diverse groups requires knowledge about the perception of seeking help. These perceptions may be strongly influenced by ethnic values, beliefs, and traditions. Thus, seeking professional help may be viewed as unacceptable as problems are perceived as shameful.

When mental health problems are considered a stigma, there is often a reluctance to seek professional help. This reluctance is magnified in those groups that have suffered discrimination and insensitivity by the health care system.

Understanding the factors that may affect help seeking is a prerequisite to action that can assist and accommodate groups. Reaching out to specific communities, educating them about services, and having providers from the same ethnic backgrounds are factors that can increase utilization. Accessibility and acceptability are critical in encouraging service utilization. Accessibility demands that the services are located within communities and that programs are affordable while acceptability means that these services reflect the beliefs and values of the group, often having staff of the same ethnic group. An example is offered by the Asian Clinic Treatment Services, located in Brooklyn, New York. Although the Clinic focuses on mental health, this is not mentioned in the clinic's name, which underscores the importance of cultural acceptability in care. The Clinic is located within the Asian community, with staff, from the same ethnic groups as the clients, furthering the compatibility and acceptance of the Clinic with the community and its residents

Understanding specific cultural backgrounds and beliefs is essential for appreciating how persons may perceive problems and counseling. Accordingly, devout Muslims may interpret mental health symptoms as a curse from God and seeking help as a sign of weakness (Abbasi & Paulsen, 2021). If they do seek help, it is more likely from a faith healer who shares the same beliefs and traditions. Moreover, many may have experienced anti-Muslim attitudes or Islamaphobia, which in itself can be potential causes of mental health problems while simultaneously acting as barriers to care (Samari et al., 2018).

Working with Jewish clients demands an understanding of anti-Semitism and how it may impact even the most assimilated individuals. The current reality of anti-Semitism in the United States, with its increasing incidence of violence, suggests that historical stereotypes remain influential and that Jewish "whiteness" does not necessarily correlate with full acceptance into society. A recent poll (ADL, 2020) found the beliefs that Jews control business and financial institutions, are likely to use shady business practices, are responsible for killing Christ, and are more loyal to Israel are held by approximately 14% of all Americans, with 61% agreeing with at least one antisemitic sentiment.

Microaggressions that include verbal, nonverbal, and environmental slights, snubs, or insults, which convey hostile, derogatory, or negative messages toward Jewish people are powerful forms of antisemitism. Remarks such as "Jewing someone down," "You don't look Jewish," or "You must be rich since you are Jew" are common examples of anti-Semitic microaggressions that can impact identity and interactions.

Working with the ultra-Orthodox Jewish community whose traditions may keep them isolated in society due to the desire to maintain pure religious practice demands specific understanding of their values and perspectives (Coleman, 2007). Due to stigma and a need for secrecy, help is usually provided by a rabbi or friend. However, culturally sensitive practitioners who offer discreet services and respect the many aspects of their life can be effective in working with them (Stolovy et al., 2012). As with many other ethnic groups, understanding how they view mental health issues, how these problems affect them, and how to work within the context of their community is a prerequisite for practice (Holiman & Wagner, 2015).

Conclusions

Ethnicity, culture, and religion continue to be powerful forces in society as they influence individual identity, interactions, and power, with each the potential target of oppression. With its focus on social justice, diversity, and human rights, it is imperative that social work continues to address and recognize the impact that these factors continue to have on individuals and society. Given the ease with which social media can spread beliefs that contribute to oppression and the threats that may ensue, efforts must be taken to challenge and confront these movements that reinforce stereotypes and often lead to violence. Confronting hate and propaganda that fuels it is critical for inclusion and a socially just society.

As discussed in this chapter, ethnicity is a complex term that continues to impact individuals and groups as it connotes distinct cultures, behaviors, and values. As such, ethnic groups may be the targets for discrimination and oppression as they are perceived as different or threats to the majority. Knowledge of ethnic values, traditions, and behaviors offers a foundation for sensitive practice and establishing relationships but must not ignore the reality of the individual. However, ethnicity is not a constant, its saliency continues to shift, and thus generalizations based on ethnicity may not be sensitive to any individual's unique experiences.

Culture refers to the ideas, traditions, and behaviors of individuals and can be an important force in influencing interactions and expectations within ethnic groups. Through culture, persons learn what to expect from each other and how they themselves should behave and interact. Similar to ethnicity, the influence of culture on any individual cannot be assumed, as it is also a dynamic concept whose significance in a person's life can vary with interactions and experiences.

This fluidity does not minimize the importance of cultural knowledge for effective practice. Understanding and sensitivity to values and traditions that may influence behavior and perceptions are critical to relationships and even the access and utilization of services. Awareness of the ways in which values and beliefs may be embedded in the helping process, both in the perception of problems and the roles of professionals, is central to practice. Equally important is the concept of cultural humility, which implies that one clearly sees the world through the experiences of others and not through their own values, biases, and positions.

Religion continues to play a defining role in the lives of many people. For many, it provides a sense of identity, tradition, and values. At the same time, religious persecution continues throughout the world without regard to the individual or their actual religiosity. This oppression is a direct violation of the human right to religious freedom. Understanding the role that religion may have in the lives of any individual is important for practice. However, the major challenge for the profession is to contest religious discrimination and harassment at the macro level so that religious tolerance and freedom prevail over discrimination and bigotry.

The lens model is an important tool in working with diverse groups. The lens through which practitioners view clients must be free of biases, stereotypes, and beliefs that can cause distortions in what one perceives. It is important to recognize that all of our lenses are impacted and shaped by our own uniqueness, including power and privilege, and thus to work with others, one must be able to see the world and reality from their perspective.

These distorted lenses reflect the values and perspectives of the viewer rather than the actual experiences of the client. Without clarity, it is impossible to understand the reality of another, a factor that is critical for cultural humility and effective practice.

Finally, working with diverse groups is an exciting challenge. It demands self-reflection, knowledge, sensitivity, and the understanding of many forces that continue to shape lives. Building relationships depends on trust and mutual respect, which are the foundation of all effective social work relationships. Recognizing the many factors that are associated with diversity and their roles in any individual's life offers an important foundation for practice at all levels.

Oppression remains a formidable force across the globe with those in power continuing to exclude and harass the less powerful and vulnerable, whether it be due to ethnicity, culture, or religion. Recognizing and combatting this oppression is essential for equity and social justice and for the recognition of human rights and remains a critical challenge for social work. Every group is a potential victim of bias and hate and will remain so until divisiveness is overruled by mutual respect, acceptance, and understanding. Social work can assume a major role in working toward unity as it continues to empower individuals and groups, recognizes and confronts social injustice, and contests the ideologies and beliefs that foster hatred, prejudice, and exclusion.

References

Aaronovitch, D. (2010). *Voodoo histories: The role of the conspiracy theory in shaping modern history.* New York, NY: Riverhead Books.

Abbasi, F and Paulsen, E (2021). *Working with Muslim patients.* American Psychiatric Association, Retrieved from www.psychiatry.org/psychiatrists/cultural- competency/education/best-practice-highlights/working-with-muslim-patients#:~:text=Muslims%20with%20mental%20illness%20may,demarcates%20between%20competency%20and%20incompetency.

Abe, J. (2019). Beyond cultural competence, Toward social transformation: Liberation psychology and the practice of cultural humility. *Journal of Social Work Education, 56,* 696–707.

Anti Defamation League (ADL) (2020). Jews Have Too Much Power, Retrieved from https://antisemitism.adl.org/power/

Akresh, I. (2011). Immigrants' religious participation in the United States. *Ethnic and Racial Studies, 34*(4), 643–661, DOI: 10.1080/01419870.2010.526719

Archdeacon, T. (1983). *Becoming American: An ethnic history.* New York: Free Press.

Asian American Commission. (2021). *Violence against Asian Americans.* Retrieved from www.aacommission.org/resources/anti-asian-hate-resources/

Baldwin, N. (2002). *Henry Ford and the Jews: The mass production of hate.* New York, NY: NY Public Affairs.

Blakemore, E. (2019). *Race and ethnicity: How are they different.* Retrieved from www.nationalgeographic.com/culture/topics/reference/race-ethnicity/#:~:text=Race%20 is%20defined%20as%20%E2%80%9Ca,or%20cultural%20origin%20or%20background.%E2%80%9D

Black, L., & Stone, D. (2005). Expanding the definition of privilege: The concept of social privilege. *Journal of Multicultural Counseling and Development, 33*(4), 243–255.

Boissoneault, L. (2017). How the 19th century know nothing party reshaped American politics. *Smithosonian Magazine*, January, Retrieved from www.smithsonianmag.com/history/immigrants-conspiracies-and-secret-society-launched-american-nativism-180961915/

Chaitt, J. (2021). GOP Congresswoman Blamed Wildfires on Secret Jewish Space Laser. *New York Magazine*, January 28. Retrieved from https://nymag.com/intelligencer/article/marjorie-taylor-greene-qanon-wildfires-space-laser-rothschild-execute.html

Cohen, A. (1974). *Urban ethnicity*. London: Tavistock.

Coleman, K. (2007). Researching hard-to-access, culturally insular populations: Methodological and ethical challenges. *Journal of Health, Social, and Environmental Issues, 8*(1), 11–18.

Corrigan, J (2020). *Religious intolerance, America, and the world: A history of forgetting and remembering*. Chicago, IL: Univ of Chicago Press.

CSWE. (2018). *Ten core competencies of social work practice*. Washington, DC: Author

Cox, C., & Ephross, P. (1998). *Ethnicity and social work practice*. New York, NY: Oxford

Dias, E. (2020). *Christianity will have power*. Retrieved from www.nytimes.com/2020/08/09/us/evangelicals-trump-christianity.html

Djupe, P., & Dennen, J. (2021). Christian nationalists and Qanon followers tend to be anti-Semitic: That was seen at the Capital attack. *Washington Post*. Retrieved from www.washingtonpost.com/politics/2021/01/26/christian-nationalists-qanon-followers-tend-be-anti-semitic-that-was-visible-capitol-attack/

Dominelli, L. (1997). *Anti-racist social work* (2nd edn.). London: MacMillan.

Douglas, K. M., Sutton, R. M., and Cichocka, A. (2017). The psychology of conspiracy theories. *Current Directions in Psychological Science, 26*(6), 538–542. https://doi.org/10.1177/0963721417718261

Ellis, N., and McPhillips, D. (2021). *White people are getting vaccinated at higher rates than Black and Latino Americans*. Retrieved from www.cnn.com/2021/01/26/us/vaccination-disparities-rollout/index.html

Glatfelter, C (1990). *The Pennsylvania Germans: A brief account of their influence on Pennsylvania*. University Park, PA: Historical Association.

Gordon, M. (1964). *Assimilation in American life*. New York, NY: Oxford University Press.

Hardiman, R, Jackson, B., and Griffin, P. (2007). Conceptual foundations for social justice courses. In M. Adams (Ed.), *Teaching for diversity and social justice* (2nd ed., pp. 35–66). New York, NY: Routledge

Hick, S., Fook, J., and Pozzuto, R. (2005). *Social work: A critical turn*. New York, NY: Thompson Educational

Hodge, D. (2006). Advocating for the forgotten human right, Article 18 of the Universal Declaration of Suman Rights-religious freedom. *International Social Work, 49*(4), 431–443

Holilman, R., & Wagner, A. (2015). Responsive counseling Jewish Orthodox communities. *Journal of Counselor Practice, 6*(2), 56–75.

Israel, E., and Tatalova, J. (2020). *Mexican immigrants in the United States*. Retrieved from www.migrationpolicy.org/article/mexican-immigrants-united-states-2019

Jolley, D., and Douglas, K. (2019). Conspiracy theories fuel prejudice towards minority groups. *The Conversation*. Retrieved from https://theconversation.com/conspiracy-theories-fuel-prejudice-towards-minority-groups-113508

Juby, H. L., and Concepción, W. R. (2005). Ethnicity: The term and its meaning. In R. T. Carter (Ed.), *Handbook of racial-cultural psychology and counseling, Vol. 1. Theory and research* (pp. 26–40). Hoboken, NJ: John Wiley & Sons, Inc.

Kesar, A (2002). Reconstructing static images of leadership: An application of positionality theory, *Journal of Leadership Studies, 8*, 94–109.

Kim, P. Y., Kendall, D. L., and Chang, E. S. (2016). Emotional self-control, interpersonal shame, and racism as predictors of help-seeking attitudes among Asian Americans: Application of the intrapersonal-interpersonal-sociocultural framework. *Asian American Journal of Psychology,* 7, 15–24. Doi:10.1037/aap000003

Kim, R. (2011). Religion and ethnicity: Theoretical consideration. *Religions, 2*, 312–329. Doi:10.3390/rel2030312

Kruglanski, A. W., Bélanger, J. J., and Gunaratna, R. (2019). *The three pillars of radicalization: Needs, narratives, and networks*. New York: Oxford University Press.

Lum, D. (2000). *Social work practice and people of color: A process stage approach*. Belmont, CA: Wadsworth

Mattison, T. (2014). Intersectionality as a Useful Tool, Anti-Oppressive Social Work and critical reflection. *Affilia,* 29, 8–17.

Majumdar, S. (2020). *Government restrictions on religion around the world reached new record in 2018*. Retrieved from www.pewresearch.org/fact-tank/2020/11/10/government-restrictions-on-religion-around-the-world-reached-new-record-in-2018/

Masci, C. (2019). *Many Americans see religious discrimination in U.S.-especially against Muslims*. Retrieved from www.pewresearch.org/fact-tank/2019/05/17/many-americans-see-religious-discrimination-in-u-s-especially-against-muslims/

McIntosh, P. (2012). Reflections and future directions for privilege studies. *Journal of Social Issues, 68*(1), 194–206.

Mullaly, R. (2010). *Challenging oppression and confronting privilege: A critical social work approach*. New York, NY: Oxford University Press.

NASW (2016). *Standards and indicators for social work competence in social work practice*. Washington, DC: Author.

NASW (2017). *Code of ethics*. Washington DC: Author.

Nguyen, P., Naleppa, M., & Lopez, Y. (2020). Cultural competence and cultural humility: a complete practice. *Journal of Ethnic and Cultural Diversity in Social Work*, 30, 273–281 DOI: 10.1080/15313204.2020.1753617

Ó Gráda, C. (1999). *Black '47 and beyond: The great Irish famine in history, economy, and memory*. Princeton, NJ: Princeton University Press.

Payne, M. (2014). *Modern social work theory*. New York, NY: Palgrave Macmillan.

Perry, S., & Whitehead, A. (2019). Christian American in black and white: Racial identity, religious-national group boundaries: Explanations for racial inequality. *Sociology of Religion, 8*(3), 277–98.

Pew Research Center. (2015). *The changing religious composition of the U.S.* Retrieved from www.pewforum.org/2015/05/12/chapter-1-the-changing-religious-composition-of-the-u-s/

Raphael, M. (2011). *The synagogue in America, A short history* (By Marc Lee Raphael). New York: NYU Press, pp. vii + 247.

Samari, G., Alcalá, H., & Sharif, M. (2018). Islamophobia, health and public health. *American Journal of Public Health, 108*(6): e1–e9. doi: 10.2105/AJPH.2018.304402

Scala, D. (2020). Polls and elections: The skeptical faithful: How Trump gained momentum among evangelicals. *Presidential Studies Quarterly, 50*(4), https://doi-org.avoserv2.library.fordham.edu/10.1111/psq.12642

Schragm P. (2010). *Not fit for our society: Nativism and immigration.* Berkeley, CA: University of California Press.

Sloan, l., Joyner, M., Stakeman, C., & Schmitz, C. (2018). *Critical multiculturalism and intersectionality in a complex world* (2nd ed.). New York: Oxford University Press.

Smedley, A. (1998). "Race" and the construction of human identity. *American Anthropologist, 100*, 690–702.

Spann, E. (1981). *New metropolis, New York City, 1840–1857.* New York: Columbia University Press.

Spencer, S. (2006). *Race and ethnicity: Culture, identity and representation.* Milton Park: Routledge. Doi:10.4324/9780203696828

Stolovy, T., Levy, Y. M., Doron, A., & Melamed, Y. (2012). Culturally sensitive mental health care: A study of contemporary psychiatric treatment for ultra-Orthodox Jews in Israel. *International Journal of Social Psychiatry, 59*(8), 819–823. Doi: 10.1177/0020764012461206

Straughn, J., & Feld, S. (2010). America as a Christian Nation: Understanding religious boundaries of national identity in the United States, *Sociology of Religion, 71*(3), 280–306.

Sue, S., Cheng, J. Y., Saad, C. S., & Chu, J. P. (2012). Asian American mental health: A call to action. *American Psychologist*, 67, 532–544. Doi:10.1037/a0028900

Takaki, R. (1993). *A different mirror: A history of multicultural America.* Boston, MA: Little Brown.

Trattner, W. (1994). *From Poor Law to Welfare State: A History of Social Welfare in America* (6th edn.). New York: Free Press.

Vasquez, M., and Acosta, J. (2019). *Jewish leaders outraged by Trump saying Jews disloyal if they vote for Democrats.* Retrieved from www.cnn.com/2019/08/20/politics/donald-trump-jewish-americans-democrat-disloyalty/index.html

Villa, V. (2020). *Women in many countries face harassment for clothing deemed too religious—or too secular.* Retrieved from www.pewresearch.org/fact-

Yan, M. (2008). Exploring the meaning of crossing and culture: An empirical understanding from practitioners' experience, *Families in Society, 89*(2), 282–292. Retrieved from tank/2020/12/16/women-in-many-countries-face-harassment-for-clothing-deemed-too-religious-or-too-secular/

Yancy-Bragg, N. (2021). *Stop killing us: Attacks on Asian Americans highlight rise in hate incidents amid Covid-19.* Retrieved from www.usatoday.com/story/news/nation/2021/02/12/asian-hate-incidents-covid-19-lunar-new-year/4447037001/

Zipperstein, S. (2020, August 25). The Conspiracy theory to rule them all, What explains the strange long life of the Protocols of the Elders of Zion, *The Atlantic.* Retrieved from www.theatlantic.com/politics/archive/2020/08/conspiracy-theory-rule-them-all/615550/

5 Economic Inequality and Social Justice

Rosemary A. Barbera

Introduction

In order to understand economic justice/injustice, we must take a look at the meaning and practice of economics. For far too long, economics has been presented to U.S. society as an immutable concept, particularly the view that capitalism is the only economic system that can benefit all. Markets have been treated as gospel truth; economic growth has been declared the indicator of a good life; Wall Street, which benefits a small segment of society, has been worshipped; and capitalism has been equated with democracy. But what if none of that were true? What if it were all a lie that perpetuates economic injustice? This chapter will delve into these issues by taking a short look at the history of economics as understood today. It will likewise examine the predominant economic model—free market capitalism—from a critical perspective. It will address how this model has as its basis injustice. It will look at what has not worked, and, finally, it will offer some suggestions for how we can work toward a society that puts people over profits and how social workers can be part of the movement to create this society.

As noted by the editors of this volume, social justice is an integral part of social work. At the same time, there seems to be some ambiguity around what social justice is. Is it a concept that we will know when we see it? Or can we get a handle on it today to help us guide our work? Perhaps it includes elements of both. Social justice is a manifestation of a world where human rights—individual and collective—are respected and human needs are met so that people can thrive, not just survive. This necessarily includes attention to living being rights since the quality of life of human beings is dependent upon the health of all life on the planet. Likewise, economic opportunities and just social conditions that are shared among all and an understanding of the equal worth and value of all are important elements (Reisch, 2002). A key element is the concept of equity, which goes beyond equality to recognize that while our rhetoric may say that we have equal opportunity, the reality is far from that. As a result, in order to achieve any semblance of justice we must deal with the unlevel playing field upon which we are operating. Social justice "is the absence of exploitation-enforcing

DOI: 10.4324/9781003111269-7

domination; it implies liberty, while domination-induced injustice" (Gil, 1998, 2013, p. 10) involves inequality, discrimination, inequity, and greed. "In a just world, human beings on the whole treat others fairly so that all may live in dignity without fear and with adequate means for satisfying universal needs of humankind" (Smith & Max-Neef, 2011, p. 10).

Social workers in the United States are obligated by their Code of Ethics to pursue social justice, not to know about it, not to explain it, or not to hold it only as a value but to act on it and to make it a core part of social work practice. Yet still many social workers do not engage in social justice work in their jobs; rather, social justice is what they do after hours (Bricker-Jenkins & Barbera, in press).

Social justice is the larger umbrella that includes other forms of justice such as economic and environmental justice. "The distribution of economic and financial power determines how just a society is" (Smith & Max-Neef, 2011, p. 10). In the United States, 1% of the population controls 40% of wealth and the gap is growing. At the same time, "CEO compensation has grown 740% since 1978. Typical worker compensation has grown only 12%" (Mishel & Wolfe, 2018, para 12) during that same time period. These are clear examples of how unjust the society is. Economic inequality affects all aspects of life from housing, education, community violence, to the violence of poverty (Leech, 2012). And since "politics and economics cannot be separated" (Smith & Max-Neef, 2011, p. 10), economic inequality affects the level of democracy in society. This inequality is exacerbated by the ineffective and inaccurate way that poverty is measured in the United States (Madrick, 2020), based on an emergency formula developed by Mollie Orshansky in the early 1960s, which effectively gives us a poverty rate that is about half of the actual rate of poverty. As a result, millions of people are left without access to programs that might improve their quality of life and their opportunities for a better life.

A Short History of Economics for Non-Economists

The term "economics" came from a Greek word—*"oikonomia"*—that means housekeeping (Smith & Max-Neef, 2011, p. 12) and had as its focus the concept of living well. That is, economics was a tool to be used to ensure that members of society could live a fulfilling and happy life. This changed when the focus on economics became more mathematical in nature and looked more at acquisition rather than quality of life. In order to justify the standing of economics in the wider society, the discipline saw a need to have the prestige of the natural sciences, thus the move toward a more mathematical focus (Smith & Max-Neef, 2011). This reduced the concept and practice of economics to something that did not consider the environmental factors that influence our lives and that saw itself as purely objective and by the numbers.

The invention of private versus communal property also played a hand in leading up to a focus on acquisition. In early societies where members of society saw themselves as linked and working in partnership, goods were shared so that all members could thrive. A shift occurred, precipitated by drought or another climatic event, that led to a shift in how people interacted with each other as they saw themselves as needing to protect themselves from others rather than collaborate with others. Instead of partnership, domination became the prevailing logic and private property rather than communal sharing was the basis for the structure of society (Eisler, 1987). As this shift happened, economics became less connected to the idea of housekeeping and more connected to the idea of acquisition that has become an undergirding principle of economics today. Economics was no longer about making sure that we could keep a good house—have our needs met—but about ensuring a certain societal structure and a certain vision of the world. As such, economics was born as a way to reify the status quo—that poverty and hunger are natural "and that trying to alleviate it would go against nature and disrupt the orderly state of affairs" (Smith & Max-Neef, 2011, p. 24). As Chilean economist Manfred Max-Neef explains, "[W]e have arrived at a point in human existence, the characteristic is that we *know* a lot, but we *understand* very little" (Smith & Max-Neef, 2011, p. 16) (italics in original). Max-Neef encountered this when he was working with poor Indigenous people in the altiplano of Perú. He had studied economics for years, had published, and had taught at the University of California at Berkeley, but when confronted by the poverty all around him he realized that all he knew could of no way be of service to the people he was working with. That economics had become divorced from reality and served itself and those who benefitted from the present structure. He developed what he called "barefoot economics" (Max-Neef, 1982), where the focus would be "economics as if people mattered" (Max-Neef, 1982, p. 19).

The shift in the focus of economics led to a practice where "economists had become dangerous people" (Max-Neef, 1982, p. 19) who engaged in a practice that allowed those with money and power to solidify their influence and wealth and those without to suffer. According to Max-Neef,

> Economics, originally the offspring of moral philosophy, lost a good deal of its human dimension, to see it replaced by fancy theories and technical trivialities that are incomprehensible to most and useful to none, except to their authors who sometimes win prizes with them.
>
> (1982, p. 20)

Economics has ceased to be meaningful in the day-to-day lives of the majority of people in the world. Instead it leads to a practice where "the market transfers more wealth and power to those who already have much of both" (Smith & Max-Neef, 2011, p. 11). This happens both within a nation and at the global level. Of course, many non-governmental organizations (NGOs) did arise to deal with issues of poverty and inequality, but as we will see, their influence has not been great. Since the use of international monetary policies, meant to reduce poverty, poverty and "inequality [has] only increased" (Leech, 2012. p. 1; see also Smith & Max-Neef, 2011). The time and energy devoted to economic pursuits are vastly greater than the time and energy used to eradicate, or even just ameliorate, poverty. "**There is never enough time for those who have nothing, but there is always enough time for those who have everything**" (Smith & Max-Neef, 2011, pp. 128–129) (bold in original). The next section will examine the model that has emerged from this history and that continues to benefit those who have at the expense of those who do not.

Predominant Economic Model

Social workers are accustomed to working with people who are the most affected by injustices based on many factors—economics, race, gender identity, gender, sexual orientation, ability, age, religion, and other factors. Vandana Shiva notes that "the poor are not those what have been left behind; they are the ones who have been robbed" (2005, para. 3). That is, the people who suffer injustice are not less fortunate and have not been left behind. They are the victims and survivors of societal conditions that have been the result of decisions made at various levels of society and upheld by power relations that benefit a few to the detriment of the many. The majority has been robbed and exploited, and continue to be robbed and exploited by these very deliberate structures. Since the focus of this chapter is on economic injustice, we will focus here on the economic system of capitalism that abuses people and our planet, recognizing that the intersections of race, gender, and other identities also affect how capitalism impacts people's lives. It is important to note that racism and capitalism were born together and so we cannot separate out these two forms of injustice. "Capitalism and racism did not break from the old order but rather evolved from it to produce a modern world system of 'racial capitalism' dependent on slavery, violence, imperialism, and genocide" (Kelley, 2017, para. 5).

"The distribution of economic and financial power determines how just a society is" (Smith & Max-Neef, p. 10). The present system of capitalism[1] maintains power in the hands of a few, exacerbating the already unjust structures in society. It accepts human suffering and unemployment as given in order to uphold both the economic model and the current arrangement in society (Leech, 2012) such that millions of people have lost their jobs during the COVID-19 pandemic in the United States, while CEOs have seen their wealth and pay increase (Choe, 2021). Unemployment is a necessary feature of the economic model in order to create conditions of competition and to maintain low wages and production costs. People are valued not as humans but only in their role as workers and producers in society. This is not just true of business, it is also true of philanthropy. One of the largest philanthropies, the Bill and Melinda Gates Foundation, succinctly states this on their webpage: "Guided by the belief that every life has equal value, the Bill & Melinda Gates Foundation works to help all people lead healthy, productive lives" (Gates Foundation, n.d.). People are not valued because they are living beings who have rights but because they produce and participate in the market. If they do not produce, then their value is diminished. Value is only conceived as coming from usefulness in the market.

Capitalism has risen to the level of theology. To question the current economic structure is to question the underlying core beliefs and values of society (Joseph, 2017). However, from a social justice and human rights perspective, underlying capitalism is not value but unvalue—*desvalores* in Spanish. These are intransigent negative values that place profits above people and the planet. Capitalism is a myth that has been legitimized and perpetuated and equated with democracy. We learn that the reality is that there is not enough to go around in the market economy and that scarcity exists (Joseph, 2017) even though the problem is not scarcity but distribution and a lack of will to equitably distribute the necessities of life. We are taught this from a young age and often religion is misused to perpetuate the myth. For example, in the Christian tradition, people quote the words of Jesus of Nazareth out of context in order to justify poverty and suffering by repeating that "the poor you will always have with you" (Matthew 26:11). In other realms, we are taught the benefits of the present arrangement from an early age through marketing and schooling.

One of the most successful elements of capitalism is how it is able to get people who suffer its effects to buy into it. We could ask why people who are suffering are still supporters of capitalism? One of the reasons is that they have bought into the myth that capitalism and democracy are the same and that capitalism will allow all boats to rise, even though that has never happened. Another reason is social control, sometimes obvious and other times subtle. Antonio Gramsci noted that the system has been able to get people to buy into this belief system by social control and by introducing small changes that really do not disrupt the status quo (Leech, 2012). For example, a minimal rise in the minimum wage or a minimal increase in a benefit of some sort. Messages of capitalism's benevolence dominate the media and the discourse. Children learn early to compete with one another and that independence, not interdependence, will be rewarded. They learn that they should be self-sufficient and not trust others. They also learn that they "should look out for number 1." In other words, they learn that their own self-interest is more important than the interests of the collective. Also, the way the term "free market" is used to discuss capitalism gives the overt implication that capitalism and freedom are connected. These messages, shared generation after generation and repeated often, make capitalism function.

Another element of capitalism that has risen to the level of myth is the concept of economic growth. We have built a system that measures success based on how fast and how far the economy grows. In truth, economic growth allows those who are already well-off to accumulate more. "After several centuries of economic growth the majority of the world's population still has less in the way of housing, food, and infrastructure" (Smith & Max-Neef, 2011, p. 69) to live a dignified life. There is also the problem that economic growth depends on use of natural and raw materials, which are finite, and it creates pollution. Their extraction leads to climate change and destruction of the natural world. However, since value is related to how useful something is to the market, raw materials have no value on their own apart from what they can earn in the market. This has created a situation where we are addicted to growth under the guise of having a healthy economy. However, human beings created this measure of what it means for an economy to be healthy. It can be changed.

Social workers see the results of this economic system on a daily basis. They see the structural violence and inequality that capitalism imposes in society; as Gandhi said, "[P]overty is the worst form of violence." Structural violence is violence exerted systematically—that is—indirectly—by everyone who belongs to a certain social order. . . . In short, the concept of structural violence is intended to inform the society of the social machinery of oppression" and to reinforce who has value and power. There is also a link between structural violence and behavioral violence, in that those societies with the most economic inequality have the highest rates of violence (Wilkinson & Pickett, 2009). Violence happens both directly and indirectly (Leech, 2012, Gil, 1998/2013) by the following ways:

- Depriving people of what they need to survive and thrive
- Abuse of power—through direct abuse and covert abuse
- Acts of violence
- And, "the daily violence of economic exclusion" (Davis, 2006, p. 202)

In the next section, we will unpack this a bit more.

Rising Inequality and Inequity

As noted earlier, today in the United States the gap between the wealthiest and the poorest continues to grow as income is distributed upward to those at the top rather than toward the bottom and those who need it most. The work of noted economists Thomas Piketty and Emmanuel Saez (Matthews, 2017) have examined this phenomenon. The top 10% of persons in the United States have steadily increased their wealth and income, while the bottom 90% have stayed in relatively the same place over time. The quality of life for the bottom 90% varies greatly from the quality of life for the top (Matthews, 2017; Saez, 2008). According to Komlos (2015) and others, inequality begins in the womb in the United States since structural inequality is part of the system. This structural inequality leads to death and suffering—"violence is inherent in the internal logic of capital and, therefore, it is a permanent feature of the capitalist system" (Leech, 2012, p. 2) that has serious implications for quality and longevity of life. "More than ten million people die globally each year from hunger and from preventable and treatable diseases" (Leech, 2012, p. 6), which can be connected to the logic of capital, which stresses competition and corporate profits over the quality of life of people. This emphasis leads to hunger, starvation, death by preventable disease, and other preventable sufferings. It also affects learning in children since when children are hungry "cognitive abilities are seriously reduced" (Madrick, 2020, p. 5).

Mental health is another area affected by economic inequality (Ferguson, 2017). While living in poverty, people experience higher levels of mental distress and anxiety, which then have an effect on their mental health. To be clear, mental health problems have always existed, but they have been significantly exacerbated by economic injustice (Ferguson, 2017). Poverty "leads to stress, anxiety, abuse, poor nutrition, infrequent doctor visits or no visits at all" (Komlos, 2015, para. 4). Mental health issues often follow the existing inequalities in society and so in order to improve mental health, it is necessary to go beyond the individual level. The structural inequality and economic injustice in society create an increase in stress and trauma (Shade, 2021). It creates situations that require people to constantly be on guard. It forces people to live in a constant state of vigilance. And it also requires people to be resilient to things that should not exist in the first place. In order to deal with all of that, we must address the structural level or we are just putting band-aids over the wounds.

> We must create a society where people can thrive: a society where people have their basic needs of food, housing, healthcare, and job security met, but also a society where people feel loved and valued, and where people have free time for pursuits that make their lives meaningful.
>
> (Shade, 2021, para. 9)

Also affected by economic injustice is climate destruction, which disproportionately affects people of color and poor people. "Capitalism threatens the well-being of people and planet" (Smith & Max-Neef, 2011, p. 11) because of its constant need for economic growth, which requires using more and more raw materials. The economic growth mentality relies on constant accumulation and greed and "one cannot be in favour of both greed and justice at the same time" (Smith & Max-Neef, 2011, p. 12). Climate change affects access to clean water, healthy food, and safe living conditions. Water across the world has been polluted through manufacturing and mining; it has been privatized for profit so many people cannot afford access to clean water. Water is a human right according to the United Nations, but not according to the CEO of Nestle, a company known to steal the clean water supplies of communities around the world. "Those dying from dehydration, water-transmitted disease, and starvation in the world perish due not to the actual lack of food or water, but to societal inefficiencies that allow (or create) such deprivation" (Joseph, 2017, p. 263). It is a choice to engage in practices that disrupt and ruin the environment, which means it is a choice to permit massive death from dehydration, starvation, water-transmitted disease, and pollution.

As Martin Luther King noted, "Whatever affects one directly, affects all indirectly. I can never be what I ought to be until you are what you ought to be. This is the interrelated structure of reality" (King, 1963, p. 5). As social workers, we are made aware of the connections between and among us on a daily basis. Part of our role is to educate others on these connections and to fight against the inhumane practices that perpetuate the inequity. We must see ourselves as part of the same garment (King, p. 1963).

It is true that many people have studied this situation. There have been interventions attempting to lessen the negative effects; yet, things have not changed. In the next section, we will look at what has been tried and has not worked. We will then look at some suggestions for change and implications for social work practice.

A Wolf in Sheep's Clothing. Or Solutions That Do Not Get to the Root of the Problem

Solutions to poverty and economic inequality have abounded over the years. Yet, the problems persist.

> There have been attempts to humanize and improve capitalism, but they are intra-systemic, and it is like caressing the shark's teeth, deluding oneself that one will eliminate its aggressiveness. Capitalism is inherently inhumane, because the priority, the number one value is the private appropriation of wealth, which gives the few the freedom to own a lot and prevents the many from having anything.
>
> (Vitorria, 2021, para. 7)

More often than not, those ideas proposed as solutions have been developed by those who know but do not understand (Smith & Max-Neef, 2011), or do not want to understand so that they do not have to be inconvenienced. Many of these so-called solutions keep "hope alive by helping some people get ahead" (Kivel, 2000, p. 8) while most stay behind. This provides the illusion that everyone can get ahead, but they are not designed to make the profound changes necessary for society to change.

With the realization of ongoing and increasing economic inequality and economic injustice, national and international organizations have called for programs and policies to mitigate the effects of an economy based on profit. These calls have come from within the system, however, without questioning the mythology and structure of the system itself. International financial institutions (IFIs) such as the World Bank Group (WBG) and the

International Monetary Fund (IMF) have funded programs around the world. Oxfam has pointed out that these programs often benefit those at the top rather than the poor and exploited. Money from IFIs is often distributed to banks and private equity firms with the belief that the funds will trickle down and that economic growth will increase (Geary, 2015). There are two problems with this line of thinking: first, as discussed earlier, using the model of economic growth to measure the health of the economy has devastating effects on the planet and on the most exploited, who suffer because of pollution and climate change, and trickle down has never happened. Aid that is sent from wealthy countries also does not make an impact since most of the funds allocated are actually spent in the country of origin. The United States spends less than 1% of its overall budget on foreign aid (Oxfam, 2018) and some of that funding is military. Much of U.S. foreign aid money is spent in the United States itself through funding of the U.S. Agency for International Development (USAID) and purchasing goods and services from U.S.-based corporations. And a good deal of foreign aid money goes to countries that the United States has been involved in militarily such as Afghanistan, Iraq, and Colombia. So instead of these funds going to create economic justice, they are used to mitigate some of the effects of U.S. intervention.

Microcredit and microfinance have been cited as a possible solution to extreme poverty. The idea of microcredit was conceptualized by Bangladeshi economist Muhammad Yunus, who was awarded the Noble Peace Prize for founding Grameen Bank. Microcredit offers small loans to people living in poverty who would not typically be able to borrow from a bank. There have been a number of critiques of the concept of microcredit, however, since more than to alleviate poverty its purpose is to integrate poor people into the market and make them dependent upon market forces (Muhammad, 2009). This has permitted the financial sector to grow at the expense of the exploited. In Bangladesh, for example, microcredit was introduced just as the government pulled out of providing health care for people. Most people who then used their microcredit money for health care expenses (Muhammad, 2009). Others used the money "to meet their basic nutritional needs" (Bello, 2006, para. 3). Another concern about microcredit is that it does nothing to challenge or transform the structural inequalities that exist in the present model: "by rejecting the notion that poverty has structural causes, they deny the need for collective responses" (Feiner & Barker, 2006, para. 1). Grameen Bank publicizes that its borrowers are able to leave poverty behind as a result of their microcredits. But a close examination of the numbers tells a different story: "[W]hen it comes to people's lives and economic scenario the success rate drops to 13.74% (education) and for poverty reduction to only 2.26 %" (Muhammad, 2009, para. 17). Another study that examined microfinance and conducted "by the Bangladesh Institute of Development Studies (BIDS) and the World Bank, found that less than 5% of borrowers could lift themselves out of poverty by borrowing from a microfinance programme" (Muhammad, 2009, para. 23). Also significant is that only about 1% of the overall population has access to microfinance, to begin with. Sometimes, the ways numbers are presented do not tell the whole story. Oftentimes, macroeconomic indicators tell a story of success but when examined closely the quality of people's lives has not changed discernably.

Another approach has been to appeal to morality by asking people to be concerned with the fate of others and to dig deep to help them. But that would necessitate that those who benefit most from the system, and who hold the power, would agree to significant change. It is more likely that they will "naturally find cognitive dissonance with the idea of altering the very mechanism that has rewarded them so disproportionately" (Joseph, 2017, p. xxi). It is not in their interests to change the structures that benefit them; they are more apt to focus on approaches such as microcredit, where they could increase their own wealth, rather than dismantling the structures that perpetuate economic injustice.

Charity and philanthropy are also not solutions to economic injustice. In fact, charity is part of the problem. Charity does not question the underlying structures that cause oppression, injustice, and exploitation. "Charity is the humanitarian mask hiding the face of economic exploitation" (Žižek, 2008, p. 21), the band-aid that covers the scars without letting them heal. Charity can create the climate "creating an atmosphere of 'progress'" (Kivel, 2000, p. 6) without really changing anything. Charity is designed to be essentially temporary, responding to a fleeting need. It does not dig deep to look at the root causes of what is going on and therefore cannot confront injustice and transform it. By its nature it is noncontroversial. Any solution to injustice would by definition have to upset the status quo, being controversial. In the words of Brazilian Bishop Dom Helder Camara: "When I give food to the poor they call me a saint. When I ask why the poor have no food they call me a communist." Charity makes rich people and corporations look generous while upholding and legitimizing the systems that concentrate wealth" (Spade, 2020, p. 23). Justice is long-term, recognizing that the path to transformation will be long, and it must dismantle the systems that concentrate wealth. And philanthropy operates from a charity mindset, where the ones awarding the money set the agenda without a true understanding of what is at stake in people's lives. Often philanthropists, who are wealthy people themselves, engage in philanthropic work as a way to support their wealthy friends (Spade, 2020) and move money around.

Finally, providing more services is not a solution to economic injustice. The goal of social justice should not be more programs and more services; it should be the eradication of the need for so many programs and services, to begin with. This is particularly true in a neoliberal environment, which keeps non-profit organizations under-resourced and fighting for funding (Barbera, 2006). Creating more "professionals in providing social services without necessarily producing greater social justice or equality of opportunity" (Kivel, 2000, p. 6) will not bring about the change we need.

Suggestions for Moving Forward

According to the International Federation of Social Workers (IFSW), "Social work is a practice-based profession and an academic discipline that facilitates social change and development, social cohesion, and the empowerment and liberation of people" (2018). As such, social workers should engage in practice that brings about change rather than perpetuate the status quo. This requires action for change. "Philosophers have hitherto only interpreted the world in various ways; the point is to change it" (Karl Marx as quoted by Leech, 2012, p. 1). In order to effectively fight against economic injustice, social workers must learn how the economy functions and push back (Barbera, 2006). The way the economy is structured in society system was created. "Capitalism and colonialism created structures that have disrupted how people have historically connected with each other and shared everything they needed to share" (Spade, 2020, pp 7–8).

The current structure benefits a small group of people. The structure can be changed, and social workers should be part of that change. We can work along with social movements of poor and exploited people to call for policies that serve people and the planet, not people serving the economy (Baptist et al., 2012). And we should be connecting the people we work with to social movements, as well.

> When people get together they build community by establishing projects, organizations, friendships, connections, coalitions, alliances, and understanding of differences. They do not acquiesce to, but rather fight against the agenda of the ruling class. They are in a contentious relationship to power.
>
> (Kivel, 2000, p. 10)

This includes social service agencies and social workers who have worked in such a way as to perpetuate the status quo rather than fight against it. Social and economic systems have created the ongoing crisis of economic inequality; we need "collective coordination to meet each other's needs, usually from awareness that systems we have in place are not going to meet themselves" (Spade, 2020, p. 7).

One example of a social movement is the Poor People's Campaign—A National Call for Moral Revival (www.poorpeoplescampaign.org). This campaign, led by those most affected by poverty and exploitation, continues the work of Rev. Dr. Martin Luther King, Jr. to build a social movement for social change. The Poor People's Campaign has created a moral budget and a series of policy proposals to bring about social, economic, and environmental justice. Social workers across the country have been engaged as members of the Poor People's Campaign. The national organization Social Welfare Action Alliance has partnered with the Poor People's Campaign as well.

Social workers should support efforts to build the solidarity economy, which is not based on profit or accumulation, but on meeting the needs of people and helping them thrive. The principles of a solidarity economy are "solidarity, sustainability, equity in all dimensions, participatory democracy and pluralism" (Kawano, 2009, p. 13). Examples include working to build either worker- or member-owned cooperatives. Worker-owned cooperatives can ensure a living wage, adequate benefits, and fair working conditions. The region of Emilia Romagna in Italy or the Mondragón co-op in Spain are examples of thriving cooperatives that have grown to include all areas of economic activity, including housing, food, education, and health care. The solidarity economy places collaboration over competition and solidarity over individualism. In Philadelphia, cooperatives exist for things like groceries, energy, bicycle repairs, power tools, pet food, and others.

Another example is to support efforts at mutual aid. One of the clearest examples of the power of mutual aid has been during the COVID-19 pandemic. All over the world instances of mutual aid have sprung up as neighbors join together to help each other through the pandemic. Likewise, during times of disaster, the first responders are always the people themselves who come to the aid of each other (Solnit, 2009). These mutual aid efforts are based on the concept of horizontalism and solidarity—people working together without hierarchy where people and communities empower themselves (Sitrin, 2006). Horizontalism is about protagonism—people and communities being the agents for change in their own lives and not relying on outside and outdated structures for change to happen. "Mutual aid projects work to meet survival needs and build shared understanding about why people do not have what they need" (Spade, 2020, p. 9). They are not charity since the element of critical consciousness, like the work of the Black Panther Party and the Young Lords, is integral to the work. "Charity programs are set up in a way that make it stigmatizing and miserable to receive help" (Spade, 2020, p. 23). "Mutual aid projects mobilize people, expand solidarity, and build movements" (Spade, 2020, p. 12) and social workers should be in the trenches as partners.

Another suggestion is to change how we measure economic activity. For years, the country of Bhutan has not measured economic activity through GDP or economic growth; they have measured it through happiness. They have even influenced the United Nations, which now publishes the World Happiness Report each year (n.d.). This report measures things like health, mental health, equal opportunity, and quality of life. The measures are not set to the whims and interests of the wealthy but to the well-being of all persons in society. Part of happiness includes low rates of economic inequality.

> In societies where income differences between rich and poor are smaller, the statistics show that community life is stronger and levels of trust are higher. There is also less violence, including lower homicide

> rates; physical and mental health tends to be better and life expectancy is higher.
>
> (Wilkinson & Picket, 2009, p. 145)

The economy should be at the service of human rights and human needs.

Conclusion and Implications for Social Work Practice

We need an economic system "as if people mattered" (Max-Neef, 1982, p. 19). Social workers can be part of this by embracing and advancing economic human rights in their practice. Only if we have our rights respected and our needs met can we live lives of dignity, so these rights must be the cornerstone of a social work practice committed to economic justice. We have to understand that we do not want a "more just world." Such a thing does not exist as it implies that injustice will remain, which means justice will not be realized. As social work scholar Mary Bricker-Jenkins says: "[W]hich of your children would like to remain in poverty when we have more justice, but not complete justice?".

Social and economic systems have created the ongoing crisis of economic inequality; we need "collective coordination to meet each other's needs, usually from awareness that systems we have in place are not going to meet" (Spade, 2020, p. 7) our needs. Social workers have skills that could be useful in the movement for economic justice, but only if we move beyond the mentality of seeing people as clients and engage people as partners. As Chilean economist Manfred Max-Neef (in Smith & Max-Neef, 2011) says,

> [W]hen we realize that knowledge is not the road that leads to understanding, because the port of understanding is on another shore and requires a different navigation, we will then be aware that we can attempt to understand only that of which we become a part. That understanding is the result of integration, while knowledge has been the result of detachment. That understanding is holistic, while knowledge is fragmented.
>
> (p. 17)

We must move beyond knowledge to understanding and solidarity by integrating ourselves into movements to end poverty, racism, and other forms of exploitation. That means we may need to do away with comfortable practices like charity that in actuality increase injustice. We must recognize that many social work practices and organizations are disempowering; we need to relearn how we interact with those we often call clients in order to truly collaborate. And we must be explicitly committed to ending economic exploitation and developing programs and practices that intentionally demonstrate this commitment.

Note

1 Capitalism is sometimes referred to as free market capitalism and/or neoliberalism. While there are slight nuances between these, they all rely on the supremacy of the market and they all perpetuate economic inequality.

References

Baptist, W., Barnes, S., & Caruso, C. (2012). *The right not to be poor: The growing global struggle for economic human rights*. New York, NY: Kairos Center for Religions, Rights, and Social Justice. Retrieved from https://kairoscenter.org/publications-research/

Barbera, R. A. (2006). Understanding globalization through short-term international field experiences. *Journal of Baccalaureate Social Work, 12*(1), 287–302.

Bello, W. (2006). *Microcredit, macro issues*. Retrieved from www.tni.org/es/node/11361

Bricker-Jenkins, M., & Barbera, R. A. (in press). *Radical social work*. Encyclopedia of Macro Social Work.

Choe, S. (2021). *CEO pay has risen again. Typical package: $12.7 million*. Retrieved from www.inquirer.com/business/ceo-average-pay-2020-coronavirus-pandemic-20210528.html

Davis, M. (2006). *Plant of slums*. Davis: Verso. "the daily violence of economic exclusion, p. 202

Esiler, R. (1987). *The chalice and the blade: Our history, our future*. HarperSanFrancisco.

Feiner, S. F., & Barker, D. K. (2006). Microcredit and Women's Poverty. *Dollars and Sense*. Retrieved from www.dollarsandsense.org/archives/2006/1106feinerbarker.html

Ferguson, I. (2017). *Politics of the mind. Marxism and mental distress*. Bookmarks Publications.

Gates Foundation. (n.d.). *Foundation Fact Sheet*. Retrieved from www.gatesfoundation.org/about/foundation-fact-sheet

Geary, K. (2015). The suffering of others. Retrieved from www.oxfam.org/en/research/suffering-others

Gil, D. (1998/2013). *Confronting injustice and oppression: Concepts and strategies for social workers*. New York: Columbia University Press.

Joseph, P. (2017). *The new human rights movement: Reinventing the economy to end oppression*. BenBella Books, Inc.

Kawano, E. (2009). Crisis and opportunity: The emerging solidarity economy. In E. Kawaon, T. N. Masterson, and J. Teller-Elsberg (Eds). *Solidarity economy 1: Building alternative for people and planet* (pp. 11–24). Switzerland: Center for Popular Economics.

Kelley, R. D. G. (2017). What did Cedric Robinson mean by racial capitalism? *Boston Review*. Retrieved from https://bostonreview.net/articles/robin-d-g-kelley-introduction-race-capitalism-justice/

King, M. L. (1963). *I have a dream and letter from a Birmingham jail*. New York: Tale Blazers.

Kivel, P. (2000). *Social service or social justice*. Paul Kivel. Retrieved from http://paulkivel.com/wp-content/uploads/2015/07/socialserviceorsocialchange.pdf

Komlos, J. (2015). *In American, inequality begins in the womb*. Retrieved from www.pbs.org/newshour/economy/making-sense/america-inequality-begins-womb

Leech, G. (2012). *Capitalism: A structural genocide*. London: Zed Books.

Madrick, J. (2020). *Invisible Americans: The tragic cost of child poverty*. New York: Alfred Knopf.

Matthews, D. (2017). *You're not imagining it: The rich really are hoarding economic growth*. Retrieved from www.vox.com/policy-and-politics/2017/8/8/16112368/piketty-saez-zucman-income-growth-inequality-stagnation-chart

Max-Neef, M. (1982). *From the outside looking in: Experiences in 'barefoot economics.'* Dag Hammarskjöld Foundation.

Mishel, L., & Wolfe, J. (2018). *CEO Compensation has grown 940% since 1978. Typical worker compensation has risen on 12% during that time*. Retrieved from www.epi.org/publication/ceo-compensation-2018/

Muhammad, A. (2009). Grameen & microcredit: A tale of corporate success. *Economic and Political Weekly*, *44*(35), 35–42.

Oxfam. (2018). *Myths about foreign aid*. Retrieved from www.oxfamamerica.org/explore/stories/myths-about-foreign-aid/

Reisch, M. (2002). Defining social justice in a socially unjust world. *Families in Society*, *83*(4), 343–354.

Saez, E. (2008). *When income grows, who gains?* Retrieved from http://www.econ.berkeley.edu/~saez/TabFig2008.xls

Shade, C. (2021). *Mental health is a political problem*. Retrieved from https://tribunemag.co.uk/2021/02/mental-health-is-a-political-problem?fbclid=IwAR0G7LmNSfyAWE8SCrP4DrIRd7H7i4BkKRlILTizx43COIK-eh1KK57ZbGc

Shiva, V. (2005). New emperors, old clothes. *The Ecologist*. Retrieved from https://theecologist.org/2005/jul/01/new-emperors-old-clothes

Sitrin, M. (2006). *Horizontalism. Voices of popular power in Argentina*. AK Press.

Smith, P., & Max-Neef, M. (2011). *Economics unmasked: From power and greed to compassion and the common good*. Devon: Green Books.

Solnit, R. (2009). *A paradise built in hell: The extraordinary communities that arise in disaster*. New York: Viking.

Spade, D. (2020). *Mutual aid: Building solidarity during this crisis (and the next)*. New York: Verso.

United Nations. (n.d.). *World Happiness Report*. Retrieved from https://worldhappiness.report/

Vittoria, P. (2021). *Paulo Freire's Brazil: Return to 'Grassroots popular Education.'* Retrieved from https://portside.org/2021-04-17/paulo-freires-brazil-return-grassroots-popular-education?fbclid=IwAR1x-ZM5jC8M-HoX-kHvlJj01-aG2KnZ-Z3umLST4w399k2FPNmz8ANc4Um4

Wilkinson, R., & Pickett, K. (2009). Equality is better—for everybody. In D. Ransom and V. Baird (Eds.), *People first economics*. New York: New Internationalist Publications.

Žižek, S. (2008). *Violence*. Picador. https://unesdoc.unesco.org/ark:/48223/pf0000187610

Resources

Busted—America's Poverty Myths Poverty Map—https://povertyusa.org/data

Institute for Policy Studies

Center for Economic & Policy—cepr.net www.youtube.com/watch?v=QPKKQnijnsM

How is poverty measured—www.irp.wisc.edu/resources/how-is-poverty-measured/#:~:text=in%20your%20browser.-,Official%20Poverty%20Measure,and%20adjusted%20for%20family%20size.

6 Environment, Social Work, and Environmental Justice

Julie L. Drolet, Wasif Ali, and Nicola C. Williams

Environmental degradation, unsustainable development, and the impacts of climate change have localized and global implications that demand attention to the complex relationship between people and their natural and physical environment. Environmental concerns and issues are dynamic and will continue to influence how social work addresses human rights and social justice at all levels. It is recognized that the global climate crisis threatens most people and their human rights, with profound implications for individuals, communities, societies, and the planet (Levy & Patz, 2015). This chapter considers the environment, social work, and environmental justice through a social development perspective that integrates the social, economic, and environmental dimensions of human wellbeing. Rights-based and social justice principles and perspectives are considered using an integrated approach for transforming systems that create injustices and inequities at a societal level that directly affect individual and community wellbeing. The social work profession is at an important developmental milestone in determining what constitutes social work practice from a human rights and global justice perspective, to ensure justice and equality as well as civil, political, environmental, economic, social, and cultural rights (Maschi et al., 2019). Extreme weather events, climate change impacts, vulnerability to climate risks, environmental and climate justice, and transformation are considered. The integration of social, economic, and environmental justice requires a holistic and integrated approach that considers all aspects of society and the environment to inform and to guide social work practice at all levels.

Over the past few decades, it has been increasingly recognized that environmental justice is part of social work (Erickson, 2018). Many communities affected by environmental injustices are the same communities where social workers deliver services and practice at the individual, family, and community levels (Teixeira & Krings, 2015). Environmental problems, from water scarcity and pollution to biodiversity loss and global warming, have the capacity to affect all of us. However, as many contemporary struggles demonstrate, people are not affected equally or in the same ways. Further, people do not have equal power to seek solutions to these problems or to take the necessary action to solve them. This unequal and differentiated positioning,

DOI: 10.4324/9781003111269-8

which tends to place the heaviest burdens upon marginalized, disadvantaged, at-risk, and less powerful populations, forms the central premise of the problem of environmental injustice and the hope for environmental justice as its solution (Holifield et al., 2017). Low-income countries and poor people in high-income countries are disproportionately affected by the environment and climate crisis, which profoundly affect human rights and social justice (Levy & Patz, 2015). Environmental justice and activism have included a wide array of concerns including environmental hazards and pollution; rampant industrialization; resource depletion; energy use; consumption patterns; food systems; access to environmental amenities; and public policies affecting minority, Indigenous, and low-income communities, other vulnerable groups such as disabled, immigrant, and linguistically isolated populations, as well as the impact for future generations (Holifield et al., 2017).

Environment and Environmental Justice

There are multiple definitions and meanings of the terms "environment" and "environmental justice." In the social work profession, the "person in environment" (PIE) approach traditionally focused on individual problems in the context of the social environment or ecosystems approach (Coates & Gray, 2012; Zapf, 2009). While PIE, or ecosystems approach, has guided social work to engage in the empowerment of the individual and society, it has been critiqued for its exclusion of the natural world (Norton, 2012). The need to address the natural and physical environment in social work has undergone a renewal, with a paradigm shift that embraces the role of social workers in environmental and social justice advocacy (Teixeira & Krings, 2015).

A review of the various definitions of environmental justice spans the conceptualization of "justice" as:

1. Political and attainable through legitimate frameworks of adjudication (Shoelandt & Gaus, 2018);
2. Justice as ethical and distributive (Rawls, 2001); and
3. Justice as inalienable rights connected to human capabilities (Nussbaum, 2011); cumulatively characterizing justice as equality, equity and human dignity.

Schlosberg (2007) articulates that environmental justice is a messy intersection of all components and that efforts to propose a singular universal definition may be futile in a context where plurality is inevitable. Schlosberg (2007) asserts that environmental justice movements "often employ multiple conceptions of justice simultaneously and accept both the ambiguity and the plurality that come with such heterogeneous discourse" (p. 5). Lewis (2012) states that "environmental justice is concerned with the fair and equal distribution of environmental burdens and benefits at local, national and international levels" (p. 65). Further, Nesmith and Smyth's (2015) definition adds to this understanding by considering participation where "there is equal inclusion in decision-making processes that result in environmentally related policies and actions" (p. 485). It is at this juncture that social work practice negotiates the tensions that exist at the level of the community reality and its intersection with national and transnational policies. Social work practitioners are on the frontline of the impact of global policies and the point of connection or disconnection from local realities. Social workers traverse the continuum of individual, group, community, national, and international responses. In situations where the national and/or international measures do not reflect the micro experiences of individuals and communities, social workers act to restore fit through working alongside communities to advocate for change (Dominelli, 2012).

The question of "justice for whom" has contributed to complex understandings as the expansion of environmental justice has evolved, from a focus on inequitable distributions of waste and pollution to a wide variety of substantive problems, struggles, and aspirations. For example, the changing understanding of the relationships between human and nonhuman nature has important implications for environmental justice.

The Indigenous prayer phrase "all my relations" captures a relational ontology (Temper, 2019). Indigenous environmental justice is grounded in Indigenous philosophies, ontologies, and epistemologies in order to reflect the Indigenous conceptions of what constitutes justice, given the challenges of the ecological crisis and the various forms of violence and injustices experienced specifically by Indigenous peoples (McGregor et al., 2019). A number of human rights are specifically accorded to Indigenous peoples under international law, which can be adversely affected by environmental harm (Lewis, 2012). Globally, Indigenous communities are at the forefront of struggles against land dispossession and environmental degradation (Temper, 2019).

The Council on Social Work Education (CSWE) officially launched a committee on environmental justice in February 2015 to explore the history of green social work, environmental justice, and social work practice related to environmental issues. The committee adopted the following definition of environmental justice:

> Environmental justice occurs when all people equally experience high levels of environmental protection and no group or community is excluded from the environmental policy decision-making process, nor is affected by a disproportionate impact from environmental hazards. Environmental justice affirms the ecological unity and the interdependence of all species, respect for cultural and biological diversity, and the right to be free from ecological destruction. This includes responsible use of ecological resources, including the land, water, air, and food.
>
> (CSWE, 2015, p. 20)

CSWE included environmental justice in the competencies and practice behaviors of social work education, identifying an ongoing commitment to growing, and understanding social work and environmental justice (CSWE, 2015). Social work students are expected to apply their understanding of social, economic, and environmental justice to advocate for human rights at the micro and macro level as well as engage in practices that advance social, economic, and environmental justice (CSWE, 2015, p. 7). Social work is uniquely situated to respond to and collaborate at the intersections of the social, political, economic, and natural environments that surround individuals, groups, communities, and societies, thus locating itself at the crux of an interdisciplinary milieu for advancing the global agenda for environmental justice and human rights.

The Environmental Movement

In the history of the environmental movement, there have been four waves of environmentalism. Erickson (2018) reviews these waves to show how environmentalism and environmental justice have emerged and merged over the years:

- First wave—Late 1800s—mid-1900s: traditional environmental movement focused on preservation of the natural environment.
- Second wave—Mid-1900s: environmental movement begins to question consumption, reconsiders notions of progress and the environmental impact of some modern conveniences.
- Third wave—1970s—1990s: environmental movement adopts radical rethinking of how culture and the environment intersect to impact the lives of people and nature; the third wave considers environmental racism and ecofeminism alongside other social movements.
- Fourth wave—2000s—Present Day: environmental movement critically addresses human and environmental inequities with a focus on environmental justice (see Erickson, 2018).

In the early years of the mainstream environmental movement, social justice, and inequality issues were ignored and continue to be debated by some despite the proliferation of research that has documented unequal exposures by race, ethnicity, and economic class (Mohai et al., 2009). Ecofeminism and feminist standpoint place women's lives in social and ecological contexts, amplifying "the feminist slogan that the 'personal is political'- and ecological too" (Gaard, 2017, p. 74). Today, green social work and ecological social work theories and approaches fit in the fourth wave of environmentalism (Erickson, 2018). Environmental justice is a social movement and discourse that influenced how climate justice has been conceptualized and understood (Scholsberg & Collins, 2014).

Climate change is one of the greatest social and ecological challenges of the 21st century (Dietz et al., 2020). With the release of the Fourth

Assessment Report of the Intergovernmental Panel on Climate Change (IPCC) in 2007, more public and political discussions affirmed that there is and will be human-induced climate change (Frommer, 2013). Article 1 of the United Nations (UN) Framework Convention on Climate Change (UNFCC) defines climate change as "a change of climate, which is attributed directly or indirectly to human activity that alters the composition of the global atmosphere and which is in addition to natural climate variability observed over comparable time periods" (UNFCC, 1992, p. 4). Climate justice is local and global and concerned with the causes and consequences of climate change, and the inequitable impacts of climate change. Globally, low-income countries that produce the least greenhouse gases (GHGs) are more adversely affected by climate change than high-income countries, which produce substantially higher amounts of GHGs (Levy & Patz, 2015). Climate change raises many ethical challenges, especially on the issue of climate justice. Environmental disasters such as Hurricane Katrina in 2005 revealed how pre-existing injustices like poverty, racial discrimination, segregation, a poor education system, substandard housing, and a lack of community preparation were exacerbated by extreme weather events (Scholsberg & Collins, 2014). Environmental justice movements are environmental social movements confronting diverse issues and embedded in other social movements, including movements for racial equality, the rights of Indigenous peoples and the poor, farmers, workers, and many others (Sicotte & Brulle, 2017).

The Global Sustainable Development Report 2019 (GSDR) states that unless there is a fundamental—and urgent—change in the relationship between people and nature, and a significant reduction in inequalities between and inside countries, any "development" progress of the past two decades risks being undone (United Nations Publications, 2019). The GSDR 2019 stresses the need to transform key areas of human activity, which could otherwise lead to systems failure—including food, energy, consumption and production, and cities—and increase resilience to economic shocks and disasters caused by natural and human-made hazards, through active implementation of the Sendai Framework (United Nations Publications, 2019). There are a number of international frameworks to consider in this respect.

The Sustainable Development Goals (SDGs)

An essential tangible outcome of the UN efforts is the global development agenda currently enshrined in the Sustainable Development Goals (SDGs) adopted in 2015. The SDGs elaborate upon the eight (8) Millennium Development Goals that were created to reduce extreme poverty by 2015. The Sustainable Development Agenda lists 17 goals and 169 targets for charting the path to sustainable development across the globe. All 17 goals have implicit or explicit targets that are aligned with the Global

Agenda for Social Work as well as the Universal Declaration of Human Rights (UDHR). Choondassery (2017) argues that the United Nations' Transforming Our World: The 2030 Agenda for Sustainable Development is undeniably human rights-based. Advocates of a rights-based approach identify three principal areas:

1 The right to a clean and safe environment
2 Access to information and public participation in decision-making
3 The right to promote and defend the protection of the environment and human rights (Choondassery, 2017)

The Global Agenda for Social Work and Social Development is both an outcome and an ongoing process that began in 2004 to articulate and align the global efforts of social work practitioners. The Global Agenda (2010–2020) included four pillars: (1) promoting social and economic equalities; (2) promoting dignity and worth of peoples; (3) working toward environmental sustainability; and (4) strengthening human relationships. The Agenda captures the work by social work practitioners and provides direction for the role of the profession in eradicating inequalities across the globe. This will be accomplished by social workers acting as implementers and leaders in shaping global policy for sustainable development (Jones & Truell, 2012).

The critical role of developmental social work practice has been highlighted and recognized by UN partners as a vital contributor toward global sustainable development. Helen Clark, in speaking of the acceptance of the Global Agenda for Social Work and Social Development, acknowledged that "for more than a century, the social work profession has been at the forefront of promoting human rights and supporting people to realize their full potential" (Clark, 2012, para 8). She further stated that,

> As indicated in the Global Agenda, social workers can help build and strengthen interaction between governments and their citizens, bring the concerns of the vulnerable to the fore, and help local authorities to be more responsive to citizens and accountable for the services they deliver.
>
> (Clark, 2012, para 19)

The Global Agenda for Social Work (2010–2020) comprise four (4) objectives, which align with the SDGs and the entitlements safeguarded by the UDHR.

Internationally, the numerous interconnections between the environment and human rights are well established, and it is understood that environmental issues (e.g., pollution, deforestation, or the misuse of resources) can impact on individuals' and communities' enjoyment of fundamental rights, including the right to health, the right to an adequate standard of living, the right to self-determination, and the right to life (Lewis, 2012). The right to a healthy environment is a basic human right that is connected to sustainable development. This is particularly important in communities most in need of such a right. Boyd (2012) argues that most countries are better off if they adopt a constitutional right to a healthy environment, that recognize environmental rights as human rights. Woods (2017) considers environmental human rights in the growing inclusion of environmental issues in both human rights theory and practice that point to a significant shift in our collective understanding of the relationship between human beings and nonhuman nature. Social workers are often on the frontline, working with populations who are the focus of the sustainable development agenda (Lombard, 2015). Furthermore, their efforts are legitimized by the objectives of the Global Agenda for Social Work and Social Development (Jones & Truell, 2012) and the social development approach which addresses structural inequalities that are both antecedents and outcomes of social and environmental injustice.

Social Development

Social development is a process that involves all levels of institutions, from national governments to diverse civil society organizations, to build an equitable and just society through the apportion of economic opportunities and social services, while addressing power imbalance (United Nations, 2005). Social development utilizes and/or changes the processes of societal institutions and systems, through policies and programs, to strengthen the capabilities and capacities of individuals, families, and communities (Drolet & Sampson, 2014). A social development approach recognizes that social and ecological systems are interconnected and intrinsically linked to human rights, social justice, and environmental justice (Drolet & Sampson, 2014; Miller et al., 2012). In social work, a social development approach is recognized as a viable response to many of the existing social injustices (Banerjee, 2005; Todd & Drolet, 2020). Also, social justice encompasses economic and environmental justice (Lombard & Twikirize, 2014). Development social work is a form of social work in low- and middle-income countries that adopts a social development approach.

The goal is to shift from an unsustainable development model to a risk-informed one that restores and regenerates natural systems to ensure that "no ecosystem is left behind." The resilience and stability of natural ecosystems, their restoration and regeneration are of paramount importance for systemic risks to be managed effectively. Within this context, the vision of a resilient society gains relevance as the concept of resilience comprises three components important to cope with environmental (climate) change. These are the capacity (1) to resist and (2) to recover from disturbances and shocks and (3) to adjust functioning—prior to or following—changes and disturbances (Frommer, 2013). Adaptations to climate change will have transformational effects on humans and societies at every level from the local to the global.

The Sendai Framework on Disaster Risk Reduction clearly articulates the need to improve understanding about disaster risks and vulnerability to hazards. In the preamble, the expected outcomes emphasize the implementation of inclusive economic, environmental, social, and structural measures to prevent and reduce vulnerability to disasters. Adopted by the United Nations member states in 2015, the Sendai Framework succeeded the Hyogo Framework for Action (2005), which articulated a strategic response to improving global resilience to hazards. The Sendai Framework along with the SDGs calls for action in all aspects of society that intersect human, social, and economic wellbeing with the natural environment and its management. The Sendai Framework advocates four priority areas:

1 Understanding disaster risks
2 Strengthening disaster risk governance to manage disaster risks
3 Investing in disaster risk reduction for resilience and
4 Enhancing disaster preparedness for effective response and to "Build Back Better" in recovery, rehabilitation and reconstruction (UNDRR, 2015).

The guiding principles of the Sendai Framework along with the SDGs underscore the need for public and private investments to protect vulnerable communities and to protect the environment in post-disaster responses and to foster sustainable development. Priority theme three of the Sendai Framework clearly advocates the sustainable and just use of eco-systems for environment protection and disaster risk reduction. It also encourages investments, insurances, and financial protection for urban and rural communities. Priority theme four advocates disaster preparedness at all levels and considers climate change and associated disaster risks as a threat to vulnerable people and communities. The Sendai Framework identifies the need to empower women, persons with disabilities for a gender-focused, equitable, and universally accessible disaster response. The concept to "Build Back Better" calls for greater cooperation among all people, communities, and stakeholders at all levels. This community-focused cooperation requires collective action based on awareness, policy, planning, and training to develop inclusive and collective responses to the impacts of climate change and environmental disasters for a sustainable and resilient future (UNDRR, 2015).

Green Social Work

Green social work, as defined by Lena Dominelli (2012), is a

> practice that intervenes to protect the environment and enhance people's well-being by integrating the interdependencies between people in their socio-cultural, economic and physical environments, and among

> peoples within an egalitarian framework that addresses previously structural inequalities and on. Equal distribution of power and resources.
>
> (p. 8)

Green social work challenges the neoliberal model of global capitalism by the demand for environmental justice.

> Green social workers promote environmental justice and resist environmental injustice by helping people mobilize and organize activities that protect their physical environment . . . green social work practice affirms human rights and social justice to enhance the well-being of people and the environment for today and the future.
>
> (Dominelli, 2013, p. 437)

Dominelli (2012) explains that environmental injustice is threatening the sustainability of global society. Unequal distribution of natural resources is a common failure of modern society. The present industrialization model is not working and social workers need to play an important role to formulate alternative models for the well-being of human society. However, the challenge is that the social work profession in many countries is part of, and dependent upon, the unsustainable neoliberal industrial model and its power structures.

Environmental Justice and Human Rights

Environmental justice is inextricably linked to human rights concerns across the globe. The impacts of climate change and the climate crisis threaten the right to security and the right to a standard of living adequate for health and well-being, including food, clothing, housing, medical care, and necessary social services rights (United Nations, 2021). Civil and political rights are threatened such as "the inherent right to life" and rights related to culture, religion, and language (International Covenant of Civil and Political Rights). Economic, social, and cultural rights (International Covenant on Economic, Social, and Cultural rights) and the rights of women (Convention on the Elimination of all Forms of Discrimination against Women) are also threatened (Levy & Patz, 2015). The United Nations Declaration on the Rights of Indigenous Peoples (2007) recognizes the importance of the environment to Indigenous peoples in article 29:

> Indigenous peoples have the right to the conservation and protection of the environment and the productive capacity of their lands or territories and resources. States shall establish and implement assistance programmes for indigenous peoples for such conservation and protection, without discrimination.
>
> (p. 21)

Social workers often find themselves at the crux of brokering the connection to the financial and technical support enshrined in global governance frameworks, holding governments accountable, and bridging gaps in access to resources at the community level while enhancing community capacity to define their justice needs and act to protect the environment. Social workers must therefore interpret and apply lofty ideals and facilitate practical grassroot responses, through championing national policies and the establishment of institutions and mechanisms for appropriately operationalizing the global agenda. One critical environmental issue that is demonstrably a universal concern and necessitates an understanding of the interaction among human rights, environmental justice, and social work is access to clean water. This issue continues to be exacerbated by global climate change and associated natural hazard events. Access to water is by definition a human right (article 25 in the UDHR) and operationalized by SDG goal 6 for ensuring access to water and sanitation.

Water Justice in Pakistan

Pakistan is facing water scarcity, and it is predicted that by 2025 the country will face absolute water scarcity (Jamil, 2019). Water justice is defined as a combination of social and environmental justice that applies to water allocation and management (Boelens et al., 2018) examines not only the distribution of outcomes but also the processes that underpin them (Boelens et al., 2018)"the land of five rivers" (Sutlej, Beas, Ravi, Chenab, and Jhelum), and historically served as the food capital of south and central Asia, it is currently facing a severe water crisis. The water crisis is due, in part, to rising temperatures, human-made transboundary water agreements, industrialization, changes in weather patterns, and inequities in access and control over available water resources (Hussain et al., 2020).

In the Punjab region, 75% of the population lives in villages and directly depends on agriculture for their economic needs and food security. The lack of water lowers income and earnings, creating serious challenges to meet livelihoods in the prevailing environmental crisis (Khan et al., 2021). Large agricultural businesses with the means to procure water have access to and use up a significant amount of water. Further, large corporations often have more access to water than small independent farms. Inefficient irrigation practices significantly contribute to water wastage because poor communities are not in a position to afford the more efficient modern technologies (Hassan and Hassan, 2017). Crop contamination is also a major source of concern in this region. When contaminated water is used to irrigate crops, the water becomes a part of the food, and people unknowingly consume contaminated foods which can cause serious health problems (Bakhsh and Hassan, 2005).

Many communities face waterborne diseases due to contaminated water, specifically drinking arsenic-contaminated water, and UNICEF has designated certain areas of the Punjab region as red zones (Zakar et al., 2020).

Because arsenic is an odorless, colorless, and tasteless poison, it is one of the leading causes of cancer in this region. It has also been discovered that boiling the contaminated water makes it even more dangerous, demonstrating the far-reaching impact of water quantity and quality problems (Rasool et al., 2016).

Lahore is the capital city of Punjab, one of the largest cities in South Asia with a population of 14 million. Lahore is dependent on underground water to meet human daily needs. In the early 2000s, the people of the Punjab region would dig deep wells approximately 40–60 feet deep to access underground water; however, due to water scarcity, the wells are deeper at 600 feet in order to reach the underground water (Ali, 2018). While it has become increasingly difficult to access water, there is a threat that underground water sources will soon be dry. All urban centers will be at risk of having no access to drinking water in the future (Khan et al., 2021).

The gender dimension of water is an important consideration for water justice, given women's gendered role that attributes women responsible for the use of water at the household level. This is evidenced in women's responsibilities for cooking, washing clothes, and cleaning. Women are disproportionately affected by water scarcity and exposure to toxins in the water (Rauf et al., 2015). In cases where water is unavailable at home, women are responsible for the transportation of water from a nearby place to the household. Often, women carry water, perform extra domestic work and labor to fulfill the water needs in the household. The availability and quality of drinking water have implications for women's health, contributing to higher child mortality and maternal mortality rates in the region (Scheelbeek et al., 2016).

Water justice considerations for drinking, sanitation, and productive uses must be identified, understood, and assessed in relation to a wide range of social and political factors, including gender, income, indigeneity, and race (Harris et al., 2017). Social workers in Punjab are engaged in community development initiatives to address water challenges. A community water supply and sanitation project aims to address the water quantity and quality challenge, with social workers directly engaged with vulnerable communities using community mobilization strategies for water conservation. Strategies include planning, designing, and executing health and hygiene campaigns for the well-being of communities (Padawangi, 2010). Adequate water quantity, quality, risk considerations, and changing governance practices are all concerns that require careful consideration through an environmental justice lens (Harris et al., 2017). Access to housing and security of tenure are important considerations in remediating human rights issues and facilitating environmental justice.

Housing Justice in Jamaica

Jamaican history is marked by the poorer class having insecure land tenure post emancipation when newly freed slaves had to move away from plantation settlements, having previously been unable to own land (Besson, 1984).

The informal nature of settlement continued post independence as persons moved closer to urban centers in search of economic opportunities with many settling on unproductive crown land and near the coastline (Brooks, 2016). The topographical features of Jamaica as a small island state renders the island vulnerable to natural hazards, including hurricanes and earthquakes. Consequently, citizens residing on marginal land with substandard housing stock are at a greater risk of loss of property and life. This risk has continued to increase as climate variability and natural hazards have increased in occurrence and severity (Peduzzi, 2019). In 1994, the Government of Jamaica launched the Programme for Resettlement and Integrated Development Enterprise (PRIDE). The program had the stated objectives of addressing shelter needs of low-income Jamaicans, improving environmental and living conditions, and mobilizing resources to improve livelihoods and overall national development (Housing Agency of Jamaica, n.d.). While the objectives are desirable ends for persons living in poor housing conditions, as the program unfolded, the historical factors intersected with social, economic, and political conflict challenged the implementation of the project. Reports of beneficiaries' needs not being met by the program, cost overrun, as well as allegations of corruption and nepotism dominated the process with an eventual merger of the program in 1998 with the National Housing Development Corporation (NHDC) to rebrand the initiative. This rebranding effort was unsuccessful and community development practitioners working alongside the initiative felt that a lack of respect for the residents led to external stakeholders using their circumstances for partisan gains rather than facilitating the improvement of their standard of living. The community development practitioners also felt betrayed by the government as they believed their work and relationship with the community were exploited by the government stakeholders and set back their efforts to work with communities toward strengthening grassroot capacities for sustainable community development. The question of how the state should respond to informal (squatter) settlements continues to be a polarizing issue bereft of a critical exploration of the socio-economic and historical forces, which continue to dictate land tenure and access to adequate housing in Jamaica.

Article 25 of the UDHR addresses the right to adequate housing that affords a standard for adequate health and wellbeing. This is operationalized by SDG 11 charting an agenda for sustainable communities and cities. This brings into focus the reality of vulnerable groups that inhabit marginal land and informal (squatter) settlements that are not outfitted with the amenities necessary for health, water, and sanitation. Despite the neoliberal economy situating house and land as an investment asset, quality housing is an entitlement for all human beings and essential to their wellbeing (Foy, 2012). However, displacement as a result of socio-economic forces and poor housing policies has resulted in the emergence of informal (squatter) settlements as housing solutions. Informal (squatter) settlements tend to be characterized by poor housing stock, inadequate access to safe water and sanitation, overcrowding within households, and insecure land tenure catalyzed by existing challenges to securing affordable housing in established communities (Konadu-Agyemang, 1991; Jones, 2016). Furthermore, social and environmental injustice that the SDGs seek to remedy is evident in societies where persons with less wealth are residing in communities with greater environmental risks and vulnerabilities (Foy, 2012).

This case highlights some of the key considerations and challenges in advancing human rights and environmental justice. As social workers and other development practitioners work with vulnerable groups, confounding factors such as history and political agenda can facilitate or undermine efforts toward sustainable ends. This must be negotiated by social work practitioners to ensure the best possible outcome for all stakeholders while maintaining the focus on sustainable development and ensuring that human rights entitlements are afforded to all.

Extreme Weather Events and Disasters

Since 1950, many changes have been observed in extreme weather and climate events, some of which are due to human influences, and include a decrease in cold temperature extremes, an increase in warm temperature extremes, an increase in extreme high sea levels, and an increase in the number of heavy precipitation events in a number of regions (IPCC, 2014, p. 7). Many extreme weather events have and will become more frequent and more intense due to climate change. The number of climate-related disasters has tripled in the last 30 years (Oxfam, 2020). The cumulative effect of disasters produces a significant personal, material, and economic strain on individuals, communities, and the fiscal capacity of all levels of governments (Drolet, 2019). In Canada, extreme weather and climate events contributed to the 2016 wildfires in the province of Alberta, which is recognized as the worst disaster in Canadian history. The 2016 wildfire spread quickly, resulting in a mandatory evacuation of all 88,000 residents in Fort McMurray. Research on the roles and responsibilities of social workers in the 2016 wildfires found social work practice offered a unique contribution in disaster contexts (Drolet et al., 2021). By focusing on the social dimensions of disasters and drawing from social work values and the code of ethics, social workers recognized the importance of client self-determination, working to advance human dignity and respect, social justice, and provide assistance in a professional manner (Drolet et al., 2021). Yet their role and contributions were not acknowledged or well understood by emergency and disaster management officials, and many were disappointed that they were not used to their full capacity during the wildfire.

In Canada, social work practice responds to the needs of individuals, families, groups, and communities and addresses barriers and injustices in organizations and society (CASW, 2020). The 2016 Alberta wildfire and ensuing recovery period demonstrate that disasters are multi-layered and have long-term effects, which intersect with other social, economic, health, and environmental challenges (Drolet et al., 2021). Social support systems and services are crucial to long-term recovery, and social workers are unique in considering the needs of vulnerable populations and intervening at the micro, mezzo, and macro level (Drolet et al., 2021). In order to build more resilient communities and systems, there is an important role for social work practitioners and human service professionals to mitigate risks and to reduce adverse impacts.

Climate risks are unevenly distributed between groups of people and between regions, affecting disadvantaged people and disadvantaged communities in greater ways. This is particularly important in the social work profession as vulnerable and marginalized populations and communities are increasingly affected by extreme weather events and climate impacts. The human, social, and structural dimensions are central in addressing vulnerabilities, as people's health and well-being suffer as a result of inequalities, poverty, and unsustainable development practices (Drolet et al., 2013). Differences in vulnerability and exposure arise from non-climatic factors and from multidimensional inequalities often produced by uneven development processes. These differences shape differential risks from climate change. People who are socially, economically, culturally, politically, institutionally, or otherwise marginalized are especially vulnerable to climate change. This heightened vulnerability is rarely due to a single cause but intersecting social processes that result in inequalities in socio-economic status and income, as well as in exposure. Such social processes include, for example, discrimination on the basis of gender, class, ethnicity, age, and (dis)ability (IPCC, 2014, p. 54). The COVID-19 pandemic has brought to light the importance of addressing collective problems in a collective manner, and the need for collaboration and cooperation.

Many governments favor climate change and disaster policies that promote "community resilience." Community resilience is defined as a community or region's capability to prepare for, respond to, and recover from significant multi-hazard threats, with minimum damage to public safety and health, the economy, and national security (Colten et al., 2008, p. 38). Benefits from adaptation can already be realized in addressing current risks, which can be realized in the future for addressing emerging risks (IPCC, 2014, p. 18). For at least two decades, governments have adopted neoliberalism by giving priority to market forces over social benefits, resulting in reduced government interventions, a decline in infrastructure, and an expectation that people and communities will become more self-reliant (Alston & Kent, 2009). The environmental crisis has called into question contemporary social and economic systems, and related production and consumption patterns, that depend on the unsustainable exploitation of natural resources (UNRISD, 2015). Yet, political ideology continues to influence how social-economic-environment relationships are imagined.

The COVID-19 pandemic in 2020 has brought to the forefront how racial bias is present at all levels in society, with the "Black Lives Matter" movement and anti-racism demonstrations in many parts of the world. These interconnected crises—climate change, COVID-19, systemic racism—are severely affecting racialized and Indigenous communities, calling for transformative change and justice (Cooper, 2020). A holistic and integrated approach that considers all aspects of society and the environment is needed to inform and to guide social work practice at all levels.

Conclusion

Social work is a field not only of direct practitioners but also of leaders, change agents, activists and community builders, and social workers are positioned to advance human rights and environmental justice (Schmitz et al., 2012). Collaboration, networking, advocacy, community development, and capacity building are found in the scope of social work practice around the world. At the macro level, social work is engaged in advocacy, policy making, and promoting environmental justice. At the mezzo level, social work is engaged in community development and working in organizational environments. At the micro level, social workers conduct assessments and interventions and can enhance human-nature connections (Norton, 2012).

Social work has its roots in human rights and social justice (Nesmith & Smyth, 2015), thus environmental injustice is relevant to the social work profession. The growing recognition of environmental human rights, in both theory and practice, may represent a powerful tool in the struggle for environmental justice (Woods, 2017). Developmental social work practice heralds the global commitments by way of the UDHR and the SDGs, to human wellbeing and environmental justice. Through the guidance provided by the Global Agenda for Social Work and Social Development, it is apparent that there is more work to be done to promote resilience, foster sustainable development, and eradicate inequities. Therefore, social work practitioners must continue to collaborate with stakeholders at all levels of society to facilitate accountability for human wellbeing and responsibility for the natural and physical environment.

References

Ali, W. (2018). *Social construct of water scarcity: A challenge for the sustainability of ground water in Lahore* [Unpublished doctoral dissertation]. University of the Punjab.

Alston, M., & Kent, J. (2009). Generation X-pendable: The social exclusion of rural and remote young people. *Journal of Sociology, 45*(1), 89–107.

Bakhsh, K., & Hassan, S. (2005). Use of sewage water for radish cultivation: A case study of Punjab, Pakistan. *Journal of Agriculture and Social Science, 4*, 322–326.

Banerjee, M. M. (2005). Social work, Rawlsian social justice, and social development. *Social Development Issues, 27*(1), 7–14.

Besson, J. (1984). Land tenure in the free villages of Trelawny, Jamaica: A case study in the Caribbean peasant response to emancipation. *Slavery & Abolition, 5*(1), 3–23. https://doi.org/10.1080/01440398408574862

Brooks, S. (2016). Informal settlements in Jamaica's tourism space: Urban spatial development in a small island developing state. *Urban Island Studies, 2*, 72–94. https://doi.org/10.20958/uis.2016.4

Boelens, R., Vos, J., & Perreault, T. (2018). Introduction: The multiple challenges and layers of water justice struggles. In R. Boelens, T. Perreault, & J. Vos (Eds.), *Water justice* (pp. 1–32). Cambridge: Cambridge University Press. doi:10.1017/9781316831847.001

Boyd, D. R. (2012). *The right to a healthy environment: Revitalizing Canada's constitution Press*. Vancouver: UBC Press.

Canadian Association of Social Workers [CASW]. (2020). *CASW scope of practice statement*. Retrieved from www.casw-acts.ca/en/Code-of-Ethics%20and%20Scope%20of%20Practice#:~:text=CASW%20Scope%20of%20Practice%20Statement&text=Social%20work%20focuses%20on%20the,families%2C%20groups%2C%20and%20communities

Choondassery, Y. (2017). Rights-based approach: The hub of sustainable development. *Discourse and Communication for Sustainable Education, 8*(2), 17–23.

Clark, H. (2012, March 26). *Opening remarks on the occasion of world social work day*. Retrieved from www.undp.org/content/undp/en/home/presscenter/speeches/2012/03/26/helen-clark-opening-remarks-on-the-occasion-of-world-social-work-day.html

Coates, J., & Gray, M. (2012). The environment and social work: An overview and introduction. *International Journal of Social Welfare, 21*, 230–238.

Colten, C. E., Kates, R. W., & Laska, S. B. (2008). Three years: Lessons for community resilience. *Environment, 50*, 36–47.

Cooper, R. (2020, June 29). *On climate, COVID, and race*. Retrieved from www.psychiatrictimes.com/view/on-climate-covid-and-race

Council on Social Work Education (CSWE). (2015). *Accreditation standards and policy*. Retrieved from www.cswe.org/getattachment/Accreditation/Standards-and-Policies/2015-EPAS/2015EPASandGlossary.pdf.aspx

Dietz, T., Shwom, R. L., & Whitley, C. T. (2020). Climate change and society. *Annual Review of Sociology, 46*, 135–158.

Dominelli, L. (2012). *Green social work: From environmental crises to environmental justice*. Cambridge, UK: Polity Press.

Dominelli, L. (2013). Environmental justice at the heart of social work practice: Greening the profession. *International Journal of Social Welfare, 22*, 431–439.

Drolet, J. (Ed.). (2019). *Rebuilding lives post disaster*. New York City, NY: Oxford University Press.

Drolet, J., Lewin, B., & Pinches, Al. (2021). Social work practitioners and human service professionals in the 2016 Alberta (Canada) wildfires: Roles and contributions. *British Journal of Social Work, 51*(5), 1663–1679. https://doi.org/10.1093/bjsw/bcab141

Drolet, J. L., & Sampson, T. (2014). Addressing climate change from a social development approach: Small cities and rural communities' adaptation and response to climate change in British Columbia, Canada. *International Social Work, 60*(1), 61–73. London, England: Sage Publications.

Drolet, J., Sampson, T., Jebaraj, D., & Richard, L. (2013). Social work and environmentally induced displacement. A commentary. *Refuge: Canada's Journal on Refugees, 29*, 55–62.

Erickson, C. L. (2018). *Environmental justice as social work practice*. Oxford: Oxford University Press.

Foy, K.C. (2012). Home is where the health is: The convergence of environmental justice, affordable housing, and green building. *Pace Environmental Law*

Review, 30(1). Retrieved from https://digitalcommons.pace.edu/cgi/viewcontent.cgi?article=1707&context=pelr

Frommer, B. (2013). Climate change and the resilient society: utopia or realistic option for German regions. *Natural Hazards, 67*, 99–115.

Gaard, G. (2017). Feminism and environmental justice. In R. Holifield, J. Chakraborty, and G. Walker (Eds.), *The Routledge handbook of environmental justice* (pp. 74–88). New York, NY: Routledge.

2Harris, L. M., McKenzie, S., Rodina, L., Shah, S. H., & Wilson, N. J. (2017). Key concepts, debates and research agendas. In R. Holifield, J. Chakraborty, and G. Walker (Eds.), *The Routledge handbook of environmental justice* (p. 338). New York, NY: Routledge.

Hassan, G. Z., & Hassan, F. R. (2017). Sustainable use of groundwater for irrigated agriculture: A case study of Punjab. *Pakistan. European Water, 57*, 475–480. https://doi.org/10.1007/978-3-319-29948-8_10

Holifield, R., Chakraborty, J., & Walker, G. (2017). Introduction: the worlds of environmental justice. In R. Holifield, J. Chakraborty, and G. Walker (Eds.), *The Routledge handbook of environmental justice* (pp. 1–11). New York, NY: Routledge.

Housing Agency of Jamaica. (n.d.). *Operation PRIDE—Building Jamaica one community at a time.* Retrieved from www.hajl.gov.jm/operation-pride/

Hussain, S., Malikb, S., Cheemac, M. J. M., Ashrafd, M. U., Waqase, M. S., & Iqbalf, M. M. (2020). An overview on emerging water scarcity challenge in Pakistan, its consumption, causes, impacts and remedial measures. *Big Data in Water Resources Engineering (BDWRE), 1*, 22–31.

IPCC. (2014). *Climate Change 2014: Synthesis report. Contribution of working groups I, II and III to the fifth assessment report of the intergovernmental panel on climate change.* Retrieved from www.ipcc.ch/report/ar5/syr/

Jamil, M. (2019). *Running dry: Water scarcity in Pakistan.* Naval Postgraduate School Monterey United States.

Jones, D. N., & Truell, R. (2012). The global agenda for social work and social development: A place to link together and be effective in a globalized world. *International Social Work, 55*(4), 454–472. https://doi.org/10.1177/0020872812440587

Jones, P. (2016). Informal urbanism as a product of socio-cultural expression: Insights from African cities: The case of Kumasi, Ghana. *Urban Studies, 28*(1), 139–151.

Khan, M. A. A., Ashraf, I., & Siddiqui, M. T. (2021). A qualitative insight into the factors behind water scarcity in Punjab, Pakistan. *Pakistan Journal of Agricultural Sciences, 58*(1).

Konadu-Agyemang, K. O. (1991). Reflections on the absence of squatter settlements in west the island Pacific. *Dynamics and Resilience of Informal Areas*, 165–181.

Lewis, B. (2012). Human rights and environmental wrongs: Achieving environmental justice through human rights law. *International Journal for Crime and Justice, 1*(1), 65–73.

Levy, B., & Patz, J. (2015). Climate change, human rights, and social justice. *Annals of Global Health, 81*(3), 310–322.

Lombard, A. (2015). Global agenda for social work and social development: A path toward sustainable social work. *Social Work/Maatskaplike Werk, 51*(4). https://doi.org/10.15270/51-4-462

Lombard, A., & Twikirize, J. M. (2014). Promoting social and economic equality: Social workers' contribution to social justice and social development in South Africa and Uganda. *International Social* Work, *57*(4), 313–325.

Maschi, T., Rees, J. Leibowitz G., & Bryan, M. (2019). Educating for rights and justice: a content analysis of forensic social work syllabi. *Social Work Education: The International Journal, 38*(2), 177–197.

McGregor, D., Whitaker S., & Sritharan, M. (2019). Indigenous environmental justice and sustainability. *Current Opinion in Environmental Sustainability*, *43*, 35–40.

Miller, S. E., Hayward, R. A., & Shaw, T. V. (2012). Environmental shifts for social work: A principles approach. *International Journal of Social Welfare*, *21*(3): 270–7.

Mohai, P., Pellow, D., & Roberts, J. T. (2009). Environmental justice. *Annual Review of Environment and Resources*, *34*, 405–430.

Nesmith, A., & Smyth, N. (2015). Environmental justice and social work education: Social workers' professional perspectives. *Social Work Education: The International Journal*, *34*(5), 484–501.

Norton, C. L. (2012). Social work and the environment: An Eco social approach. *International Journal of Social Welfare*, *21*, 299–308.

Nussbaum, M. C. (2011). *Creating capabilities: The human development approach*. Cambridge, MA: Harvard University Press.

Oxfam. (2020). *5 natural disasters that beg for climate action*. Retrieved from www.oxfam.org/en/5-natural-disasters-beg-climate-action

Padawangi, R. (2010). Community-driven development as a driver of change: Water supply and sanitation projects in rural Punjab, Pakistan. *Water Policy*, *12*(S1), 104–120.

Peduzzi, P. (2019). The disaster risk, global change, and sustainability nexus. *Sustainability*, *11*(4), 957. https://doi.org/10.3390/su11040957

Rasool, A., Xiao, T., Farooqi, A., Shafeeque, M., Masood, S., Ali, S., . . ., & Nasim, W. (2016). Arsenic and heavy metal contaminations in the tube well water of Punjab, Pakistan and risk assessment: A case study. *Ecological Engineering*, *95*, 90–100.

Rauf, S., Bakhsh, K., Hassan, S., Nadeem, A. M., & Kamran, M. A. (2015). Determinants of a household's choice of drinking water source in Punjab, Pakistan. *Polish Journal of Environmental Studies*, *24*(6), 2751–2754.

Rawls, J. (2001). *Justice as fairness: A restatement*. Cambridge, MA: Harvard University Press.

Scheelbeek, P. F., Khan, A. E., Mojumder, S., Elliott, P., & Vineis, P. (2016). Drinking water sodium and elevated blood pressure of healthy pregnant women in salinity-affected coastal areas. *Hypertension*, *68*(2), 464–470.

Schlosberg, D. (2007). *Defining environmental justice*. In *Defining Environmental Justice: Theories, Movements, and Nature* (pp. 3–10). Oxford: Oxford University Press. https://doi.org/10.1093/acprof:oso/9780199286294.003.0001

Schlosberg, D., & Collins, L. B. (2014). From environmental to climate justice: Climate change and the discourse of environmental justice. *Wiley Interdisciplinary Reviews: Climate Change*, *5*(3), 359–374.

Schmitz, C., Matyók, T., Sloan, L. M., & James, C. (2012). The relationship between social work and environmental sustainability: Implications for interdisciplinary practice. *International Journal of Social Welfare*, *21*, 278–286.

Sicotte, D. M., & Brulle, R. J. (2017). Social movements for environmental justice through the lens of social movement theory. In R. Holifield, J. Chakraborty, and G. Walker (Eds.), *The Routledge handbook of environmental justice* (pp. 25–36). Routledge.

Teixeira, S., & Krings, A. (2015). Sustainable social work: An environmental justice framework for social work education. *Social Work Education*, *34*(5), 513–527.

Temper, L. (2019). Blocking pipelines, unsettling environmental justice: from rights of nature to responsibility to territory. *Local Environment*, *24*(2), 94–112.

Todd, S., & Drolet, J. (Eds.) (2020). *Community practices and social development*. Springer Nature.

United Nations. (2021). *Universal declaration of human rights 1948*. Retrieved from https://www.un.org/sites/un2.un.org/files/2021/03/udhr.pdf

United Nations. (2005). *The social summit ten years later.* Retrieved from www.un.org/esa/socdev/publications/SocialSummit-10YearsLater.pdf

United Nations. (2005, January 22). *Hyogo framework for action 2005–2015: Building the resilience of nations and communities to disasters.* Retrieved from www.unisdr.org/2005/wcdr/intergover/official-doc/L-docs/Hyogo-framework-for-action-english.pdf

United Nations. (2007). *United Nations declaration on the rights of Indigenous peoples.* Retrieved from www.un.org/development/desa/indigenouspeoples/wpcontent/uploads/sites/19/2018/11/UNDRIP_E_web.pdf

United Nations Publications. (2019). *Global sustainable development report 2019: The Future is now-Science for achieving sustainable development.* Retrieved from https://sustainabledevelopment.un.org/content/documents/24797GSDR_report_2019.pdf

United Nations Framework Convention on Climate Change. (1992, May 9). *United Nations Framework Convention on Climate Change.* Retrieved from https://treaties.un.org/doc/Treaties/1994/03/19940321%200456%20AM/Ch_XXVII_07p.pdf

United Nations Office for Disaster Risk Reduction (UNDRR). (2015). *Sendai framework for disaster risk reduction 2015–2030.* Retrieved from www.undrr.org/publication/sendai-framework-disaster-risk-reduction-2015-2030

United Nations Research Institute for Social Development (UNRISD). (2015). *Research for social change: Transformations to equity and sustainability.* UNRISD. https://doi.org/10.1093/oxfordhb/9780199645121.013.34

Van Shoelandt, C., & Gaus, G. (2018). Political and distributive justice. In S. Olsaretti (Ed.), *The Oxford handbook of distributive justice* (pp. 283–305). New york: Oxford University Press. https://doi.org/10.1093/oxfordhb/9780199645121.013.34

Woods, K., Holifield, J. Chakraborty, & G. Walker (2017). *Environmental human rights.* In R. Holifield, J. Chakraborty, and G. Walker (Eds.), *The Routledge handbook of environmental justice* (pp. 149–159). Routledge.

Zakar, M. Z., Zakar, D. R., & Fischer, F. (2020). Climate change-induced water scarcity: a threat to human health. *South Asian Studies, 27*(2).

Zapf, M. K. (2009). Social work and the environment: Understanding people and place. Toronto: Canadian Scholars' Press.

7 Social Work and Health Equity

An Examination of the Five Dimensions of Access

Rachelle Ashcroft and Keith Adamson

Introduction

Understanding health as a human right creates an obligation to ensure timely, acceptable, and affordable access to health and social care (World Health Organization (WHO), 2017). The WHO Constitution establishes the right to health as the right to "the highest attainable standard of health as a fundamental right of every human being" (WHO, 2017). Attaining a high standard of health for every human being means striving for greater health equity using a multifaceted approach that spans multiple sectors. The person-in-environment perspective from social workers brings a crucial understanding of the disparities and inequities that manifest as health and mental health conditions for many of the individuals, families, and communities with whom we work. Although we write this chapter from the perspective of two academics in a Canadian context, we believe the underlying tenets of human rights, health equity, and access presented in this chapter are applicable across contexts. In addition, both authors have extensive clinical experience working as social workers in various Canadian healthcare settings. We know first-hand that social workers hold a unique role in health and mental health settings and have the potential to provide leadership to interdisciplinary teams, organizations, and communities on health equity initiatives.

What Is a Health Equity?

Health equity is a foundational principle to reduce and eliminate unfair and avoidable disparities in health (Braveman, 2014; WHO, 2013). Horizontal equity refers to the principle that individuals with similar needs should receive similar levels of services; whereas, vertical equity refers to the principle that those individuals with the greatest need should receive higher priority and attention for services (Bayoumi, 2009). A commitment to health equity means pursuing the highest standard of health for all people and attending to the needs of individuals, families, and communities at greatest risk of poor health because of the social conditions that are underlying

DOI: 10.4324/9781003111269-9

disparities (Braveman, 2014; WHO 2013). The United States Department of Health and Human Services (2008) defines health disparity as:

> a particular type of health difference that is closely linked with social or economic disadvantage. Health disparities adversely affect groups of people who have systematically experienced greater social or economic obstacles to health based on their racial or ethnic group, religion, socioeconomic status, gender, mental health, cognitive, sensory, or physical disability, sexual orientation, geographic location, or other characteristics historically linked to discrimination or exclusion.
>
> (p. 28)

There is a long-standing recognition of the connection between eliminating health disparities by attending to social determinants and health (Ashcroft, 2010; Raphael, 2019). Social determinants of health are the political, social, behavioral, and economic factors that shape the health of individuals and communities (Raphael, 2019). These non-medical factors profoundly influence health outcomes (WHO, 2013). *Risk conditions* rather than *risk factors* are of utmost importance from a social determinants of health perspective. There is a long-standing historical awareness of the role that social conditions have on health outcomes. For example, it was back in the 19th century when Rudolph Virchow and Frederich Engels named political, social, and economic forces as key influencers on health, disease, and mortality (Raphael, 2019). Current examples of social determinants of health that can influence health equity include income, social protection, education, unemployment and job security, working conditions, food insecurity, housing quality, social inclusion, non-discrimination, early childhood development, and access to affordable high-quality health and social services (WHO, 2013).

The range of social determinants of health extends across three main levels. First, the distal level determinants refer to public policies and social conditions such as poverty and racism (Walters et al., 2016; Warnecke et al., 2008). Second, the intermediate level determinants refer to immediate physical and social contexts where distal level determinants are realized. For example, such contexts include institutions, social relationships, places, and settings where distal determinants are experienced and actualized (Walters et al., 2016; Warnecke et al., 2008). The final level is the proximal determinants, which refers to the individual-level factors such as changes that occur across one's developmental lifecycle from experiences of trauma (Gehlert, 2014; Walters et al., 2016). In addition, health behavior and demographic characteristics are also examples of proximal determinants (Walters et al., 2016; Warnecke et al., 2008). The political economy perspective, however, provides an additional understanding for addressing health inequities.

The political economy perspective adds a critical view to the social determinants of health. Taking a more critical approach to the political and economic structures influencing health disparities, the political economy perspective views disparities between populations resulting from inequitable power and structural relations (Ashcroft, 2010). The critique of predominant structures also calls attention to inequitable structures inherent in healthcare that may be perpetuating "social control, reinforcing racism and patriarchy" (Lupton, 2013, p. 7). This is not to discount the value of healthcare but instead to highlight the need for critical assessment of medical and other healthcare structures as potential sources of inequities for individuals, families, and communities (Ashcroft, 2010; Lupton, 2013). For example,

> marginalized groups, such as women, people from non-English-speaking backgrounds, non-whites, the aged, the unemployed and members of the working class, [who] tend to endure greater social and economic disadvantage than those from privileged groups, have restricted access to health care services and suffer poor health as a result.
>
> (Lupton, 2013, p. 5)

Addressing the broad range of social determinants of health is fundamental, as is attending to the proximal, intermediate, and distal structures related to healthcare, to alleviating health disparities.

Why Is Health Equity Important to Social Workers?

Social workers are crucial to the pursuit of health equity (Ashcroft, Lam et al., 2021). Social work's foundational values of social justice, human rights, respect for diversity, and collective responsibilities mean that social work has an inherent commitment to strive for health equity and alleviate existing and future disparities (Ashcroft, 2010; Hermans & Roets, 2020; Walters et al., 2016). Health was one of the first fields of practice for social work and remains one of social work's largest practice domains (Beddoe, 2013; de Saxe Zerden et al., 2018). Social workers have a long-standing history of practice in a wide range of health settings—in hospitals, primary health care, public health, community mental health, social services, non-profit organizations, and elsewhere—and are well positioned to attend to the risk conditions of people's lives. In these and other settings, social work brings a unique lens of situating health in relation to people's social, environmental, economic, and political contexts (International Federation of Social Workers (IFSW), 2008). From this vantage point, health is understood as social experiences that impact people's identities, opportunities, and relationships (IFSW 2008). Social workers have the necessary lens to identify the social determinants of health and related factors that perpetuate health inequalities (Ashcroft, 2010; Ashcroft et al., 2021). In health settings, social workers bring a recognition that health is holistic, multi-dimensional, relational, and dynamic (Ashcroft et al., 2017). Inevitably, social work's view of health recognizes the social determinants of health, and, in practice, witnesses first-hand the implications for individuals, families, and communities.

Social work's systems perspective can guide change across the micro-, mezzo-, and macro-levels, which is an asset to the pursuit of health equity. Micro-level includes individual psychosocial, behavioral, and material risk conditions; mezzo-level refers to organizational and institutional structures; while the macro-level encompasses societal level characteristics such as health care policy, societal norms, and income distribution (Richter & Dragano, 2018). The socio-political function of social work's guiding values of social justice and human rights implies that social work interventions and strategies need to bridge across these various levels (Hermans & Roets, 2020). Addressing health disparities means that "social work strategies might involve individual-, community-, and policy-oriented work, so long as they also attend to the socioenvironmental issues influencing health" (Ashcroft, 2010, p. 252). This is a unique distinction that social workers bring to interdisciplinary health and mental health settings.

The diverse skills combined with the systemic understanding that social workers bring are important contributions to the health and wellbeing of individuals, families, and communities. Social workers fulfill many roles in health and mental health settings. Some of these roles include psychosocial assessments, behavioral health prevention and treatment, crisis management, advanced care planning, individual and group therapy, service coordination, case management, problem-solving, discharge planning, systems navigation, resource allocation, community mobilization, and policy development (Ashcroft et al., 2019; de Saxe Zerden et al., 2018; Walter-McCabe, 2020).

Prioritizing the social determinants of health and working toward health equity is a complex and multifaceted endeavor that requires collaboration across a wide range of stakeholders within and beyond the health sector (WHO, 2013). Social workers in health and mental health settings often work as members of interdisciplinary teams (Ashcroft et al., 2018; de Saxe Zerden et al., 2018). Interdisciplinary collaborative teams that bring together a range of healthcare providers—including social workers—are considered an important means of promoting health equity (Walters et al., 2016).

The COVID-19 pandemic created devastating social and economic conditions that illuminated and widened disparities. Individuals, families, and communities have experienced major unexpected financial pressures, economic hardships, job loss, precarious housing and living conditions, food insecurity, discrimination, racism, isolation, and profound grief. Older adults, children and youth, racialized communities, people with reduced access to socioeconomic resources, and those with disabilities have suffered disproportionately during the COVID-19 pandemic. Social workers have been active across a broad range of practice settings, fighting for social justice, particularly against these drastic disparities and increases of racism during the COVID-19 pandemic (Miller & Lee, 2020; Walter-McCabe, 2020). The pandemic demonstrated the need for social work's involvement to help address some of the inequitable structural systems and social determinants of health issues emerging during the pandemic health crisis (Truell, 2020; Walter-McCabe, 2020). Despite the dire need for support and care during the pandemic, there were incidences of reduced access to much-needed health and social services (Abrams & Szefler, 2020; Ashcroft, Sur et al., 2021; Walter-McCabe, 2020).

What Can Social Workers Do?

Social work practice takes on many different forms. We recognize that addressing health disparities is complex and requires multifaceted approaches (Ashcroft, 2010). Strengthening social work's capacity to improve access to services is an essential first step for meeting individuals, families, and community's needs for services and fostering health equity (Bayoumi, 2009). In this section, we aim to illustrate what access is and how social workers can improve access. We chose to focus on access because those with greatest social vulnerabilities and are at greatest risk of experiencing health disparities are those who are more likely to experience difficulties accessing health and social services (Haggerty et al., 2020). As well, service accessibility is essential for assuring social justice and working toward individual and societal change in the pursuit of health equity (Wronka, 2017).

Although the development of the accessibility framework comes from a health systems perspective, we believe Levesque et al.'s (2013) framework has significant value for social workers in all settings. The person-centered accessibility framework sees access as being an interaction between people's ability to perceive, seek, reach, afford, and engage with service providers—like social workers—with five dimensions of organizational accessibility (Haggerty et al., 2020; Levesque et al., 2013). According to this framework, many individuals who require health and social services will experience problematic access unless providers—in our case, social workers—and organizations have made care *approachable*, *acceptable*, *available and accommodating*, *affordable*, and *appropriate* (Haggerty et al., 2020; Levesque et al., 2013). "Inequitable access occurs when access varies according to personal and social factors rather than according to need" (Haggerty et al., 2020, p. 2). We review each of the five dimensions of access to define and demonstrate how each dimension applies, from a social work perspective, so that social work can use this framework to improve access to our own services. In addition, the Levesque et al. (2013) framework acts as a useful reflective tool for social workers to scrutinize, examine, and inform organizational structures and processes within which we operate. For each of the five dimensions, we provide examples of interventions at the clinical level (micro), interventions at the organizational level (mezzo), and interventions at the societal level (macro) to illustrate how social workers promote access to health care.

Approachability

Approachability refers to the awareness of health services from people with health needs as well as people's perception of these services. As such, approachability is not just about how services can be reached electronically or physically, but to a further extent, whether a service is deemed potentially useful or not by a particular group of people or prospective clients. From a social work perspective, approachability answers three questions: (i) Are people within a given marginalized group able to identify the services that exist for a particular health concern?; (ii) Are the services available and/or easy to engage with?; and (iii) Are services perceived as helpful or potentially not helpful by the marginalized group? Answers to these questions will help determine access to appropriate healthcare services for marginalized groups.

Approachability means that services are known across various social and geographical population groups. For example, ensuring transparency, sharing information regarding available treatments and services, and conducting outreach activities enhance approachability of services. It is also important to note that access to services starts by people recognizing that there is a need for care. Levesque et al.'s (2013) framework emphasizes that the ability to perceive the need for care among populations is crucial. The ability to perceive is influenced by important factors such as an individual's or groups' *health literacy* level, whether or not the *health beliefs* of an individual or group align with the healthcare services, and whether or not the individual or group *trusts* their health care provider(s).

Health literacy refers to

> the achievement of a level of knowledge, personal skills and confidence to take action to improve personal and community health by changing personal lifestyles and living conditions. Thus, health literacy means more than being able to read pamphlets and make appointments. By improving people's access to health information, and their capacity to use it effectively, health literacy is critical to empowerment.
>
> (WHO, 1998, p. 10)

Health beliefs refer to the meaning individuals attach to their health-related issues. Positive beliefs about a health condition can help people adopt a healthy lifestyle and engage in behaviors deemed useful, while negative or false beliefs about an illness can be potentially harmful to patient care and outcomes (Cai et al., 2016). Finally, *trust* refers to a way of being that inspires confidence from clients. When a social worker exhibits trust, they are honest about what they know, they do what they say they will do, and they are consistent in their ability to nurture and support clients.

Approachability—Clinical

At the clinical level, social workers need to understand a client's health literacy level, health beliefs about their health condition, and attend to the development of a strong therapeutic relationship built on trust. These three elements should be included in a comprehensive psychosocial assessment completed during the first few meetings with the client and included in social work recommendations.

HEALTH LITERACY

Social workers providing individual services needed to emphasize and deliver interventions that increase health literacy and assist clients in accessing quality treatment and becoming empowered advocates for their own care (Mendenhall & Frauenholtz, 2013). For example, the processes and paperwork required to engage in the healthcare system, to provide health and social histories, and to complete consent forms are daunting to many. Navigating these processes can be particularly daunting for clients who do not speak the dominant language that services are offered. Some clients prefer having services in concordant language because it is easier for them to relay information and have a shared meaning with their provider (Ashcroft et al., 2021).

Social workers need to enhance clients' confidence and ability to engage in services without creating conditions that further marginalize them. For example, research has demonstrated that individuals experience fear of displeasing health care providers (Sundler, Raberus, & Holmstrom, 2020). As well, research has also demonstrated how problematic it is that clients report the need to learn and adopt medical jargon in order to gain respect from healthcare providers, instead of using the words and vernacular that are most meaningful to them (Ashcroft et al., 2021). These examples are concerning as they may further perpetuate health inequities. Social workers play a critical role in ensuring that individuals, families, and the interdisciplinary team are communicating effectively and in ways that are most meaningful to clients. Social workers negotiate the understanding of the healthcare context with the client's needs and preferences as central driving forces. It also requires facilitating the client's and family's understanding of health information and supporting the removal of barriers in preparation for patient discharges (Warren et al., 2017). Social workers provide interventions that aim to empower clients to advocate as much as possible for themselves.

HEALTH BELIEFS

Health beliefs are important elements to consider in any psychosocial assessment. There are many models that speak to the importance of beliefs. For example, the Health Belief Model facilitates predictions of health-promoting conducts to develop preventive strategies and improve patients' health behaviors, exploring individuals' beliefs of health conditions (Smith & Mercado-Sierra, 2021). A second model that may be more consistent with social work is the Health/Illness Belief System developed by Browne (Browne & Gehlert, 2019). Browne (Browne & Gehlert, 2019) suggested that it is crucial that social workers inquire about key family beliefs that shape family illness narratives and coping strategies. The inquiry should consider (i) assumptions about what caused an illness and what will influence its course and outcome; (ii) meanings attached by family, ethnic group, religion, or wider culture to symptoms; and (iii) beliefs about normative assumptions, and internal (members can affect the outcome of a situation) versus external (outcomes are not in the control of the family member) locus of control. An assessment of the congruence of health beliefs within the family and its various systems and subsystems as well as between the family and the healthcare system and wider culture may be necessary to ensure that the services are most aligned with the individual and family's needs.

TRUSTING RELATIONSHIPS

Every clinical relationship should start with establishing trust as part of the therapeutic intervention in healthcare. Trusting relationships are essential (Ashcroft et al., 2021). In a study by Brinkley- Rubinstein et al. (2015), it was suggested that social workers consider trust as a subcomponent upon which health literacy is founded. They emphasized that the development of health literacy requires an initial connection or relationship between the client and the social worker. After rapport is established, the social worker is better able to assess the client's capacities to understand and use various types of health-related materials. Similarly, they add that a client is increasingly likely to reveal sensitive information that may inform the best ways to develop health literacy.

Approachability—Organizational

There is a growing demand for healthcare organizations to better meet the needs of individuals with all levels of health literacy. Annarumma and Palumbo (2016) describe how health care organizations can nurture health literacy. The authors stated that since healthcare organizations host most of the interactions between patients and healthcare professionals, health organizations should be considered as the most fitting context to enhance the ability of professionals to handle health information and to properly help clients navigate the health system. They added that to boost individual and collective levels of health literacy, healthcare organizations are urged to include health literacy within their strategic planning, assuming that it is a core value that drives their operational imperatives.

To identify the key features of organizational-level interventions for health literacy, Brach et al. (2012) suggested ten attributes of health literate health care organizations. They state that healthcare organizations that embody the following attributes create an environment that enables people to access and benefit optimally from a range of healthcare services:

1) Health literacy is integral to its mission, structure, and operations.
2) Integrates health literacy in planning, evaluation measures, patient safety, and quality improvement endeavors.
3) Prepares their workforce to be health literate.
4) Includes populations served by the organization in the design, implementation, and evaluation of health information and services.
5) Meets the needs of populations with a range of health literacy skills.
6) Uses health literacy strategies in interpersonal communication and confirms understanding at all points of contact.
7) Provides easy access to health information and services and navigation assistance.
8) Designs and distributes print audio-visual and social media content that is easy to understand and act on.
9) Addresses health literacy in high-risk situations, including care transitions and communications about medicines.
10) Communicates clearly what health plans cover and what individuals will have to pay for services.

Approachability—Societal

Social workers are central actors in the fight to advance a health literacy agenda. Social workers should be aware of the impact of the political arena on practice and should advocate for changes in policy and legislation to improve social conditions to meet basic human needs and promote social justice (Ashcroft et al., 2021; Miller et al., 2017). Health literacy is gaining increasing attention as a means of promoting individual-, community-, and population-level health and is key to delivery of health services in emerging and advanced healthcare systems around the world (Rowlands, 2018). Even more interesting is that health literacy has been used as a vehicle to address macro-level policies and mezzo-level actors to sustain health outcomes effects at the micro-level (Okan et al., 2018). It has been noted that health literacy has been used primarily to augment the efficacy and effectiveness of health promotion and prevention efforts (Smith & Mercado-Sierra, 2021). Ultimately, increasing health literacy empowers individuals and communities to be informed, active participants in their healthcare and can improve the health of marginalized populations through prevention and proactive interventions.

Acceptability

Acceptability refers to cultural and social factors that facilitate clients' ability to engage in the service. If a service is tailored to the cultural and social characteristics of a particular population, then the uptake in accessing the service should be greater, compared to if the service was offered without taking user needs into consideration. The population is composed of people who come from different social locations, who have different social and personal values, as well as various intersecting identities. Individuals from all communities have a human right to access health services that are relevant and appropriate to their groups' health and mental health needs. In the Levesque et al. (2013) framework, the ability to seek health care relates to concepts of personal autonomy and the capacity to choose to seek care. Practitioners and organizations are encouraged to submit resources to understanding and meeting the needs of vulnerable individuals and groups, as well as ensuring culturally relevant and sensitive care. Investments into ensuring acceptability of services may intentionally avoid discrimination against a given marginalized group, as well as persuade vulnerable groups to seek care. Ultimately, acceptability is about setting up the optimal conditions for individuals and groups to favorably engage with a service.

Acceptability—Clinical

Social workers encounter individuals from vulnerable and marginalized populations in all areas of their practice and across all service user groups. Social workers all over the world have committed to championing social justice and honoring diversity. According to the International Association of Schools of Social Work (IASSW): Social workers have a responsibility to engage people in achieving social justice, in relation to society generally, and in relation to the people with whom they work. This means challenging discrimination and institutional oppression. The IASSW's statement of ethics continues to further delineate that social workers challenge discrimination, which includes but is not limited to age, capacity, civil status, class, culture, ethnicity, gender, gender identity, language, nationality (or lack thereof), opinions, other physical characteristics, physical or mental abilities, political beliefs, poverty, race, relationship status, religion, sex, sexual orientation, socioeconomic status, spiritual beliefs, or family structure (International Federation of Social Workers (IFSW & IASSW, 2004).

Social workers on interdisciplinary teams need to ensure that they advocate for client preferences and that they take the time required to ensure patient concerns are addressed within the team. In practice, a great deal of messages about a service's receptiveness to different groups is reflected in the way that clients from marginalized groups are received from health care professionals and social workers within the organization. For example, George et al. (2020) studied the reasons why some cultural communities typically struggle with accessing healthcare services. One perspective emerged that the understanding of healing and disease in most formal education of providers follows a biomedical framework where health and illness are defined primarily from an individualistic and objectivist standpoint. Yet, on the other hand, there are multiple ways of defining health (George et al., 2020). Some individuals and communities take a more holistic approach to life and health, which is rooted firmly in their cultural tradition (George et al., 2020). Social workers need to be open to multiple ways of knowing and must include healing strategies that are culturally relevant and appropriate to the clients they serve.

Driven by their professional code of ethics, social workers need to be non-judgmental and practice cultural humility. According to Gunn (2019), cultural humility is an individual commitment to self-evaluation and critique. She added that by allowing others to practice their ways without projecting personal views, cultural respect is maintained. In a study by Duby et al. (2018), where he contextualized healthcare access for men who have sex with men, female sex workers, and people who use drugs in two south African cities, healthcare worker behaviors played a huge role in preventing access to care. Health workers described their own attitudes toward marginalized populations and demonstrated a lack of relevant knowledge, skills, and training to manage the health needs and vulnerabilities facing key populations. The marginalized populations in the study described their experiences of stigmatization, and related feelings of guilt, shame, and a loss of dignity because of discrimination by healthcare providers and other community members. The authors' findings suggest that the uptake and effectiveness of health services among marginalized populations are limited by internalized stigma, reluctance to seek care, unwillingness to disclose risk behaviors to healthcare workers, combined with a lack of knowledge and understanding on the part of the broader community members, including healthcare workers (Duby et al., 2018).

Acceptability—Organizational

Sensitization training of healthcare workers has been a strategy used in attempts to reduce prejudice and discrimination (Duby et al., 2018). Kaminsky and Hoglund (2019) investigated healthcare managers' views on gender inequity. They found that although most of the managers interviewed expressed a lack of awareness in inequity, they also expressed an openness to learning more about equity. The authors added that while this openness may have reflected a desire to show political correctness, it also pointed out a need for educational training to increase the awareness of inequity issues in healthcare among healthcare managers. Duby et al. (2018) suggested that focusing equity training interventions at the management level within healthcare organizations was critical because managers supervise and influence the work of healthcare employees and set expectations for employees. Healthcare organizations have a responsibility to ensure that the professionals who are providing care to patients are competent and knowledgeable about what they know and about what they do. What clinicians know must include an understanding of culture, not just a perspective of culture that refers to the traditions within a particular ethnic group but culture in a more general sense where clinicians are trained to be curious about a patient's "normal ways of being in the world." In other words, it is an exercise in cultural humility. Furthermore, cultural humility is a way of being with the patient that ensures respectful, compassionate, and equitable interactions, and healthcare organizations must be open to this fact.

Organizations are also making concerted efforts to increase access of particular client's groups by proving specialty services within healthcare organizations or by becoming specialty healthcare organizations. For example, Women's College Hospital in Canada is a leading academic, ambulatory hospital, and a world leader in women's health. The hospital advances and advocates for the health of women and improves healthcare options for all by developing, researching, teaching, and delivering new treatments and models of integrated care. In organizations such as these, Jenkins and Newman (2021) have implied that incorporation of sex and gender differences go into daily practices that involve the consideration of whether there are known sex or gender differences in the disease presentation, diagnosis, treatment, and/or prognosis of gender bias in the delivery of patient care. A consideration of gender and sex will become a natural part of a clinician's approach to patient care. Any clinician in a specialized setting for women's health would be familiar with sex and gender differences and will be able to challenge potential bias by asking patients the impacts of sex and gender, which in turn will ultimately contribute to providing the best evidence-based, individualized care possible. Specialized services usually also tend to market solely on the specialized nature of their services and tend to attract those within a particular group seeking care.

Acceptability—Societal

Health equity advocates must be vigilant and skilled in their ability to identify legislation or policies that deter people from marginalized or vulnerable groups from seeking care (Ashcroft, Lam et al., 2021). For example, the Government of Ontario (2020) in Canada eliminated the practice of birth alerts. A birth alert was the practice of child welfare agencies notifying a hospital and birth centers of safety concerns before a baby was born. Those concerns might be due to previous involvement with child welfare, drug use, issues surrounding mental health, or other challenges that are perceived to be potential factors that may impact their parenting. Birth alerts are a practice that can result in a baby being immediately taken away from its mother after being born. Policy makers have suggested that the practice was never looked at critically. Policy decision-makers never reflected on its long-term impact on the infant or their mother, or that the other components of the baby's safety, for example, their emotional, spiritual, and intellectual safety, were compromised in those situations. Furthermore, it was reported that the practice of birth alerts disproportionately affected racialized and marginalized mothers and families. Expectant mothers could be deterred from seeking prenatal care or parenting support while pregnant, due to fears of having a birth alert issued (Government of Ontario, 2020). Oliver et al. (2019) noted that when doing policy work, it is incumbent on all stakeholders to think about and imagine the unintended consequences that may fall most heavily on the most disenfranchised. Furthermore, they suggested that thinking carefully about who is likely to be affected by new or existing policies is a question of equity and one which can be addressed through mindful stakeholder engagement.

Availability and Accommodation

Availability and accommodation refer to the fact that health services (either the physical space or people working in health care roles) can be reached physically and in a timely manner. Levesque et al. (2013) contend that availability constitutes the physical existence of health resources with sufficient capacity to produce services, to the point of appropriately meeting the needs of the population it is intended to serve. He adds that availability and accommodation result from characteristics of facilities (e.g., density, decentralization of services, distribution of services, transportation to facilities, and building accessibility), as well as characteristics of the health care provider (e.g., presence or absence of trained health professionals, professional qualifications, and chosen modes of service provision—face to face or virtual care). Levesque et al. (2013) also contends that if individuals do not have tangible supports that permit them to obtain physical and/or virtual healthcare spaces, then that connotes a lack of access. He calls this "the ability to reach" healthcare, which is connected to the idea of personal mobility, the availability of transportation, the flexibility to leave work if necessary to seek an appointment, and knowledge about health services that would enable a person to physically reach service providers.

Availability and Accommodation—Clinical

Social work's primary role in increasing availability of services to marginalized individuals lies in facilitating access to timely, effective care. Social workers must consider each patient's unique circumstances and initiate care where possible that limits the burden of an individual's opportunity to accessing care; in other words, removing barriers that may be connected to transportation, restricted mobility, employment status, referral to specialty care, and other barriers. For example, health social workers work with individuals to provide education about health conditions and to promote lifestyle adjustments to support the individual's increased participation in life. However, social workers also assist individuals with transportation to and from appointments. This reflects the need for social workers to consider where a client lives in relation to the availability of resources and the client's ability to access services. In a study about emerging competencies for rural social work practice, Riebscheger et al. (2015) suggested that for parents who are involved in their child's care, poverty can be a barrier to meeting the goals of a treatment plan. Riebscheger et al. (2015) stated that parents' ability to pay for services or having to leave work to attend appointments for counseling and visits with children who need care are barriers to successfully completing a treatment plan. Riebscheger et al. (2015) add that lack of public transportation options and lack of access to a vehicle are also barriers for these families. They concluded that it is important for social workers to be aware of these barriers when writing their treatment goals and plans or assisting families to find resources that are flexible with work schedules or that even exist in rural communities.

Availability and Accommodation—Organizational

Most healthcare organizations around the world are looking for ways to improve access to quality care. Access within healthcare organizations can be answered by asking five operational questions (QHR Health, 2021): (i) How many clients can the providers in a service or clinic see in a week? (ii) How are those appointments distributed daily or weekly? (iii) What is the current utilization of appointments? (iv) What volume patterns are evident and when are the typical peaks of service in demand? (v) What access barriers have clients identified? These questions may appear to be simple, but there are complex operational processes. For example, understanding peak patterns means that the organization needs to align supply with demand—the number of patients requiring care against the number of healthcare providers that are present to provide care at a given time. If there is more demand than supply, then invariably, issues about long waitlists, insufficient time for each person's appointment, or issues about heavy workloads and staff fatigue may affect the quality of care provided. Organizations need to ensure that they provide "the right care at the right time by the right provider." Other ways that organizations continually try to improve access is to ensure that they offer extended hours and flexible operating hours.

Availability can also be influenced by technical innovation. The COVID-19 crisis brought to the fore significant challenges for healthcare organizations in service delivery. With social distancing guidelines and shelter-in-place orders to reduce the spread of the virus, traditional in-person services could not be delivered for many clients, who had medical concerns other than COVID infections. Already because of COVID-19, many healthcare organizations had rapidly moved to using telehealth (i.e., treatment that is delivered either by audio and/or by video call) in place of in-person contact (Ashcroft, Sur et al., 2021; Donnelly et al., 2021; Taylor et al., 2020). Organizations are increasingly realizing the benefits of implementing patient portals (electronic personal health records that are connected to institutional health records), which are recognized as a promising mechanism to support greater patient engagement. Irazarry et al. (2015) stated that a client's ability to use patient portals is strongly influenced by personal factors such as age, ethnicity, education level, health literacy, health status, and role as caregiver. They add that health care delivery factors mainly provider endorsement and patient portability also contribute to patient's ability to engage through and with the patient portal. Regrettably, COVID-19 has exposed the limitation of access to care for those clients or individuals who do not have Internet access. Overwhelmingly, studies around the world show that Internet access is now vital for improvements in access to health and healthcare (Barry, 2020).

Availability and Accommodation—Societal

Systematic disparities exist in the provider networks between urban and rural settings: an urban setting is akin to a city or a big town, whereas rural denotes a location in the county side or outside of the city (Hart et al., 2005). One challenge that exists for policy makers is knowing how to attract specialized healthcare professionals to rural areas. Traditionally, a higher proportion of professionals establish themselves in the city and a smaller percentage move and work in rural areas. This uneven distribution of providers may negatively impact access to care within non-urban areas (Cyr et al., 2019).

One solution with the limited availability of health providers involves expanding a health professional's scope of practice. Expanding the scope of practice means allowing more procedures, actions, and processes that a healthcare provider is legally permitted to do. For example, there are current debates in the state of Alabama in the United States about unrestricting nurse practitioner's authority in rural and low-income areas because it has been associated with greater access to primary care (Hart et al., 2020). Nurse practitioners are registered nurses who have met additional education, experience, and exam requirements set by the professional regulatory board. They are often authorized to diagnose, order, and interpret diagnostic tests, and prescribe medication and other treatments (College of Nurses of Ontario (CNO), 2021). The basis of the argument for the change to the legislative landscape is based on the idea that unrestricted access to nurse practitioner services has been associated with fewer emergency department visits, increased access to primary care, and lower costs of healthcare with no sacrifice in quality. It is also important to note that expansions of scopes of practice within other disciplines have improved healthcare access (Serban, 2020).

Affordability

Affordability refers to whether individuals can cover the costs attached to accessing healthcare services and/or that healthcare costs are publicly funded. If costs prohibit an individual from seeking a healthcare service, then services are not accessible. Levesque et al. (2013) contend that affordability means the ability to pay for healthcare—which implies that the ability to generate economic resources to pay for health services without expenditure of resources required for necessities. However, Levesque et al. (2013) extend the understanding of affordability to include the opportunity costs related to loss of income. These include secondary costs involved in reaching the appointment like travel and child-care and the opportunity costs of seeking care, like missing work.

Affordability—Clinical

Social workers in the field of healthcare will undoubtedly encounter situations where a client's lack of financial resources puts the client at risk for poor healthcare outcomes. Social workers should have knowledge about government health programs and policies, have expertise in eligibility for government-sponsored financial programs, and connect clients with available resources. Understanding the nature and scope of services that exist helps overcome persistent barriers that result from a client's lack of knowledge or misinformation about government financial programs. For example, social workers working in the field of disability should understand the state or provincial Assistive Devices programs that support clients with long-term physical disabilities with funding for customized equipment, like wheelchairs and hearing aids. In a study by Liddy et al. (2019), clinical interventions that supported economically vulnerable clients to accessing their prescribed medication included specific instructions on how to access the prescription through the drug benefits program without incurring cost to the client. It is important to note that alongside some of the more formal governmental programs that provide financial assistance to clients, social workers should also be aware of the informal resources that can be accessed to help support clients with financial needs, including family and various community supports. There are non-profit organizations and drug manufacturers that provide patient assistance programs (PAPs) to help ensure that patients receive critical care that they may not otherwise be able to afford (Therigy, 2021).

Affordability—Organizational

Organizational level interventions should focus primarily on those actions that not-for-profit healthcare organizations can make to support their economically disadvantaged clients. In a difficult economic environment, healthcare organizations are increasingly aware of the links between a client's health outcome and a client's income. For organizations that understand the impact of health disparities in access, costs, quality, and outcomes, there should be a particular interest in what can be called a viable financial safety net for their clients. For example, an initiative funded by the hospital foundation at one of Canada's largest children's rehabilitation hospitals created what was known as a Family Support Fund. The Family Support Fund offers financial support to the organization's clients and families during a time of transition or stress. The fund may provide financial compensation for equipment, medication, recreational activities, and respite services during the client's and family's journey at the hospital. In fact, the Family Support Fund was among the first hospital-based funds in Canada to respond to the financial crisis brought on by COVID-19. The Foundation's generous increase to the Fund's annual budget made it possible for the organization to respond to emergent needs arising from COVID-19 and directly impact the lives of kids, youth, and families more than ever before (Holland Bloorview, 2021). Internal funding programs such as these within healthcare organizations demonstrate a sensitivity to equity issues as well as demonstrate concrete actions to narrow the gap between the social determinants of health and positive health outcomes.

Affordability—Societal

Universal health care exists in some countries and means that there is a national insurance plan for each citizen in that country whereby most medical interventions are covered publicly without any costs to the beneficiary. Those social workers who work in countries where there is no national health insurance plan may observe that clients with no or inadequate insurance coverage may experience late diagnosis and treatment, poor health status and outcomes, and inappropriate use of health services, such as the emergency rooms (Browne & Gehlert, 2019). Those social workers who work in countries where there is a universal health insurance plan for all, need to focus explicitly on progressively eliminating geographical, economic, sociocultural, and gender barriers, supported by interventions for action on social determinants of health (Ashcroft, 2010). It is imperative that any initiatives be paired with approaches based on human rights to facilitate effective deployment of resources to advance equity. For example, Richmond and Cook (2016) have suggested that in Canada, the persistence and growth of Indigenous health and social inequity signals that Canada is at a critical public health juncture that fails the contemporary health needs of Indigenous peoples. They add that public health policy needs to recognize and prioritize the rights of Canada's Indigenous people to achieve health equity. They end by stating that healthy public policy recognizes that the health of a population requires investment and coordination on a whole range of economic, social, environmental, and political forces. Health policy must continue to address systemic problems of access, cost, quality, and accountability.

Appropriateness

Appropriateness refers to the fit between services and the client needs, its timeliness, the amount of care spent assessing health problems and determining the correct treatment and interpersonal quality of the services provided. Appropriateness also speaks to the types and the quality of services that are provided. Services that are of poor quality deter optimal access. A large component of appropriateness centers around client engagement in the care process. Levesque et al. (2013) stated that the ability to engage in health care relates to participation and involvement of the client in decision-making and treatment decisions, which is in turn are strongly determined by capacity and motivation to participate in care and commit to its completion. He ends by stating that the access to optimal care requires a person to be fully engaged in care, and this is seen as interacting with the nature of the services offered and provided.

Appropriateness—Clinical

Promoting shared decision-making in health care situations is a key and central role for social work. Appropriateness includes the client's role in decision-making, situated within a healthcare team, as a collaborator in triaging and learning about available health care options. This is an endeavor that can lead to the client receiving healthcare. In the ideal world, effective treatment options should be based on what is best for clients, since many factors influence treatment preference, including psychological, social, cultural, and spiritual history, that influence the healthcare encounter, histories that are sometimes ignored in the health and mental health encounter (Peterson, 2012). Social workers have the knowledge base and skillset to ensure a holistic approach to engaging clients, and partnering meaningfully with patients, in order to provide collaborative decision-making.

Social workers in healthcare settings should also rely on culturally appropriate evidence-based interventions to ensure the provision of optimal client care. Evidence-based practice is a process for making practice decisions in which practitioners integrate the best research evidence available with their practice expertise and with client attributes, values, preferences, and circumstances (Rubin & Bellamy, 2012). According to Hays (2019), a culturally responsive approach begins long before the start of social worker's work with clients. She states that it begins with the therapist's attention to those areas in which social workers may hold biases. She ends by indicating that all social workers have biases, and the first step in recognizing them is to acknowledge and recognize the role that biases play in contributing to systems of privilege and oppression.

Social workers must be aware of their bias toward certain populations and the health disparities that exist for those populations. It has been suggested that successfully addressing the possibility of clinician bias begins with awareness of the pervasiveness of disparities, the ways in which bias can influence clinical decision-making and behavior, and a commitment to acquiring the skills to minimize these processes (Williams & Wyatt, 2015). An example of how clinician bias can impact appropriateness of services for clients was described in a seminal article by Williams (2002) with respect to race, ethnicity, and mental health services. She reported that in Canada, research evidence indicated that there were specific problems with providing health services to ethnoracial and ethnocultural groups.

Williams (2002) concluded the following: First, many ethnic and racial minority people never access mental health care. They "fall through the gaps" while mental health problems are prolonged and unaddressed. A persistent disengagement between service providers and ethnoracial communities has prevented both sides from gaining an understanding of when help is needed and how it should be provided. Second, racial and ethnic minorities receive inadequate care. Racial minority clients receive less care than other clients do. They often seek help but withdraw from mental health and social services after their initial contacts. During these first contacts, clinician's failure to communicate in ways that can lead to shared understanding of problems is a significant barrier to receiving care. Third, racial and ethnic minorities receive improper and inappropriate care. Racial stereotyping has also been associated with inappropriate use of treatment (tranquilizing medications, restraints, containment) to deal with the presumption of danger from racial minority patients. This is but one example that demonstrates the challenges of accessing services for a vulnerable group based on race and ethnicity. This example could be reiterated for many other "hierarchies of oppression." By recognizing the barriers to health and mental health care for individuals, social workers can attend to barriers in the institutions in which they practice. It has also been suggested that social workers look inward to ensure that they are not indirectly contributing to a hostile environment or a professional encounter that adversely prejudices the individual for their personal or social characteristics (Williams, 2002).

From a social work perspective, individualized care is foundational to client advocacy. According to Baker et al. (2021) individualized responses to the clinical and psychosocial needs of patients in acute care, subacute care, home health, and other outpatient settings have been guided by well-established case management process of screening, assessing, planning, implementation, follow-up, transitioning, and evaluating. In addition, they suggested that health professionals and social workers should be guided by values of advocacy, ensuring access to the right care and treatment at the right time: autonomy, respecting the right to self-determination, and justice, promoting fairness and equity in access to resources and treatment.

Appropriateness—Organizational

Health equity for vulnerable patients requires organizations to have strong engagement with patient stakeholders. Agencies and agents in health care need to be equipped with the knowledge and tools needed to cultivate modern attitudes, policies, and practices that enable the appropriateness of services (Davison et al., 2021). Some have suggested that educating staff about health disparities is a practice that pushes the organization forward in providing competent care to equity-seeking groups. However, patient engagement has become a top priority for healthcare organizations (Bombard et al., 2018). Fiscella and Sanders (2016, p. 385) implied that organizations could address the appropriateness of their healthcare care services successfully if:

1) Routine monitoring of healthcare disparities was a core element of organizational quality improvement. Monitoring requires the routine, standardized collection of patient data on various equity dimensions with linkage to quality measures.
2) Organizational commitment to the identification and elimination of health care disparities as an integral component of quality improvement. Diversity across organizations, including leadership can improve sensitivity and commitment to health care disparities.
3) Use of quality improvement structures and processes to identify healthcare disparities and corresponding breakdowns in care processes. Teams should include relevant technical and cultural expertise including the voices of patients when seeking improvements in care.
4) Design of appropriate interventions based on the care processes and the emerging literature on successful interventions. Many interventions require multilevel approaches including community engagement. Use of approaches such as user-centered design can help ensure intervention is acceptable, appropriate, and feasible for those affected.
5) Steps to ensure sustainability of the intervention. Sustainability depends on implementation factors (acceptability, adoption, appropriateness, feasibility, and cost), the level of integration into routine care, and continued organizational prioritization.

Appropriateness—Societal

At the societal level, social workers can inform creative service delivery models and integrated care programs that respond to the needs of vulnerable or marginalized populations. Much attention has been given to primary health care models, to support the appropriateness and relevance of services for marginalized populations in various parts of the world (Ashcroft et al., 2017, 2018). Primary health care organizations bring together family physicians, nurse practitioners, registered nurses, social workers, dietitians, and other professionals who work together to provide a range of health, behavioral, and mental health services for their community. They ensure that people receive the care they need in their communities, as each team is set up based on local health and community needs. Primary care teams expand access to comprehensive services service delivery models that emphasize interdisciplinary care, as well as community outreach and involvement in service decisions, facilitate positive client outcomes, and increased accessibility.

References

Abrams, E. M., & Szefler, S. J. (2020). COVID-19 and the impact of social determinants of health. *The Lancet Respiratory Medicine*, *8*(7), 659–661. https://doi.org/10.1016/S2213-2600(20)30234-4

Annarumma, C., & Palumbo, R. (2016). Contextualizing health literacy to health care organizations: Exploratory insights. *Journal of Health Management*, *18*(4), 611–624. https://doi.org/10.1177/0972063416666348

Ashcroft, R. (2010). Health inequities: Evaluation of two paradigms. *Health & Social Work*, *35*(4), 249–256. https://doi.org/10.1093/hsw/35.4.249

Ashcroft, R., Kourgiantakis, T., Fearing, G., Robertson, T., & Brown, J. B. (2019). Social work's scope of practice in primary mental health care: A scoping review. *The British Journal of Social Work*, *49*(2), 318–334. https://doi.org/10.1093/bjsw/bcy051

Ashcroft, R., Lam, S., Kourgiantakis, T., Begun, S., Nelson, M., Adamson, K., Cadell, S., Walsh, B., Greenblatt, A., Hussain, A., Sur, D., Sirotich, F., & Craig, S. (2021). Preparing social work to address health inequities emerging during the COVID-19 pandemic by building capacity for health policy: a scoping review protocol. *BMJ Open*, *11*, e053959. https://doi: 10.1136/bmjopen-2021-053959

Ashcroft, R., McMillan, C., Ambrose-Miller, W., McKee, R., & Brown, J. B. (2018). The emerging role of social work in primary health care: A survey of social workers in Ontario family health teams. *Health & Social Work*, *43*(2), 109–117

Ashcroft, R., Sur, D., Greenblatt, A., & Donahue, P. (2021). The impact of the COVID-19 pandemic on social workers at the frontline: A survey of Canadian social workers. *British Journal of Social Work*, 1–23. https://doi.org/10.1093/bjsw/bcab158

Ashcroft, R., & Van Katwyk, T. (2017). Joining the global conversation: social workers defining health using a participatory action research approach. *British Journal of Social Work*, *47*(2), 579–596.

Ashcroft, R., Van Katwyk, T., & Hogarth, K. (2017). An examination of the holism paradigm: A view of social work. *Social Work in Public Health*, *32*(8), 461–474. https://doi.org/10.1080/19371918.2017.1360818

Baker, M., Nelson, S., & Krsnak, J. (2021). Case management on the front lines of COVID-19: The importance of the individualized care plan across care settings. *Professional Case Management*, *26*(2), 62–69. https://doi.org/10.1097/NCM.0000000000000484

Barry, J. J. (2020, May 26). COVID-19 exposes why access to the internet is a human right. *OpenGlobalRights*. Retrieved from www.openglobalrights.org/covid-19-exposes-why-access-to-internet-is-human-right/

Bayoumi, A. M. (2009). Equity and health services. *Journal of Public Health Policy*, *30*(2), 176–182. https://doi.org/10.1057/jphp.2009.9

Beddoe, L. (2013). Health social work: Professional identity and knowledge. *Qualitative Social Work*, *12*(1), 24–40. https://doi.org/10.1177/1473325011415455

Bombard, Y., Baker, G. R., Orlando, E., Fancott, C., Bhatia, P., Casalino, S., Onate, K., Denis, J. L., & Pomey, M. P. (2018). Engaging patients to improve quality of care: a systematic review. *Implementation Science, 13*, 98.

Brach, C., Keller, D., Hernandez, L. M., Baur, C., Parker, R., Dreyer, B., Schyve, P., Lemerise, A. J., & Schillinger, D. (2012). *Ten attributes of health literate care organizations*. Institute of Medicine. Retrieved from https://nam.edu/wp-content/uploads/2015/06/BPH_Ten_HLit_Attributes.pdf

Braveman, P. (2014). What are health disparities and health equity? We need to be clear. *Public Health Reports, 129*(1_suppl2), 5–8. https://doi.org/10.1177/00333549141291S203

Brinkley-Rubinstein, L., Bethune, M., & Doykos, B. (2015). Health literacy as a process: Caseworker perspectives on HIV health literacy. *Social Work in Public Health, 30*(3), 250–259. https://doi.org/10.1080/19371918.2014.994724

Browne, T., & Gehlert, S. (2019). *Handbook of health social work*. Hoboken, NJ: John Wiley & Sons.

Cai, D., Stone, T. E., Petrini, M. A., & McMillan, M. (2016). 'An exploration of the health beliefs of Chinese nurses' and nurse academics' health beliefs: A Q-methodology study': Nurses' health beliefs: A Q methodology study. *Nursing & Health Sciences, 18*(1), 97–104. https://doi.org/10.1111/nhs.12251

College of Nurses of Ontario (CNO). (2021). *Nurse practitioner* [No. 41038]. College of Nurses of Ontario. www.cno.org/globalassets/docs/prac/41038_strdrnec.pdf

Cyr, M. E., Etchin, A. G., Guthrie, B. J. *et al.* Access to specialty healthcare in urban versus rural US populations: a systematic literature review. *BMC Health Serv Res* 19, 974 (2019). https://doi.org/10.1186/s12913-019-4815-5

Davison, K., Queen, R., Lau, F., & Antonio, M. (2021). Culturally competent gender, sex, and sexual orientation information practices and electronic health records: Rapid review. *JMIR Medical Informatics, 9*(2), e25467. https://doi.org/10.2196/25467

de Saxe Zerden, L., Lombardi, B. M., Fraser, M. W., Jones, A., & Rico, Y. G. (2018). Social work: Integral to interprofessional education and integrated practice. *Journal of Interprofessional Education & Practice, 10*, 67–75. https://doi.org/10.1016/j.xjep.2017.12.011

Donnelly, C., Ashcroft, R., Bobbette, N., Gill, S., Mills, C., Mofina, A., Tran, T., Vader, K., Williams, A., Miller, J. (2021). Interprofessional primary care during COVID-19: The provider perspective. *BMC Family Practice, 22*, 31.

Duby, Z., Nkosi, B., Scheibe, A., Brown, B., & Bekker, L.-G. (2018). 'Scared of going to the clinic': Contextualising healthcare access for men who have sex with men, female sex workers and people who use drugs in two South African cities. *Southern African Journal of HIV Medicine, 19*(1). https://doi.org/10.4102/sajhivmed.v19i1.701

Fiscella, K., & Sanders, M. (2016). Racial and Ethnic Disparities in the Quality of healthcare. *The Annual Review of Public Health, 37*, 375–394.

Gehlert, S. (2014). Forging an integrated agenda for primary cancer prevention during midlife. *American Journal of Preventive Medicine, 46*(3 Suppl 1), S104–S109. https://doi.org/10.1016/j.amepre.2013.12.004

George, M. S., Davey, R., Mohanty, I., & Upton, P. (2020). "Everything is provided for free, but they are still hesitant to access healthcare services": Why does the indigenous community in Attapadi, Kerala continue to experience poor access to healthcare? *International Journal for Equity in Health, 19*, 105.

Government of Ontario. (2020, July 14). *Ontario eliminating the practice of birth alerts* [News Release]. Retrieved from https://news.ontario.ca/en/release/57580/ontario-eliminating-the-practice-of-birth-alerts

Gunn, J. A. (2019). President's message: Cultural humility. *Journal of Transcultural Nursing, 30*(5), 530–530. https://doi.org/10.1177/1043659619854519

Haggerty, J., Levesque, J.-F., Harris, M., Scott, C., Dahrouge, S., Lewis, V., Dionne, E., Stocks, N., & Russell, G. (2020). Does healthcare inequity reflect variations in peoples' abilities to access healthcare? Results from a multi-jurisdictional interventional study in two high-income countries. *International Journal for Equity in Health, 19*(1), 167. https://doi.org/10.1186/s12939-020-01281-6

Hart, L. G., Larson, E. H., & Lishner, D. (2005). Rural definitions for health policy and research. *American Journal of Public Health, 95*(7), 1149–1155.

Hart, L., Ferguson, R., & Amiri, A. (2020). Full scope of practice for Alabama nurse practitioners: Act now. *The Journal for Nurse Practitioners, 16*(2), 100–104. https://doi.org/10.1016/j.nurpra.2019.10.016

Hays, P. A. (2019). Introduction. In G. Iwamasa & P. A. Hays (Eds.), *Culturally responsive cognitive behavior therapy: Practice and supervision* (2nd ed., pp. 3–24). New York: American Psychological Association.

Hermans, K., & Roets, G. (2020). Social work research and human rights: Where do we go from here? *European Journal of Social Work, 23*(6), 913–919. https://doi.org/10.1080/13691457.2020.1838086

Holland Bloorview. (2021). *Holland Bloorview Family Support Fund*. Retrieved from https://hollandbloorview.ca/our-services/family-workshops-resources/holland-bloorview-family-support-fund

International Federation of Social Workers (IFSW). (2008, August 1). *Health*. Geneva, Switzerland.

International Federation of Social Workers (IFSW) & International Association of Schools of Social Work (IASSW). (2004). *Ethics in social work, statement of principle*. International Federation of Social Workers and International Association of Schools of Social Work. Retrieved from www.iassw-aiets.org/wp-content/uploads/2015/10/Ethics-in-Social-Work-Statement-IFSW-IASSW-2004.pdf#:~:text=International%20Federation%20of%20Social%20Workers%20%28IFSW%29%20International%20Association,of%20the%20professional%20practice%20of%20social%20workers.%20

Irizarry, T., DeVito Dabbs, A., & Curran, C. R. (2015). Patient portals and patient engagement: A state of the science review. *Journal of Medical Internet Research, 17*(6), e148. https://doi.org/10.2196/jmir.4255

Jenkins, M., & Newman, C. B. (Eds.). (2021). *How sex and gender impact clinical practice: An evidence-based guide to patient care*. Elsevier. New York, NY.

Kaminsky, E., & Höglund, A. T. (2019). Swedish healthcare direct managers' views on gender (in)equity: Applying a conceptual model. *International Journal for Equity in Health, 18*(1), 114. https://doi.org/10.1186/s12939-019-1011-5

Levesque, J.-F., Harris, M. F., & Russell, G. (2013). Patient-centred access to health care: Conceptualising access at the interface of health systems and populations. *International Journal for Equity in Health, 12*(18), 1–9. https://doi.org/10.1186/1475-9276-12-18

Liddy, C., Joschko, J., Guglani, S., Afkham, A., & Keely, E. (2019). Improving equity of access through electronic consultation: A case study of an eConsult service. *Frontiers in Public Health*, 7(279), 1–10. https://doi.org/10.3389/fpubh.2019.00279

Lupton, D. (2013). *Medicine as culture: Illness, disease and the body* (3rd ed.). New York, NY: SAGE Publications Ltd. https://rbdigital.rbdigital.com

Mendenhall, A. N., & Frauenholtz, S. (2013). Mental health literacy: Social work's role in improving public mental health. *Social Work, 58*(4), 365–368. https://doi.org/10.1093/sw/swt038

Miller, D. P., Angela, R. B., Allen, H. L., Martinson, M. L., Salas-Wright, C. P., Jantz, K., Crevi, K., & Rosenbloom, D. L. (2017). A social work approach to policy: implications for population health. *American Journal of Public Health, 107*(S3), S243–S249.

Miller, V. J., & Lee, H. (2020). Social work values in action during COVID-19. *Journal of Gerontological Social Work, 63*(6–7), 565–569. S243–S249.

Okan, O., Sørensen, K., & Bauer, U. (2018). Health literacy policy-making for effective child and adolescent health promotion and prevention strategies. *European Journal of Public Health, 28*(suppl_4). https://doi.org/10.1093/eurpub/cky213.072

Oliver, K., Lorenc, T., Tinkler, J., & Bonell, C. (2019). Understanding the unintended consequences of public health policies: The views of policymakers and evaluators. *BMC Public Health, 19*(1), 1057. https://doi.org/10.1186/s12889-019-7389-6

Peterson, K. J. (2012). Shared decision making in health care settings: A role for social work. *Social Work in Health Care, 51*(10), 894–908. https://doi.org/10.1080/00981389.2012.714448

QHR Health. (2021). *How your healthcare organization can improve patient access.* Retrieved from https://qhr.com/resources/how-your-healthcare-organization-can-improve-patient-access/

Raphael, D. (2019). Chapter 6: Social determinants of health. In D. Raphael and G. Teeple (Eds.), *Staying alive: Critical perspectives on health, illness, and health care* (3rd ed.). Toronto, ON: Canadian Scholars' Press.

Richmond, C. A. M., & Cook, C. (2016). Creating conditions for Canadian aboriginal health equity: The promise of healthy public policy. *Public Health Reviews, 37*(1), 2. https://doi.org/10.1186/s40985-016-0016-5

Richter, M., & Dragano, N. (2018). Micro, macro, but what about meso? The institutional context of health inequalities. *International Journal of Public Health, 63*(2), 163–164. https://doi.org/10.1007/s00038-017-1064-4

Riebschleger, J., Norris, D., Pierce, B., Pond, D. L., & Cummings, C. (2015). Preparing social work students for rural child welfare practice: Emerging curriculum competencies. *Journal of Social Work Education, 51*(sup2), S209–S224. https://doi.org/10.1080/10437797.2015.1072422

Rowlands, G. (2018). Health literacy policy to promote public health in Europe. *European Journal of Public Health, 28*(suppl_4). https://doi.org/10.1093/eurpub/cky212.833

Rubin, A., & Bellamy, J. (2012). *Practitioner's guide to using research for evidence-based practice* (2nd ed.). Wiley.

Serban, N. (2020). *Healthcare system access: Measurement, inference, and intervention.* Hoboken, NJ: John Wiley & Sons.

Smith, M., & Mercado-Sierra, M. (2021). Health beliefs as a predictor of screening behaviors among college students. *Social Work in Public Health, 36*(4), 460–473. https://doi.org/10.1080/19371918.2021.1905130

Sundler, Darcy, L., Råberus, A., & Holmström, I. K. (2020). Unmet health-care needs and human rights—A qualitative analysis of patients' complaints in light of the right to health and health care. *Health Expectations : an International Journal of Public Participation in Health Care and Health Policy, 23*(3), 614–621. https://doi.org/10.1111/hex.13038

Taylor, C. B., Fitzsimmons-Craft, E. E., & Graham, A. K. (2020). Digital technology can revolutionize mental health services delivery: The COVID-19 crisis as a catalyst for change. *International Journal of Eating Disorders, 53*(7), 1155–1157. https://doi.org/10.1002/eat.23300

Therigy. (2021). *Blog: Patient financial assistance programs for specialty healthcare—A list of resources*. Retrieved from www.therigy.com/resources/blog/patient-financial-assistance-programs-for-specialty-healthcare-a-list-of-resources

Truell, R. (2020). News from our societies—IFSW: COVID-19: The struggle, success and expansion of social work—Reflections on the profession's global response, 5 months on. *International Social Work, 63*(4), 545–548. https://doi.org/10.1177/0020872820936448

U.S. Department of Health and Human Services. (2008). *Phase I report: Recommendations for the framework and format of healthy people 2020* (Secretary's Advisory Committee on Health Promotion and Disease Prevention Objectives for 2020). U.S. Department of Health and Human Services. Washington, DC, USA.

Walters, K. L., Spencer, M. S., Smukler, M., Allen, H. L., Andrews, C., Browne, T., Maramaldi, P., Wheeler, D. P., Zebrack, B., & Uehara, E. (2016). *Health equity: Eradicating health inequalities for future generations* (Working Paper No. 19; Grand Challenges for Social Work Initiative Working Paper No. 19). American Academy of Social Work and Social Welfare. London England.

Walter-McCabe, H. A. (2020). Coronavirus pandemic calls for an immediate social work response. *Social Work in Public Health, 35*(3), 69–72. https://doi.org/10.1080/19371918.2020.1751533

Warnecke, R. B., Oh, A., Breen, N., Gehlert, S., Paskett, E., Tucker, K. L., Lurie, N., Rebbeck, T., Goodwin, J., Flack, J., Srinivasan, S., Kerner, J., Heurtin-Roberts, S., Abeles, R., Tyson, F. L., Patmios, G., & Hiatt, R. A. (2008). Approaching health disparities from a population perspective: The national institutes of health centers for population health and health disparities. *American Journal of Public Health, 98*(9), 1608–1615. https://doi.org/10.2105/AJPH.2006.102525

Warren, S., Puryear, E., Chapman, M., Barnett, T. M., & White, L. S. (2017). The role of social work in free healthcare clinics and student-run clinics. *Social Work in Health Care, 56*(10), 884–896. https://doi.org/10.1080/00981389.2017.1371097

Williams, C. (2002). A rationale for an anti-racist entry point to anti-oppressive social work in mental health services. *Critical Social Work, 3*(1), 20–31.

Williams, D. R., & Wyatt, R. (2015). Racial bias in health care and health: Challenges and opportunities. *JAMA, 314*(6), 555. https://doi.org/10.1001/jama.2015.9260

World Health Organization. (1998). *Health promotion glossary*. Geneva: World Health Organization. Retrieved from www.who.int/healthpromotion/about/HPR%20Glossary%201998.pdf

World Health Organization. (2013). *Closing the health equity gap: Policy options and opportunities for action*. Geneva: World Health Organization. Retrieved from www.afro.who.int/sites/default/files/2017-06/SDH-closing-health-equity-gap-policy-opportunities-for-action-WHO2013.pdf

World Health Organization. (2017). *Human rights and health*. World Health Organization. Retrieved from www.who.int/news-room/fact-sheets/detail/human-rights-and-health

Wronka, J. (2017). *Human rights and social justice: Social action and service for the helping and health professions* (2nd ed.). New York, NY: SAGE.

Part 3

Vulnerable Populations

Vulnerable populations are specific groups of people who are at an increased risk of having their rights denied by societies that tend to ignore them or create barriers to their inclusion. In this section's opening chapter, we build awareness about the vulnerability of children and youth. In general, children and youth are vulnerable because of their dependence on others for their development and well-being, and perhaps the most vulnerable are those who become involved in the formal child welfare system for their development and well-being. Assuring that these children thrive is a major task for policy, services, and social work practice. The authors of this chapter describe the experiences of these children in Canada while also presenting a new framework for more effective social work involvement.

Older adults are a vulnerable population across the globe as they struggle with poverty, health issues, and changing family structures, and the rights of older adults take up the focus of the next chapter. The recent COVID-19 pandemic, which had a devastating impact on the mortality of older people in every country, is a vivid example of their vulnerability. As people age, their human rights, as they pertain to independence, autonomy, and participation, are also at risk. Social workers can play key roles in supporting and strengthening older adults through interventions that enhance and empower them. At the macro level, their involvement as advocates for policy change, often working in conjunction with older adults, can be a powerful tool for assuring both their rights and ability to live in a socially just society that both recognizes them and assures their dignity.

Gender and sexual orientation continue to be major forces impacting the rights and opportunities of people. The chapter on LGBTQIA+ individuals discusses the term itself as well as the history of oppression at both the individual and societal levels that this group has experienced and the challenges that they continue to face. It presents a framework based on "care and "justice" that works to promote the rights and well-being of this population, permitting them to reach their full potential while also enhancing the peace, justice, and common good of the entire society.

The chapter on disability and social justice next explores what social justice itself means in the lives of people with disabilities. Across the globe,

DOI: 10.4324/9781003111269-10

people with disabilities remain marginalized and often discriminated against with their rights threatened or ignored. As noted by the authors, the population tends to be overlooked by the social work profession and the disability perspective is ignored by policy makers. Social workers, in connection with the Disability Rights Movement, can help to assure that social justice and the rights of these persons are recognized and put into practice.

Prisoners (incarcerated persons) overwhelmingly come from disadvantaged and oppressed communities. Policies and practices that they endure in prison further limit and undermine their human rights. As covered within the ensuing chapter, prisoners are particularly subject to cumulative disadvantage, which further erodes their rights. Given the complex issues impacting incarcerated persons, the authors highlight the areas in which social workers need to be knowledgeable as well as their abilities to work with other professionals, and the important roles that they can assume as advocates for improving the lives of this population.

Gender inequalities continue to impact women and girls across the world. The authors begin the corresponding chapter with an overview of theories that help to explain the position and vulnerability of this population. The key social issues that continue to impact women and girls and act as multiple sources of oppression are discussed as well as the areas in which progress with regards to their rights and social justice has occurred. Social work can play a major role by working to support and help realize the rights of these people and assuring that the inequalities that undermine social justice for them are alleviated.

Refugees and migrants, in their movement and displacement, are commonly deprived of their human rights. The skills and values required of social workers can be important tools in assisting these persons as they struggle with new environments, often in camp settings or migrant communities. Equally important are the roles that social workers can assume as advocates for the human rights of these people insofar as they may contribute to welcoming and accepting communities that value and support them.

8 Supporting Youth Leaving Care in Rural Canada

Clinical Practice and Social Justice

Anne Marie McLaughlin, Richard Enns, Susan Gallagher, and Jesse Henton

An alarming number of youth in Canada will have contact with the child welfare system at some point in their lives. A smaller but equally significant number of these children will have prolonged contact as a result of the termination of birth parent rights. For these youth, the government, as parent, is responsible for their health and well-being and for preparing them for successful outcomes once they leave care, which could happen as early as age 18, when, in many jurisdictions, youth are presumed old enough to be deemed adults. In this chapter, we contend that social workers who encounter these youth in community-based services should be committed to social justice as an integral part of their clinical practice. We provide a multi-dimensional framework to illustrate how clinical social workers can conceptualize social justice within their practice. This conceptualization provides avenues for engagement and interventions with youth that go beyond traditional, individualized, micro-level approaches that overlook important social, economic, cultural, and historic contexts and realities. Our analysis of a composite case will highlight the importance of relationships based on respect, and considerations of resources and systems, in a multi-dimensional social justice framework—and we argue that advocacy is an important and under-valued aspect of clinical social work practice. We acknowledge and own our perspectives, biases, and unearned privileges as white settlers on the historic homeland of many First Nations and Métis[1] peoples.

Aging Out of Care

For many youth who leave care, the state has been a less-than-ideal parent. Upon their exit, youth in care face seemingly insurmountable barriers that can follow them throughout their lives. As this population is far from homogenous, special consideration must be given to individual and group differences in identified needs and available resources (Marion & Paulsen, 2019). For instance, youth aging out of care in rural communities face inequities in the availability and access to important resources when compared to urban youth (Kreitzer, 2016); sexual minority youth, as well

DOI: 10.4324/9781003111269-11

as gender-diverse/transgender youth, face additional and systemic marginalization, harassment, and discrimination (Brandon-Friedman et al 2020); and Indigenous youth who are significantly and disproportionately overrepresented among all groups of youth in care, face the loss of community, culture, and identity as they struggle to navigate added systemic burdens including jurisdictional and funding issues (Haight et al., 2018; Ma et al., 2019). Although transitioning youth have received increased attention in the literature, they are still an underserved group, with many falling through the cracks and receiving no services at all (McLaughlin et al., 2018). Social work practitioners working with these youth require compassion and a strong commitment to clinical work informed by social justice.

Research in Canadian and international contexts shows that, compared to youth who never enter government care, youth who age out of care report generally poorer outcomes on multiple indices, including poorer employment and education prospects; a stronger likelihood of lower wages through adulthood (Reid & Dudding, 2006; Rutman et al., 2007; Serge et al., 2002; Urban Institute, 2008); increased likelihood of criminal involvement (Maschi et al., 2008); poor housing security and higher incidence of homelessness (Rutman et al., 2007; Schibler, & McEwan-Morris, 2006); higher incidence of early pregnancies and sexually transmitted infections (Dworsky & Courtney, 2010; Rutman et al., 2007); and a higher prevalence of mental health issues (Fowler et al., 2009; McMillen et al., 2004; Reid & Dudding, 2006; Rutman et al., 2007; Serge et al., 2002; Southerland, 2009).

Available data indicate that the number of youth in care in Canada increased from 42,000 in 1992 to 67,000 in 2011, and roughly 10 out of every 1000 children in Canada will enter the child welfare system at some point in their lives (Popova et al., 2014). In Canada, Indigenous youth represents 7% of all adolescents between the age of 15 and 18 but make up more than 30% of youth in care in the same age range (Turner, 2016). In some jurisdictions, the rate for placement of Indigenous children is estimated to be 15 times higher than for non-Indigenous youth (Courtney et al., 2013). These numbers are likely low because accurate statistics regarding youth in care are difficult to obtain in Canada and elsewhere, as child welfare delivery is frequently local, reporting methods and what constitutes a case may vary, and the growing number of out-of-care placements such as kinship care may not be counted (Saint Girons, 2020). The significance and enormity of the challenges faced by youth leaving care call the very child welfare systems, designed to protect children and youth, into question (Haight et al., 2018). Although Canada ratified the United Nations Convention on the Rights of Children in 1991 (Noël, 2015), research indicates that progress on respecting the rights of children in care is slow. Youth in care continue to feel powerless and that their voice is not respected (Damiani-Taraba et al., 2018). Programs and systems must be reconceptualized and redesigned in ways that more adequately respect cultural contexts, protect against harms, and build on the abilities and strengths of this important population.

Emerging Adulthood

Youth aging out of government care experience improved outcomes when they remain connected to services beyond the age of 18 (Rome & Raskin, 2019; Rutman et al., 2007). The need for extended government care is supported by research with youth, caregivers, and social workers alike (Goodkind, et al., 2011; McLaughlin, et al., 2018). At the same time that youth are aging out of care, they are transitioning to adulthood. Both aging out of care and the transition to adulthood should be seen as processes that evolve over time and overlap. Avery and Freundlich (2009) identified emerging adulthood as a developmental life stage to better describe the transition between 18 and 26 years of age. This stage characteristically involves multiple exits from and returns to home as youth learn to regulate emotions and internalize social conventions (Avery, 2010). This conceptualization of transitions offers insight into the processes and challenges youth face through their late teen years, and early 20s, as they age out of care.

Mclaughlin et al. (2018) interviewed youth, social workers, and foster parents to better understand the experience of transition for youth exiting the child welfare system. Study participants reaffirmed emerging adulthood as a meaningful conceptualization for youth at this stage of the life cycle. Highlighting a distinction between chronological age and maturity, "not being ready" was a common sentiment expressed. In this study, youth left government care under very different conditions: some left abruptly and without support, rejecting help and seeking independence; some were kicked out for failure to comply with rules or expectations; and some aged out, a term used to signify the end of service provision. Regardless of the circumstances surrounding their exit, a significant number expressed anxiety and concern regarding their future.

Policies should be revised and services delivered within an extended continuum that more adequately addresses transitioning youths' unique short- and long-term needs. For example, youth who fall through system gaps at age 16 or 17, unable to meet eligibility requirements, or who withdraw from school or other programs, may find themselves ineligible for services at age 18 (McLaughlin et al., 2018). These youth would greatly benefit from transition assistance for many years but may be reluctant or unable to return to government services. Alternatively, community-based outreach services that are flexible and creative may be a more viable and attractive alternative to facilitate a successful transition through emerging adulthood (Rome & Raskin, 2019). Community-based social workers engaged with these youth require a skillset that includes knowledge of the developmental challenges, extensive understanding of the benefits and services that support transitions, and the advocacy skills to assist youth to maximize their capabilities and rights.

Social Justice and a Clinical Approach to Practice

The current imperative to integrate social justice and clinical practice for social workers—including those serving youth in care and transitioning from care—is an extension of the historical debate regarding the dual focus of social work practice: people-helping and society-changing (McLaughlin, 2002; Swenson,1998). Clinical social workers and those involved in direct practice have frequently been criticized for their alleged abandonment of the pursuit of social justice. Those whose practice is focused on the individual have been labelled as "unfaithful angels" (Specht & Courtney, 1994), too focused on pathology to recognize or attend to the structural barriers that constrain individuals. Research has shown, however, that many social workers in direct practice are committed to fairness and equity, including the elimination of racism and all forms of discrimination (McLaughlin 2011; O'Brien, 2009), and that they consider social justice to be an essential component of their practice.

Critical Clinical Practice

Contemporary theorists who link clinical social work and social justice have identified core considerations for practitioners (Asakura & Maurer, 2018; Asakura et al., 2020; Harrison et al., 2016; Maschi, 2011). A social justice perspective for clinical practice must draw from critical social theory (Salas, et al., 2010), analyse historical factors perpetuating inequity or social divisions, prioritize practitioner reflexivity and self-awareness, pay explicit attention to power, include a critical/structural approach to assessment and intervention (Dean & Poorvu, 2008; Harrison et al., 2016), take an advocacy stance for social change (McLaughlin, 2009), and embrace social work values and ethical practice (Asakura & Maurer, 2018; Asakura et al., 2020; Brown, 2021; Marsh, et al., 2018; Maschi, 2011; McLaughlin, 2011). When considering the complexities of the lived experiences of youth aging out of care, social workers should additionally consider integrating critical concepts of race, disability and queer theory, and resilience (Mountz & Capous-Desyllas, 2020; Ungar, 2011; Van Breda, 2018).

A Framework for Social Justice

Social justice is a contested concept (Solas, 2008). For some it is a process and for others it is an outcome (Bonnycastle, 2011). The Canadian Association of Social Workers' (CASW) code of ethics (2005) identifies the core value of social justice as resting on the following principles: the right of people to have access to resources to meet basic human needs; advocacy for fair and equitable access to public services and benefits; advocacy for equal treatment and protection under the law; and a commitment to challenge injustices, especially injustice that affects the vulnerable and disadvantaged. Over time scholars have focused on various and frequently conflicting aspects of the concept: individual versus group rights and obligations, social goals and outcomes versus societal processes (Reisch, 2002). Practicing social workers typically consider equity, fairness, access to resources, rights, respect, and opportunity in their definitions, (McLaughlin, 2006; O'Brien, 2009). Regardless of one's definition, confronting and combating injustice requires an integration of perspectives and strategies (Webb, 2010).

As multiple sources of injustice and oppression exist, and a singular understanding of social justice is not sufficient, then critical appraisal is required to intervene appropriately. The injustice of a society where working families are trapped in chronic poverty differs from the injustice of police violence towards young Black men, and it differs again from the injustice Indigenous peoples face when denied decision-making authority over their own lives, or when they encounter law enforcement. As injustices differ, so too must the necessary responses or interventions needed to pursue social justice. Youth aging out of care are vulnerable to multiple forms of injustice: they may have lost their culture and community, they may face stigma and social exclusion, and they face the serious probability of unemployment or underemployment, incarceration, homelessness, exploitation, marginalization, and powerlessness.

We have developed a practice framework (McLaughlin, 2011) to guide practitioners in a multidimensional approach to social justice and to help connect diverse modes of practice to the profession's commitment to social justice. The framework includes four dimensions: respect, resources, systems, and advocacy. The first three dimensions represent practitioners' tacit understanding of social justice: through **social systems**; equitable access to **resources** (income, housing, healthcare, opportunity); and **transformative respect** (a process of valuing and regarding others in an authentic and relational manner). The fourth dimension represents social justice in action through **advocacy** strategies within their daily practice. These perceptions of social justice by practitioners resonate strongly with dominant and contemporary theories of social justice and provide practitioners with an expanded understanding of social justice activities beyond those that happen outside of their daily practice—such as organizing marches and rallies, or social action protests for social change—to recognize how their daily practice can be informed and strengthened by social justice strategies even though their primary focus may be alleviating personal distress experienced by individuals, or in families or groups.

Respect

Beginning with interpersonal relationships, workers recognize the inherent centrality of ***respect*** as an important aspect of social justice. Social justice as an interpersonal and relational process requires social workers to intentionally and authentically transmit the professional value of "respect for the inherent dignity and worth of persons" (CASW, 2005, Value 1) to those they work with. ***Transformative respect*** conceptualizes the power of this interpersonal relationship and its ability to provide an alternative narrative for those whose identity has been so frequently disrespected. Respect is viewed as a central concept in contemporary critical theories of social justice, and specifically recognition theory (Fraser, 1999; Garrett, 2010; Fraser & Honneth, 2003), where individuals and groups experience injustice as disrespect and misrecognition due to devalued social identities. Respect and recognition occur within a community context of belonging and feeling valued, where one's sense of self is affirmed and validated (Glynn, 2021; van Breda, 2015). Youth who have grown up in the care of the government have experienced multiple levels of disrespect, not only by caregivers but also by the system that denies their voice or their value (Damiani-Taraba et al., 2018). The intersections of sexual orientation, race, or disability compound the disrespect youth in care may experience.

Taken-for-granted assumptions and everyday practices and processes harm individuals when they deny another's humanity based on differences including race, gender, ability, sexual orientation or identity, or socio-economic status (Dotolo et al., 2018; Young, 2006). According to Taylor (1992), the struggle for recognition is a primary concern for social justice, and a vital human need and misrecognition can induce a "crippling self-hatred" (p. 76). Recognizing the harm done by a society that disrespects youth who have been involved with the child welfare system requires that social workers make respect a priority. This includes attending to, and critically reflecting upon, the power dynamics implicit in the helping relationship, in order that the helping process itself is not oppressive (Sakamoto, 2005). This reflection must be rooted in an openness to learning from those we work with, a determination to resist oppressive relationships, and humility.

Resources

Resources are a key element of our heuristic, as social workers frequently assess injustice in the lives of those they work with in relation to an individual's or group's access to the resources needed to live a life of value—and one that clients value (McLaughlin, 2011). Distributive justice (Rawls, 1971) is concerned with how a just and fair society should distribute its presumably scarce resources in order that all members have equal opportunities to flourish. Resources can be interpreted broadly but, in general, refer to essential goods: adequate food, water, shelter, clothing, education, health, and income. Important resources also include non-material goods such as opportunity and self-respect (Nussbaum, 2005; Rawls,1971). Resource needs are high for children leaving government care as their life circumstances are precarious (Glynn, 2021). Access to resources such as secure housing, education or training, and income is fundamental to their successful transition, so too are social supports and networks (Rutman et al.,

2007). Networks support and sustain youth and promote the development of personal resources including self-confidence, self-worth, and self-esteem (Okpych, 2012). The distributive approach emphasizes providing a social minimum, below which no individual should fall. This approach to social justice is the foundation of the Western notion of a social safety net and, more broadly, social welfare programs (Fleischacker, 2005). Social disparities and resource inequality significantly and negatively impact health and well-being of youth who age out of care (Marmot, 2005, 2017), and distributive theories resonate with social workers who daily encounter the harmful impact of resource inequities.

Social Systems

The third component of our social justice heuristic is ***social systems***. Frequently, "the system" is used euphemistically to refer to government systems and institutions that provide social services such as income support, child welfare, health care, education, social housing, and settlement services. Rawls (1971) proposed that the main concern of social justice is the "basic structure of society" (p. 7). This structure comprises the major political, economic, and social systems that distribute primary social goods and resources. These systems deliver "social welfare" programs but are also the source of systemic injustice and inequities and need to be a focus of attention for social workers motivated by social justice. For example, the child welfare system has been designed to protect vulnerable children and youth from neglect and abuse. Yet this same system has removed Indigenous, Black, and other racialized children from their homes and families in disproportion to non-racialized families and has inflicted trauma across generations (Dettlaff & Boyd, 2020).

Advocacy

A final consideration of the multi-dimensional framework is social work advocacy. Undoubtedly, social workers most frequently associate social justice with advocacy work and, on a daily basis, social work practitioners find themselves advocating for those they serve (McLaughlin et al., 2017).

Clinical social workers employ advocacy strategies that can be categorized as practical, educational, or instrumental. Advocacy strategies are considered practical when they focus on meeting immediate or short-term needs and may require the social worker to be hands-on, for example, accompanying a youth to an interview for admittance to a school program or to an assistance appeal board meeting, or assisting in the completion of forms and applications. Advocacy strategies are educational when clinical social workers intentionally and deliberately educate youth about rights that should be afforded them. They also frequently need to educate colleagues and other professionals they interact with about client rights and society's obligations.

Educational advocacy might also include public education to reduce stigma and increase awareness. Finally, advocacy strategies are instrumental when they include efforts to obtain longer-term goals, including advocating for systemic change or accountability within systems; for example, advocating for extended benefits or services for youth aging out of care; advocating for easier and open access to a youth's historical case file information; or advocating for changes to the child welfare practice with Indigenous families. Understanding that youth are bearers of rights, and worthy of recognition and inclusion in decision-making processes, supports and strengthens social workers' advocacy interests.

Case Study

In this section, we present Anthony, a composite of youth we have met through our work and research. Anthony has experienced many, but not all, of the struggles and challenges that youth aging out of care encounter. As you read his story, consider his experiences in light of the multi-dimensional conceptualization for social justice described earlier and consider what avenues for advocacy there may be.

Anthony is a young Indigenous man, 21 years of age. He lives in a rural northern community of 7,000 people in a western province of Canada. He has recently "aged out" of government care and currently shares an apartment with two roommates. He has been a permanent ward of the government for 14 years, since the age of 7. Anthony reported that he had lived with his mother and his grandmother until then. He has a vivid memory of sirens and bright lights as the police, aided by two social workers, entered his house one evening and took him and his two younger siblings away. He wonders what led to his apprehension but he knows his mother struggled with addictions before dying of an overdose when Anthony was 10 years old. He has had no connection with his father, who was not Indigenous, for many years. Anthony has recently reconnected with a younger sibling. He understands that one other sibling is living on the streets in a nearby city.

Anthony was placed in many foster homes before entering group care at the age of 12. This was deemed to be a more stable environment for Anthony, although staff turnover was high, and between the ages of 12 and 16 Anthony was placed in three different group homes. While there were frequently other Indigenous youth in the group homes, staff were predominantly non-Indigenous. Cultural activities were occasionally organized by staff at the group home, yet Anthony felt disconnected and conflicted about his identity as an Indigenous youth. He resisted attempts to connect with his culture, including members of his mother's community from a small northern reserve. His maternal grandmother called him from time to time. He ran away on several occasions and spent time on the streets but eventually returned to group care. When Anthony turned 16, he entered a supported independent living (SIL) program. He struggled with living on his own, frequently overwhelmed with managing daily tasks and the expectations of his government workers. Anthony reports that from ages 16 to 18 he spent a lot of his time partying, drinking, and, occasionally, fighting; he described himself during those years as lonely, angry, often depressed, and even suicidal. He did well in school but his attendance was sporadic and he fell behind in his studies. He does report being encouraged by teachers, and he hopes to go to college someday. He had multiple social workers over this time, few of whom he felt connected to. He also longed to learn to drive and wanted a part-time job, but he was discouraged from these activities due to his workers' strict priority that he attend school. Currently, he is only a few credits short of receiving his high school diploma, after a few bumpy years as a teenager.

Anthony was referred to the local mental health community clinic by his last child welfare social worker. She felt that, since government supports for him were ending, he needed to connect with some adult services to assist in the transition to adulthood. Although Anthony wants to be out from under the control of the government, he is anxious about being on his own.

Case Discussion

Drawing from our own practice and research experiences we will discuss some important contextual issues relative to Anthony's experiences before moving on to apply the framework. But first, we must recognize that as non-Indigenous, cis-gendered, settler-practitioners in a rural mental health social work practice, we have unearned privileges and only a partial ability to fully understand the lived experience of Anthony or to appreciate the opportunities and challenges of service provision in unique communities. However, although our understanding is partial and the unique practice setting may influence which interventions are possible, it does not reduce the ethical and professional imperative to advocate for social justice, and to reflectively and critically, use privilege to that end.

In rural parts of western Canada, publicly funded community health clinics are available where multi-disciplinary teams of health care providers, including mental health professionals, serve the health needs of the community. This hypothetical community health agency serves a large geographical area and is the service hub for many small communities, including several Indigenous communities. In this clinic, effort and attention have been paid to the *Calls to Action* (2015) issued by Canada's Truth and Reconciliation Commission (TRC) after its investigation into the impact of Canada's residential school system on Indigenous students and their families. In an effort to close the gap in health outcomes between Indigenous and non-Indigenous people (McNally & Martin, 2017), health care leaders have recently begun to respond to the particular *Calls* related to health care outcomes (Williams et al., 2019). Among the recommendations followed by the clinic is a commitment to education concerning Indigenous rights, the legacy of colonialism, and the historical harms experienced by Indigenous people (TRC, 2015). Health care workers are called to develop cultural competency, collaborate with Indigenous healers and Elders, and support Indigenous healing practices when appropriate and requested (TRC, 2015, 22, 23, 24). For clinical social workers, understanding historic injustices, and embracing reconciliation in a meaningful and authentic manner, is an essential element of social justice practice. Likewise, it is important for practitioners to both participate in and advocate for the adoption of systemic change. This will require educational as well as instrumental advocacy strategies with administrators, stakeholders, and community members about reconciliation aims and processes.

As the social worker assigned to Anthony's case, there are several considerations for ensuring a social justice approach. A critical perspective that is collaborative and reflexive are essential elements (Brown, 2021). This can partially be achieved by ensuring that Anthony leads the process. Reflecting on our own social location and our potentially colonizing approaches to practice is also essential, particularly for those of us who identify as settlers. We must acknowledge the ways social work itself represents—and has maintained—oppressive structures and institutions, through our associations with the residential school system up to and including the impact of the Sixties Scoop, and the impact this association, and social work practice, has had on youth who have been in care (Brown, 2021; Mandell, 2008; Sinclair, 2007). Understanding Anthony's experiences as an individual, as well as a member of a colonized population, contextualizes his narrative rather than pathologizing him. A critical approach to clinical practice recognizes that youth leaving care have historical and cultural connections that predate their entry into the system. These historical ties to families, communities, and cultural identity are essential components in the task of identity formation in adolescence and emerging adulthood, which may be utilized to assist in interventions. However, these ties can also be sources of trauma. When working with youth, practitioners should provide safety, space, and time to explore potential feelings about these ties. By being open and informed, workers can provide opportunities to build social supports and increase respect and recognition.

Anthony possesses many strengths and the persistence to overcome obstacles: such as his willingness to seek help for his current state of distress. By contrast, many youth who have aged out of care are distrustful of government services and are not able or willing to seek the help they need (Doucet, 2020). While Anthony seeks independence, he also realizes that he cannot achieve his goals without assistance. This insight reflects research that indicates transitioning youth are more successful when transitional processes are gradual, emphasize interdependence and continuing support, and build on social capital and social networks (Propp, et al., 2003; Stein, 2008). Continuing educational connections can help with this, and Anthony's past limited success in school, along with occasional encouragement from teachers, has had a significant impact. Anthony is "future-focused" with his stated desire to attend college, and clinical social workers can build on this indicator of health and resiliency (Bond & van Breda, 2018). The World Health Organization (2021) includes the ability to achieve one's potential in its definition of health, and helping Anthony to flourish may include attention to overcoming obstacles such as bureaucratic processes to accessing funding or meeting eligibility requirements.

Anthony also has many challenges ahead of him. He reports suffering from anxiety, and occasionally depression. He feels overwhelmed by what lies in front of him, and he has ongoing questions about his past. There is ample evidence linking adverse childhood experiences to negative impacts on health and well-being, and adverse experiences in childhood are often compounded for children in care (Brown, 2021; Courtney et al., 2013; Simkiss, 2019), and Anthony's mental health concerns are similar to the concerns of many Indigenous youth ageing out of care. Anthony's pre-care experiences, coupled with several placement breakdowns and changes in living situations (numerous foster homes, several group homes), point towards cumulative and complex trauma.

Applying the Multidimensional Framework: Respect, Resources, Systems, and Advocacy

In this section, we will apply the multi-dimensional framework for social justice in direct practice to Anthony's case, remembering that social justice is embodied in both practices and processes and is a goal we commit to in practice. Clinical social workers integrate social justice into practice by focusing on issues of respect, resources, and systems. They achieve their ends through advocacy activities for positive change.

Respect

When entering into the counselling relationship, social justice-informed social workers must respect the complexities of the youth they work with. Trauma-informed practice principles align with issues of respect to create a safe, trusting, collaborative, and empowering therapeutic environment that protects clients from re-traumatization within dysfunctional power relationships (Levenson, 2017). The therapeutic stance is one of kindness, respect, curiosity, and compassion (Levenson, 2017). Understanding the impacts of historical and intergenerational trauma is an important consideration. This helps transform symptoms and experiences of youth ageing out of care into signs of resilience and internal resolve, rather than indications of pathology—as is frequently done (Fast & Collin-Vezina, 2020). Like most Indigenous people in Canada, Anthony is likely to have experienced the genocidal impacts of the residential school system through first-hand, family, and community experience—through state and church efforts to extinguish Indigenous languages, ceremonies and spirituality, and land rights (Macdonald, 2019; Starblanket, 2018). For many, the child welfare system is an extension of the residential school system and perpetuates historical violence (Blackstock, 2007). While historical as well as intergenerational trauma may be areas of focus for work with Anthony, he may also be dealing with his lived experiences of trauma. He reports clear memories of sirens and lights as he was removed from his mother's home. These recollections may indicate somatic memory of trauma. Certainly, symptoms of anxiety and depression, as well as emotional regulation issues, may indicate the need for trauma-informed care. Appropriate considerations of trauma work with Anthony must take into consideration his culture and spirituality as pathways to healing. Because of Anthony's experiences of family disruption (or destruction) alongside ongoing experiences of racism, marginalization, and stigma, social work practitioners must understand and appreciate the impact of these factors while at the same time being mindful of how their own practice assumptions may help or hinder healing.

Respect for Anthony is very much tied to issues of identity and recognition, and the misrecognition that he has experienced as an Indigenous young person. Self-confidence and self-esteem develop in relationship with others who affirm and validate. This is especially relevant within cultural communities for the formation of positive identity (Doucet, 2020). As a ward of the government and having had numerous broken and lost relationships through placement disruptions, and as an Indigenous youth with historic and current loses including loss of contact with his family, community, and culture, Anthony has suffered misrecognition and lost opportunities to develop a strong sense of self. Recognition is required for a positive and intact sense of self and the development of self-confidence and self-esteem. Clinical interventions to promote respect and to reclaim lost identities will likely require efforts to reconnect Anthony with lost family, community, and cultural connections. Narrative therapies are consistent with collaborative and trauma-informed practices that honour people's stories and help reconstruct personal narratives that constitute identities (Carr, 1998). Working with community partners, including Band members and an Indigenous Elder, will help Anthony gain comfort and familiarity with his history and identity.

Resources

Anthony identified a desire to complete his high school education as an important goal to his overall well-being and a step towards self-sufficiency and independence. This is also an opportunity to increase his personal **resources**. Considering the very real and positive impact of post-secondary education generally, this could be a priority consideration for Anthony. As Anthony's self-confidence and sense of self are developing, this might entail more practical considerations such as research into available courses and supports at the local community college. It may include research into bursaries for former youth in care and/or Indigenous youth. It may also include accompanying Anthony to interviews and appointments to explore his options and advocacy to amplify his voice in the process. This work should be collaborative, with Anthony taking the lead while recognizing that support for Anthony can come in many different forms.

Anthony feels embarrassed that he has no driver's licence even though he is 22 years old. This is an issue for many youth aging out of care in rural communities, where personal transportation is vital and a driver's licence is a rite of passage. Rural youth often learn to drive at a young age and Anthony felt some resentment that his repeated requests while in care were ignored. Now, having passed his written driving test, he needs practice driving but has a limited number of friends or contacts to supervise his practice hours. Without a driver's licence, he must rely on others and his job prospects are limited. This seemingly mundane activity of daily life takes on great importance when it marks Anthony as different from others his age—who have never been in care—and forecloses on age-appropriate opportunities that his peers enjoy, and that could contribute significantly to Anthony's overall well-being and quality of life. Working with Anthony to secure resources and obtain this goal is more than just good social work practice, it is actually an example of social justice practice in action.

Systems

A critical and structural approach to clinical social work practice is essential—recognizing that the very child welfare system that was designed to protect youth from harm is often a source of trauma—that it actually perpetuates inequity and discrimination and contributes to the ongoing marginalization of youth in care. Empowerment theory emphasizes increasing the power of marginalized individuals, groups, and communities. Power can be viewed as personal, interpersonal, or political (Turner & Maschi, 2015). Empowerment through group affiliation can increase feelings of self-efficacy and self-esteem. Raising the critical consciousness of youth is a step in the empowerment process (Turner & Maschi 2015). Connecting Anthony with other Indigenous youth who have aged out of care may increase his sense of self-efficacy and self-esteem, and affiliating with other youth who are organizing to have their voices heard to transform the child welfare system may enhance his confidence in the possibility of effecting political change while expanding his social circle.

Advocacy

Advocacy for Anthony needs to be practical, educational, and instrumental to his future success and will take place on many levels from the personal to the structural. Increasing Anthony's understanding about his rights as an

Indigenous youth, and as a youth who has aged out of care, is socially just and empowering. As an Indigenous youth ageing out of care, Anthony may be eligible for a variety of services—but access to these resources may be deliberately confusing and opaque. In Canada, child welfare is a provincial responsibility, while the federal government is responsible for Indigenous programs and funding, so helping Anthony exercise his rights requires knowledge about provincial and federal programs that support youth who have been wards of the government, especially through their post-secondary journey.

Conclusion

Effective and transformative practice with youth who have aged out of the child welfare system requires that social workers take their social justice commitments seriously. A multi-dimensional framework of social justice directs clinical social workers to attend to (a) the relational process and power of respect, (b) fair and equitable access to resources required for youth to live a good life, and (c) attention to the systems that impact the life chances for these youth—the child welfare system, and educational and healthcare systems. These very systems, purported to support the wellbeing of individuals, frequently reproduce structural inequity through practices that oppress and marginalize those who fall outside dominant heteronormative discourses. Social workers who take their social justice commitments seriously employ advocacy strategies as part of their clinical tools to educate and empower clients about their rights, whether it be to services (or to refuse service), to resources, or to respect. At the same time, they look for—and create—opportunities to confront neoliberal constraints on service provision and, in the case of Indigenous youth, to honour historic and treaty-based obligations. Advocacy practice is practical, educational, and instrumental in the pursuit of social justice.

Note

1 The Métis in what is now called western Canada emerged from post-contact unions between European fur traders and Indigenous women beginning in the 18th century. The Métis Nation of Alberta defines Métis as "a person who self-identifies as Métis, is distinct from other Indigenous peoples, is of historic Métis Nation ancestry, and who is accepted by the Métis Nation."

References

Asakura, K., & Maurer, K. (2018). Attending to social justice in clinical social work: Supervision as a pedagogical space. *Clinical Social Work Journal, 46*(4), 289–297. https://doi.org/10.1007/s10615-018-0667-4

Asakura, K., Strumm, B., Todd, S., & Varghese, R. (2020). What does social justice look like when sitting with clients? A qualitative study of teaching clinical social work from a social justice perspective. *Journal of Social Work Education, 56*(3), 442–455. https://doi.org/10.1080/10437797.2019.1656588

Avery, R. J. (2010). An examination of theory and promising practice for achieving permanency for teens before they age out of foster care. *Children and Youth Services Review, 32*(3), 399–408. https://doi.org/10.1016/j.childyouth.2009.10.011

Avery, R. J., & Freundlich, M. (2009). You're all grown up now: Termination of foster care support at age 18. *Journal of Adolescence, 32*(2), 247–257. https://doi.org/10.1016/j.adolescence.2008.03.009

Blackstock, C. (2007). Residential schools: Did they really close or just morph into child welfare? *Indigenous Law Journal, 6*(1), 72–78.

Bond, S., & van Breda, A. (2018). Interaction between possible selves and the resilience of care-leavers in South Africa. *Children and Youth Services Review, 94*(September), 88–95. https://doi.org/10.1016/j.childyouth.2018.09.014

Bonnycastle, C. R. (2011). Social justice along a continuum: A relational illustrative model. *The Social Service Review, 85*(2), 267–295. https://doi.org/10.1086/660703

Brandon-Friedman, R. A., Wahler, E. A, Pierce, B. J, Thigpen, J. W, & Fortenberry, J. D. (2020). The impact of sociosexualization and sexual identity development on the sexual well-being of youth formerly in the foster care system. *Journal of Adolescent Health, 66*(4), 439–446. https://doi.org/10.1016/j.jadohealth.2019.10.025

Brown, C. (2021). Critical clinical social work and the neoliberal constraints on social justice in mental health. *Research on Social Work Practice*. https://doi.org/10.1177/1049731520984531

Canadian Association of Social Workers. (2005). *Code of Ethics*. Retrieved from www.casw-acts.ca/files/documents/casw_code_of_ethics.pdf

Carr, A. (1998). Michael White's narrative therapy. *Contemporary Family Therapy, 20*(4), 485–503. https://doi.org/10.1023/A:1021680116584

Courtney, M., Flynn, R. J., & Beaupré, J. (2013). Overview of out of home care in the USA and Canada. *Intervención Psicosocial, 22*(3), 163–173. https://doi.org/10.5093/in2013a20

Damiani-Taraba, G., Sky, I., Hegler, D., Woolridge, N., Anderson, B., & Koster, A. (2018). The listen to me project: Creating lasting changes in voice and participation for children in care through a youth-led project. *Child & Youth Services, 39*(1), 75–95. https://doi.org/10.1080/0145935X.2018.1446825

Dean, R. G., & Poorvu, N. L. (2008). Assessment and formulation: A contemporary social work perspective. *Families in Society, 89*(4), 596–604. https://doi.org/10.1606/1044-3894.3822

Dettlaff, A. J, & Boyd, R. (2020). Racial disproportionality and disparities in the child welfare system: Why do they exist, and what can be done to address them? *The Annals of the American Academy of Political and Social Science, 692*(1), 253–274. https://doi.org/10.1177/0002716220980329

Dotolo, D., Lindhorst, T., Kemp, S. P, & Engelberg, R. A. (2018). Expanding conceptualizations of social justice across all levels of social work practice: Recognition theory and its contributions. *The Social Service Review, 92*(2), 143–170. https://doi.org/10.1086/698111

Doucet, M. (2020). All my relations: Examining nonhuman relationships as sources of social capital for Indigenous and non-Indigenous youth 'aging out' of care in Canada. *International Journal of Child and Adolescent Resilience/Revue internationale de la résilience des enfants et des adolescents,* 7(1), 139–153. https://doi.org/10.7202/1072594a

Dworsky, A., & Courtney, M. E. (2010). The risk of teenage pregnancy among transitioning foster youth: Implications for extending state care beyond age 18.

Children and Youth Services Review, *32*(10), 1351–1356. https://doi.org/10.1016/j.childyouth.2010.06.002

Fast, E., & Collin-Vézina, D. (2020). Historical trauma, race-based trauma and resilience of Indigenous peoples: A literature review. *First Peoples Child & Family Review*, *5*(1), 126–136. https://doi.org/10.7202/1069069ar

Fleischacker, S. (2005). *A short history of distributive justice*. Cambridge, MA: Harvard University Press.

Fowler, P. J, Toro, P. A, & Miles, B. W. (2009). Pathways to and from homelessness and associated psychosocial outcomes among adolescents leaving the foster care system. *American Journal of Public Health*, *99*(8), 1453–1458. https://doi.org/10.2105/AJPH.2008.142547

Fraser, N. (1999). Social justice in the age of identity politics: Redistribution, recognition, and participation. In L. Ray and A. Sayer (Eds.), *Culture and Economy after the Cultural Turn* (pages of chapter here). New York, NY: SAGE Publications. https://doi.org/10.4135/9781446218112.n2

Fraser, N., & Honneth, A. (2003). *Redistribution or recognition? A political—philosophical exchange*. London: Verso.

Garrett, P. M. (2010). Recognizing the limitations of the political theory of recognition: Axel Honneth, Nancy Fraser and social work. *The British Journal of Social Work*, *40*(5), 1517–1533. https://doi.org/10.1093/bjsw/bcp044

Glynn, N. (2021). Understanding care leavers as youth in society: A theoretical framework for studying the transition out of care. *Children and Youth Services Review*, *121*. https://doi.org/10.1016/j.childyouth.2020.105829

Goodkind, S., Schelbe, L. A., & Shook, J. J. (2011). Why youth leave care: Understandings of adulthood and transition successes and challenges among youth aging out of child welfare. *Children and Youth Services Review*, *33*(6), 1039–1048. https://doi.org/10.1016/j.childyouth.2011.01.010

Haight, W., Waubanascum, C., Glesener, D., & Marsalis, S. (2018). A scoping study of Indigenous child welfare: The long emergency and preparations for the next seven generations. *Children and Youth Services Review*, *93*, 397–410. https://doi.org/10.1016/j.childyouth.2018.08.016

Harrison, J., VanDeusen, K., & Way, I. (2016). Embedding social justice within micro social work curricula. *Smith College Studies in Social Work*, *86*(3), 258–273. https://doi.org/10.1080/00377317.2016.1191802

Kreitzer, L., McLaughlin, A. M., Elliott, G., & Nicholas, D. (2016). Qualitative examination of rural service provision to persons with concurrent developmental and mental health challenges. *European Journal of Social Work*, *19*(1), 46–61. https://doi.org/10.1080/13691457.2015.1022859

Levenson, J. (2017). Trauma-informed social work practice. *Social Work*, *62*(2), 105–113. https://doi.org/10.1093/sw/swx001

Ma, J., Fallon, B., & Richard, K. (2019). The overrepresentation of First Nations children and families involved with child welfare: Findings from the Ontario incidence study of reported child abuse and neglect 2013. *Child Abuse & Neglect*, *90*, 52–65. https://doi.org/10.1016/j.chiabu.2019.01.022

Macdonald, D. (2019). *The sleeping giant awakens: Genocide, Indian residential schools, and the challenge of conciliation*. Toronto: University of Toronto Press.

Mandell, D. (2008). Power, care and vulnerability: Considering use of self in child welfare work. *Journal of Social Work Practice*, *22*(2), 235–248. https://doi.org/10.1080/02650530802099916

Marion, É., & Paulsen, V. (2019). The transition to adulthood from care: A review of current research. In V. R. Mann-Feder and M. Goyette (Eds.), *Leaving care and the transition to adulthood: International contributions to theory, research, and practice* (pp. 107–129). Oxford University Press. https://doi.org/10.1093/oso/9780190630485.003.0007

Marmot, M. (2005). *Status syndrome: How your social standing directly affects your health.* London: Bloomsbury Publishing.

Marmot, M. (2017). Social justice, epidemiology and health inequalities. *European Journal of Epidemiology, 32*(7), 537–546. https://doi.org/10.1007/s10654-017-0286-3

Marsh, J. C., & Bunn, M. (2018). Social work's contribution to direct practice with individuals, families, and groups: An institutionalist perspective. *Social Service Review, 92*(4), 647–692. https://doi.org/10.1086/701639

Maschi, T., Baer, J., & Turner, S. G. (2011). The psychological goods on clinical social work: A content analysis of the clinical social work and social justice literature. *Journal of Social Work Practice, 25*(2), 233–253. https://doi.org/10.1080/02650533.2010.544847

Maschi, T., Hatcher, S. S., Schwalbe, C. S., & Rosato, N. S. (2008). Mapping the social service pathways of youth to and through the juvenile justice system: A comprehensive review. *Children and Youth Services Review, 30*(12), 1376–1385. https://doi.org/10.1016/j.childyouth.2008.04.006

McLaughlin, A. M. (2002). Social work's legacy: Irreconcilable differences? *Clinical Social Work Journal, 30*(2), 187–198. https://doi.org/10.1023/A:1015297529215

McLaughlin, A. M. (2006). *Clinical social work and social justice* [Doctoral dissertation, University of Calgary] ProQuest Dissertations & Theses Global. (305358907). Retrieved from https://ezproxy.lib.ucalgary.ca/login?url=https://www-proquest-com.ezproxy.lib.ucalgary.ca/dissertations-theses/clinical-social-work-justice/docview/305358907/se-2?accountid=9838

McLaughlin, A. M. (2009). Clinical social workers: Advocates for social justice. *Advances in Social Work, 10*(1), 51–68. https://doi.org/10.18060/209

Mclaughlin, A. M. (2011). Exploring social justice for clinical social work practice. *Smith College Studies in Social Work, 81*(2–3), 234–251. https://doi.org/10.1080/00377317.2011.588551

McLaughlin, A. M., Gray, E., & Wilson, M. G. (2017). From tenuous to tenacious: social justice practice in child welfare. *Journal of Public Child Welfare, 11*(4–5), 568–585. https://doi.org/10.1080/15548732.2017.1279997

McLaughlin, A. M., Enns, R., Seaward. D. (2018). Ageing out of care: The rural experience. In D. Badry, H. M. Montgomery, D. Kikulwe, M. Bennett and D. Fuchs (Eds.), *Imagining child welfare in the spirit of reconciliation* (page numbers here). Regina, SK: University of Regina Press

McMillen, J., Curtis, S., Lionel D., Zima, B. T., Ollie, M. T., Munson, M. R., & Spitznagel, E. (2004). Use of mental health services among older youths in foster care. *Psychiatric Services, 55*(7), 811–817. https://doi.org/10.1176/appi.ps.55.7.811

McNally, M., & Martin, D. (2017). First Nations, Inuit and Métis health. *Healthcare Management Forum, 30*(2), 117–122. https://doi.org/10.1177/0840470416680445

Mountz, S., & Capous-Desyllas, M. (2020). Exploring the families of origin of LGBTQ former foster youth and their trajectories throughout care. *Children and Youth Services Review, 109*, 104622. https://doi.org/10.1016/j.childyouth.2019.104622

Noël, J. F. (2015). *The Convention on the Rights of the Child.* Government of Canada. Retrieved from www.justice.gc.ca/eng/rp-pr/fl-lf/divorce/crc-crde/conv2a.html

Nussbaum, M. (2005). Beyond the social contract: Capabilities and global justice. In G. Brock and H. Brighouse (Eds.), *The Political Philosophy of Cosmopolitanism* (pp. 196–218). Cambridge: Cambridge University Press. Doi:10.1017/CBO9780511614743.014

O'Brien, M. (2009). Social work and the practice of social justice: An initial overview. *Aotearoa New Zealand Social Work, 21*(1), 3–10. https://doi.org/10.11157/anzswj-vol21iss1-2id308

Okpych, N. (2012). Policy framework supporting youth aging-out of foster care through college: Review and recommendations. *Children and Youth Services Review*, 34(7), 1390–1396. https://doi.org/10.1016/j.childyouth.2012.02.013

Popova, S., Lange, S., Burd, L., & Rehm, J. (2014). Canadian children and youth in care: The cost of Fetal Alcohol Spectrum Disorder. *Child & Youth Care Forum, 43*(1), 83–96. https://doi.org/10.1007/s10566-013-9226-x

Propp, J., Ortega, D. M., & NewHeart, F. (2003). Independence or interdependence: Rethinking the transition from "ward of the court" to adulthood. *Families in Society, 84*(2), 259–266. https://doi.org/10.1606/1044-3894.102

Rawls, J. (1971). *A theory of justice*. Cambridge, MA: Oxford University Press.

Reid, C., & Dudding, P. (2006). *Building a future together: Issues and outcomes for transition-aged youth*: Centre of Excellence for Child Welfare. Retrieved from https://cwrp.ca/sites/default/files/publications/BuildingAFutureTogether.pdf

Reisch, M. (2002). Defining social justice in a socially unjust world. *Families in Society, 83*(4), 343–354. https://doi.org/10.1606/1044-3894.17

Rome, S. H., & Raskin, M. (2019). Transitioning out of foster care. *Youth & Society, 51*(4), 529–547. https://doi.org/10.1177/0044118X17694968

Rutman, D., Hubberstey, C., & Feduniw, A. (2007). *When youth age out of care—where to from there?* Victoria, BC: Research Initiatives for Social Change Unit, University of Victoria. Retrieved from www.uvic.ca/hsd/socialwork/assets/docs/research/WhenYouthAge2007.pdf

Saint-Girons, M., Trocmé, N., Esposito, T., & Fallon, B. (2020). *CWRP Information Sheet #211E: Children in Out-Of-Home Care in Canada in 2019*. Canadian Child Welfare Research Portal. Retrieved from https://cwrp.ca/sites/default/files/publications/Children%20in%20out-of-home%20care%20in%20Canada%20in%202019_0.pdf

Sakamoto, I. (2005). Use of critical consciousness in anti-oppressive social work practice: Disentangling power dynamics at personal and structural levels. *The British Journal of Social Work, 35*(4), 435–452. https://doi.org/10.1093/bjsw/bch190

Salas, L. M., Sen, S., & Segal, E. A. (2010). Critical theory: Pathway from dichotomous to integrated social work practice. *Families in Society, 91*(1), 91–96. https://doi.org/10.1606/1044-3894.3961

Schibler B., & McEwan-Morris, A. (2006). *Strengthening our youth: Their journey to competence and independence*. Office of the Children's Advocate. Retrieved from www.gov.mb.ca/fs/changesforchildren/pubs/strengthening_our_youth.pdf

Serge L., Eberle M., Goldberg M., Sullivan S., & Dudding P. (2002). *Pilot study: The child welfare system and homelessness among Canadian youth*. National Homelessness Initiative. Retrieved from www.homelesshub.ca/sites/default/files/attachments/Pilot_Study_The_Child_Welfare_System_and_Homelessness.pdf

Simkiss, D. (2019). The needs of looked after children from an adverse childhood experience perspective. *Paediatrics and Child Health (United Kingdom), 29*(1), 25–33. https://doi.org/10.1016/j.paed.2018.11.005

Sinclair, R. (2007). Identity lost and found: Lessons from the sixties scoop. *First Peoples Child & Family Review, 3*(1), 65–82. https://doi.org/10.7202/1069527ar

Solas, J. (2008). What kind of social justice does social work seek? *International Social Work, 51*(6), 813–822. https://doi.org/10.1177/0020872808095252

Southerland, D., Casanueva, C. E., & Ringeisen, H. (2009). Young adult outcomes and mental health problems among transition age youth investigated for maltreatment during adolescence. *Children and Youth Services Review, 31*(9), 947–956. https://doi.org/10.1016/j.childyouth.2009.03.010

Specht, H., & Courtney, M. E. (1994). *Unfaithful angels: how social work has abandoned its mission*. New York, NY: Free Press.

Starblanket, T. (2018). *Suffer the little children: Genocide, Indigenous nations and the Canadian State*. Atlanta, GA: Clarity Press.

Stein, M. (2008). Resilience and young people leaving care. *Child Care in Practice, 14*(1), 35–44. https://doi.org/10.1080/13575270701733682

Swenson, C. R. (1998). Clinical social work's contribution to a social justice perspective. *Social Work, 43*(6), 527–537. https://doi.org/10.1093/sw/43.6.527

Taylor, C., & Gutmann, A. (1992). *Multiculturalism and "The politics of recognition": An essay*. Princeton University Press.

Turner, A. (2016). *Insights on Canadian society: Living arrangements of Aboriginal children aged 14 and under*. Statistics Canada. Retrieved from https://www150.statcan.gc.ca/n1/pub/75-006-x/2016001/article/14547-eng.htm

Turner, S. G, & Maschi, T. M. (2015). Feminist and empowerment theory and social work practice. *Journal of Social Work Practice*, 29(2), 151–162. https://doi.org/10.1080/02650533.2014.941282

Truth and Reconciliation Commission of Canada. (2015). *Truth and reconciliation commission of Canada: Calls to action*. Retrieved from http://trc.ca/assets/pdf/Calls_to_Action_English2.pdf

Ungar, M. (2011). Community resilience for youth and families: Facilitative physical and social capital in contexts of adversity. *Children and Youth Services Review, 33*(9), 1742–1748. https://doi.org/10.1016/j.childyouth.2011.04.027

Urban Institute. (2008). *Coming of age: Employment outcomes for youth who age out of foster care through their middle twenties*. Retrieved from www.urban.org/sites/default/files/publication/31216/1001174-Coming-of-Age-Employment-Outcomes-for-Youth-Who-Age-Out-of-Foster-Care-Through-Their-Middle-Twenties.PDF

Van Breda, A. D. (2015). Journey towards independent living: A grounded theory investigation of leaving the care of Girls & Boys Town, South Africa. *Journal of Youth Studies, 18*(3), 322–337. https://doi.org/10.1080/13676261.2014.963534

Van Breda, A. D. (2018). A critical review of resilience theory and its relevance for social work. *Social Work/Maatskaplike Werk, 54*(1), 1–18. https://doi.org/10.15270/54-1-611

Webb, S. (2010). (Re)assembling the left: The politics of redistribution and recognition in social work. *British Journal of Social Work, 40*, 2364–2379.

Williams, K., Potestio, M. L., & Austen-Wiebe V.(2019). Indigenous health: Applying truth and reconciliation in Alberta health services. *Canadian Medical Association Journal 4*(191)(Suppl), S44–S46. Doi: 10.1503/cmaj.190585

World Health Organization. (2021). *WHO urges more investments, services for mental health*. Retrieved from www.who.int/mental_health/who_urges_investment/en/#:~:text=Mental%20health%20is%20defined%20as,to%20her%20or%20his%20community

Young, I. M. (2006). Taking the basic structure seriously. *Perspectives on Politics, 4*(1), 91–97. https://doi.org/10.1017/S1537592706060099

9 Older Adults, Human Rights, and Social Justice

Carole Cox and Manoj Pardasani

The world is aging. By 2050 the global population of those 65 and older is expected to triple (United Nations, 2013). There were 703 million persons aged 65 years or over in the world in 2019 (United Nations, 2019). The number of older persons is projected to double to 1.5 billion in 2050. Globally, the share of the population aged 65 years or over increased from 6% in 1990 to 9% in 2019. That proportion is projected to rise further to 16% by 2050 (United Nations, 2019). As noted by both the International Federation of Social Workers (IFSW, 2012) and the National Association of Social Workers (NASW, 2014), this population shift has created a greater demand for professionals with specialized knowledge and expertise in aging.

As people age, they encounter transitions that affect all areas of their lives. Retirement often means changes in relationships as well as economic status. But for many older adults, retirement is not an option. For them, access to employment and healthcare is critical. Widowhood and the loss of close relatives and friends can induce intense feelings of grief that can be numbing without skilled and sensitive interventions. Physical changes can limit mobility while mental impairment can impede overall functioning. Such changes frequently impact relationships as traditional roles are altered. Similarly, the cognitive and emotional challenges related to aging also impact their quality of life. Consequently, changing family structures mean that older adults are often left with limited supports. When such changes are accompanied by lower income and poorer health, persons become vulnerable in society with their rights threatened.

The vulnerability of the older population is highlighted by the COVID-19 pandemic. Older people were disproportionately impacted by the virus. They were the most likely to contract it, become seriously ill, get hospitalized, and die from it (Centers for Disease Control, 2021). More than 95% of the people dying from the virus in Europe were 65 years and older (Human Rights Watch, 2020) while, in the United States, the percentage was 80% with the mortality rate highest for those over 85, (CDC, 2021).

Accompanying these rates was an increase in ageism, discrimination against older persons. Such discrimination is most clearly shown in efforts to ration scarce health resources on the basis of age, which underscores the

DOI: 10.4324/9781003111269-12

perspective that older people have lower social value than yo ple and are thus given less priority (Costa-Font, 2020). Acros older people were confined to long-term care facilities, whe was rampant resulting in immense mortality (Fulmer, Kolle 2020). Many in the community were left without services and programs were forced to limit funds. In some countries they to remain in their homes, movement was restricted, and nursing home denied visits (United Nations, DESA, 2020). Such restrictions are violations of basic human rights and as they are closely associated with accessibility to essential resources, they highlight the extent of social injustice confronting older people.

The following statement by the UN High Commissioner for Human Rights, Michelle Bachelet, is strong in its description of these violations and in the support of an international legal instrument, a convention, to protect the rights of older persons.

> The crisis has exposed critical human rights protection gaps for older persons, including widespread discrimination based on older age; lack of social protection—especially for women—and of access to health services; failure to uphold autonomy and participation in decision-making; and failure to ensure that older people are free from violence, neglect and abuse.
>
> (Bachelet, 2021)

The Universal Declaration of Human Rights (UDHR) passed by the United Nations in 1948 includes five core notions (Wronka, 2008): Article 1 Human Dignity; Article 2 Nondiscrimination; Articles 3–21; Civil and Political Rights Articles 22–27 Economic, Social and Cultural Rights; Articles 28–30 Solidarity Rights. The first set of rights (Articles 2–15) relates to political and individual freedoms restricting the interference of governments with the individual while Articles 16–27 focus on the right to an adequate standard of living, including health and well-being, food, clothing housing medical care, and necessary social services. The third set of rights (Articles 28 through 30) promotes intergovernmental cooperation on global issues, such as the environment and development, international peace and international distributive justice.

Rights and Needs

Human rights are frequently confused with needs although the two are clearly distinguishable. Tangible needs exist as phenomena that can be objectively identified and measured, such as needs for food, housing, support, or income (Ife, 2012). However, needs can also be subjective, wherein society decides whether they actually exist. In contrast to human rights, which are constant, social values and beliefs are influential in determining needs.

Social workers often determine needs by measuring them through "needs assessments" that decide whether supports or services are warranted and how they may or should be met Such needs are then filtered through the prism of competing resources, where one vulnerable group may benefit at the expense of another dependent upon the values and viewpoints of policy makers and providers. Additionally, implicit biases and values lead to delineation between those in need who are deserving and those who are not. An example of this would be how medical resources were prioritized for younger individuals infected with COVID-19.

In contrast to needs, the universality of human rights and their indivisibility means that they are substantiated in themselves and are not dependent on social values or perspectives. Moreover, human rights provide the mandate to fulfill human needs with social policies acting as the means for attaining them. Consequently, social workers can play major roles in assuring that policy and practice needs are reframed and treated as basic human rights to which each individual is entitled. Rights ensure that all individuals are treated with equity and dignity.

Human Rights Conventions and Older People

Subsequent to the Universal Declaration of Human Rights, several special conventions were adopted by the General Assembly of the United Nations, including the Convention on the Elimination of Discrimination Against Women the Convention on the Rights of the Child, the Convention on the Elimination of all Forms of Racial Discrimination, and the Convention on the Rights of Persons with Disability. Countries ratifying Conventions are legally bound to adhere to their standards.

To date, there has not been a Convention on the Rights of Older People. Among the arguments against a Convention are claims that existing human rights documents cover the rights of older persons (Megret, 2011), that experience shows that conventions do not lead to real social change and, therefore, advocates should focus on ensuring the implementation of existing treaties, conventions, and principles (Doron & Apter, 2010). If that were the case, there would be no conventions for any segments of the population.

In 1991, the United Nations issued The Principles of Older Persons (UN, 1991), which detailed five areas in which the rights of older people needed to be prioritized and guaranteed: Independence, Participation, Care, Self-Fulfillment, and Dignity. Regional meetings and country reports on the status of older people continue to be held and the United Nations has developed a standing committee on the rights of older people (HelpAge International, 2010).

The Madrid International Plan of Action on Aging (MIPPA, United Nations, 2002) explicates the rights of older persons, but although it has been endorsed by the General Assembly of the United Nations, in contrast to Conventions, it is not binding on member states. Governments have only a moral responsibility to adhere to its recommendations, which focus on core issues associated with the rights and quality of life of older people. These rights include governments' promoting human rights instruments and supporting decision-making among older people; enabling people to work as long as they can and choose; retiring with adequate income security; assuring that older people have access to the same preventive, curative, and rehabilitative care as others; and ensuring that older people have access to decent housing, supports, and are free from neglect, abuse, and violence. Accordingly, these rights must not be perceived as only a moral responsibility, as doing so absolves governments and societies from committing to progressive change or concrete actions (UN, 2002). Nations must be held accountable for their obligations to uphold the rights of older persons, a growing segment of their populations.

In 2010, the General Assembly of the United Nations established the Open-Ended Working Group on Ageing. The Group is charged with considering existing international frameworks of human rights of older persons, identifying gaps in policies and services, and devising ways of addressing them. Among the major challenges it is dealing with are discrimination, poverty, and violence and abuse, The Group is also exploring the possibility of developing an international legal instrument to promote the rights and dignity of older persons (Office of the High Commissioner—Human Rights, 2014).).

Based on the recent assessment of global policies and the situation of older persons, many gaps continue to exist with regard to their rights and countries' commitment to them. Many groups are working toward a Convention on the Rights of Older People that would clarify these rights, reduce fragmentation, and strengthen the accountability of governments to adhere to them.

The Rights-Based Approach in Social Work

Two values, benevolence and paternalism, play key roles in social work with older adults. Benevolence refers to kindness and promoting the good of others, while paternalism refers to interfering with an individual's right to carry out their own decisions for their own good. Both values assume that persons are worthy of assistance and that the person offering help is committed to their well-being and best interests. However, paternalism can seriously conflict with a client's right to self-determination even when the intention is to protect the person from harm. As noted by Reamer (2005), for paternalistic interference to be justifiable, social workers must demonstrate that clients would otherwise face dire, perhaps irreversible consequences.

The following section describes policies in the United States that have significant impact on the rights and well-being of older persons. Each is intended to offer support or protections but their effectiveness in doing so remains questionable.

Guardianship

No policy has greater impact on the rights of the individual for liberty and security than that of guardianship. Guardianship deems that an individual is incompetent to make decisions on his or her own behalf for their best interests, consequently, depriving the person of their basic rights. If no immediate relative or friend is available to make such decisions, courts, under the doctrine of "parens patriae" have the ability to assign guardians to protect these persons and their property.

In the United States, guardianship can be requested by anyone with state laws regulating the actions that a guardian can make on their own and those that require court approval. However, there is little monitoring of guardians and few safeguards for the older person and are few guarantees that the guardian will uphold or fulfill this role or that the interests of the ward will be supported. In fact, several horrific cases of abuse (physical, psychological, and financial) have been brought to public attention in recent times (Aviv, 2017).

A major concern in guardianship proceedings is the lack of a standardized uniform measure for assessing competency or regulations as to who can make the judgment. Thus, one may be judged incompetent in one state and competent in another. The lack of homogeneity among competency evaluations and the qualifications of persons making these assessments puts many at risk of abuse or neglect (Moye & Naik, 2011). In addition, the absence of consistent oversight of a guardian further increases these risks.

Guardianship processes vary with the states with all reflecting individual state judicial processes. The petitioner's attorney, required in many states, collects evidence and reports to the court regarding the need for a guardian. Many states also require an attorney to be appointed to represent the individual as their advocate and support their wishes (Hurme, 2021).

Although some may require only limited guardianship with regards to medical decisions or estate management, the tendency is to grant full guardianship, giving the guardian control over all aspects of the person's life. As such, the guardianship process focuses on the weaknesses and failings of the older person (Wright, 2014). By focusing on failings, the rights of human dignity, security, and participation are seriously threatened as strengths are ignored and the person loses control of his or her life. In all these cases, the older person at the center of the issue is rarely consulted or heard.

The rights-based approach offers a conceptual framework for social work involvement in the guardianship process. At the micro level, social workers can ensure that assessments explore individual strengths and resiliency of the proposed ward and that the wishes of the person are recognized. Involvement at the mezzo level can help ensure that those assuming the role of a guardian are vetted and monitored consistently and that the interests of the person are kept paramount through proper oversight by the court. Macro involvement demands that social workers become involved as advocates and provide ethical oversight working toward improving the system to ensure that it is sensitive to, and reflective of, human rights. At the mezzo and macro levels, social workers can help create structures that develop social policies and guidelines, monitor the guardian relationship, raise community awareness, and provide training for all involved.

Employment

Employment provides a vivid example of the way in which age alone can impact human rights. Employment opportunities decline with age, with older workers commonly facing discrimination in the workplace. Moreover, once unemployed, older workers are more likely to face long-term unemployment than their younger peers, and if rehired, are likely to have earnings that are lower than their previous earnings (GAO, 2012). Consequently, rights to employment are ignored and security threatened.

The ADEA (Age Discrimination in Employment Act) of 1967 applies to companies of 20 employees or more and is intended to prevent age discrimination in hiring, terminations, promotions, training, and other conditions of employment. Data on charges made under the ADEA by those 55 and older have progressively increased since 2000 with harassment, discipline, and intimidation growing from 10% of charges in 2000 to 30% in 2010 (von Schader & Nazaro, 2015). However, proving age discrimination is difficult, as the plaintiff must show that age is the motivating factor. Thus, data from the Equal Employment Opportunity Commission (EEOC) show only 2.7% of cases taken to the EEOC were found to show reasonable cause of discrimination (U.S.EEOC, 2018).

Social workers in employee assistance programs (EAP) have the opportunity not only to counsel employees but also to bridge the gap between employees and employers. They can educate employers on the impact of workplace policies and procedures on older employees and suggest changes that increase everyone's well-being (Ottenstein & Jacobson, 2006). Consequently, they can become involved in actually changing the structure and environment of an organization to make it more sensitive to discriminatory actions and more responsive to older adults.

Persons with cognitive impairment are at particular risk of discrimination in the workforce. Employers tend to make little accommodation for these employees even though they could often continue to work in varying capacities (Belleville, 2018). Instead, they frequently let go at the beginning stages of impairment, with employers often unsure of how to counsel them or discuss their symptoms (Cox & Pardasani, 2013).

The rights of employed caregivers, the majority of whom are women, are at risk due to loss of income and benefits as they reduce work hours, decline promotions, and take early retirement in order to provide care (AARP & NAC, 2015). The Family and Medical Leave Act (FMLA) remains the primary policy to support these caregivers. The Act offers up to 12 weeks of unpaid leave to employees to provide care for a parent, child, or spouse.

However, it is restricted to companies with 50 or more workers and applies only to those who have been employed for at least 12 months. With 40% of the workforce ineligible for its benefits, many are forced to struggle to combine caregiving and employee roles (www.nationalpartnership.org). However, many states in the United States have adopted consumer-directed personal care assistance programs via Medicaid (state-funded healthcare coverage for individuals living in poverty or with a chronic disability). Consumer directed means the care recipient, to an extent, can choose his/her caregiver. Many of these states allow participants to hire friends and relatives to provide the needed assistance (American Council on Aging, 2021).

Social workers at the micro level are needed to counsel employees dealing with the cognitive decline, caregivers struggling to combine care and work, and employers seeking to understand the ramifications of dementia. Mezzo level interventions may include developing workplace support groups and educational programs on dementia, as well as different work possibilities such as flextime and telecommuting. At the macro level, advocacy for policies that protect and support rights for employment and security is essential with particular attention given to the expansion of the FMLA, which can support the well-being of the entire family.

Income

Having a decent standard of living is a basic human right (UDHR, Articles 22 and 25). However, poverty among the elderly remains a reality. In 2013, half of all people on Medicare in the United States had incomes less than $23,500, which is equivalent to 200% of the poverty level for 2015 (Cubanski et al., 2015). Those older adults most likely to be in poverty are over the age of 80, women, Blacks, and Hispanics, and those with relatively poor health (Cubanski et al., 2015).

Social Security has helped to reduce poverty among older persons in the United States and is a primary source of income for 38% of the elderly in this country and the main source of income for more than one-third of African Americans and Latinos (SSA, 2014). However, these benefits do little for the economic security of these minority groups as their rates of poverty, 19% for older African Americans and 18% for older Hispanics, are more than double the 8% rate for older whites (Waid, 2016). Since social security income is based on earned income during one's lifetime, African American and Latinx older adults are more likely to receive less support.

Supplementary Security Income (SSI) is available to many older persons whose income is below the poverty line. In 2015, the maximum annual amount for an individual was $8,804 and for a couple was $13,205 (SSA, 2015). Given the cost of living in the United States, these amounts are often not sufficient to cover usual living expenses, causing many to remain economically insecure with incomes at or below 250% of the federal poverty level (NCOA, 2016).

Proposals that would reduce Social Security benefits would force even more into poverty. The absence of a Cost of Living Adjustment in 2015, the first time in 40 years, failed to recognize the buying patterns of older adults who spend more of their budgets on healthcare, food, and housing than younger persons (AARP, 2015). Raising the retirement age for full Social Security benefits would place an undue burden on vulnerable groups, especially African American men and those with poor health, most dependent on these benefits (Ghilarducci & Moore, 2015).

At the micro level, social work knowledge and counseling skills are important in educating persons about Social Security and other benefits and assisting with access when necessary. In addition to income security, many older adults need nutritional supports, home-based services, housing, transportation assistance, etc. At the mezzo level, social workers can work toward ensuring that such programs and benefits are clear and understandable to all groups of older adults so that accessibility is itself actually strengthened. However, social work contributions may be most important at the macro level as they advocate for policies that support the economic well-being of older adults. Documenting the struggles associated with limited incomes, giving public testimony at hearings on the economic hardships that many face, and supporting the advocacy efforts of associations working for the security and rights of older adults are key areas for advocacy and involvement.

Health

Health and the right to health care in the event of illness, disability, or old age are detailed in Article 25 of the UDHR. The two major programs in the United States working to ensure this right for older adults are Medicare and Medicaid.

Medicare, the national governmental health insurance programs for persons over 65, maintains an acute or short-term focus rather than addressing the chronic care needs of older adults. Part A offers hospital insurance and Part B, an optional program that persons can purchase, covers physician services and some outpatient care. Part D covers outpatient prescriptions, while Part C is a private insurance plan offered through health maintenance organizations.

Medicare's coverage of long-term care, whether in the community through home care and home nursing, or in nursing homes remains limited. In order to receive homecare, a person must be homebound, require skilled care, be certified by a physician, and receive care from a Medicare-certified agency, with care limited to 21 days or less (Medicare, 2015). In addition, assistance is offered only if the beneficiary is expected to improve, a requirement that is difficult for many older recipients with chronic illness to meet.

Medicare coverage for skilled nursing homes is limited. Eligibility depends on being admitted to a nursing home after a qualifying hospital stay with the physician documenting that daily skilled care is required by a medical condition. Full coverage is available for 21 days with partial coverage for the next 100 days. Consequently, those needing long-term care in a skilled facility are not covered, seriously jeopardizing their health and impacting their rights to appropriate health care.

Medicaid, Title XX of the Social Security Act, provides healthcare for those, including the elderly, who fall below the poverty line or live with a chronic disability. The federal government provides federal matching dollars to the states for services on behalf of those eligible with the average federal share of about 67% of program costs (KFF, 2020). In order to meet eligibility criteria, many must "spend down" their assets and savings, which can further compromise their economic well-being.

Medicaid is the principal provider of long-term health care in the United States, covering nearly 50% of all nursing home residents and 62% of all other long-term services (Commission on Long Term Care, 2013). Older persons and those with disabilities account for almost two-thirds of its spending (Paradise, 2015). Although nursing home care must be covered, other long-term care services, such as home care, are optional and decided by each state. States who offer the Medicaid Waiver Program are able to provide community-based care for those who would otherwise be in nursing homes. In comparison to those in nursing homes, persons living in the community have been found to have less depression, anxiety, and higher levels of well-being (Drageset et al., 2013).

Social work involvement in both the Medicare and Medicaid programs is necessary at all levels. At the micro level, social workers are critical to helping persons understand their benefits, eligibility, and navigate cumbersome application/re-certification processes. Social workers are important in work with families to educate and support them during the critical phases often associated with changes in health status and subsequent program eligibility. In many instances, family members may need assistance with appealing a negative decision by a nursing facility or Medicaid. At the mezzo level, social work involvement is needed to ensure that health services are available and accessible for all groups of older adults.

At the macro level, the profession must become actively involved in actual policy development. Challenging regulations and processes that impugn the rights of older adults to adequate healthcare is critical to change. Through testimonials, letter writing, and use of the media, social workers can bring attention to the impact that health care policy has on the health and rights of older adults. As the population of older adults grows exponentially, the need for home-based and skilled nursing care will increase as well. Significant investment in the funding and development of such services is critical to ensuring the rights of older adults.

Most Vulnerable Groups of Older People

Although age itself acts as a criterion for discrimination and human rights violations, within the aging population, specific subgroups are most vulnerable to having their rights violated. Among these groups are older women,

LGBT seniors, and immigrants. For each of these populations, social work involvement at the micro level through counseling and education can help to empower individuals as needs are reframed as human rights. Advocating for services, resources, and access at the community level is a key task for social workers operating at the mezzo level. At the more macro level, social work leadership and involvement can help assure that policies and institutions recognize and realize human rights.

Older Women

Throughout the lifespan, women face discrimination and this continues into their later years. The Convention on the Elimination of All Forms of Discrimination Against Women (CEDAW) which has been approved by 170 countries but not ratified by the United States, formally recognizes the global inequality that women face. This inequality becomes even more profound as they age, become marginalized, and their well-being and security thereby threatened.

Women in the United States can expect to live 15 to 20 years as a widow. They are more likely to spend their later years alone and twice as likely as their male counterparts to be poor (Women's National Law Center, 2019). Their lower-paying jobs are often without benefits or pensions causing them to rely on Social Security as a sole source of income. However, their average payments are $4,500 less than those of men (Women's National Law Center, 2019), with Social Security benefits constituting 90% of the income for women 65 and older. In comparison to their male counterparts, a much larger proportion of women, 60% as compared to 20% of retired men, have insufficient income to cover their basic needs resulting in them having less financial security and greater financial worries (Women's Naational Law Center, 2019).

Women also struggle within the healthcare sphere. As they tend to outlive men, they are more likely to develop chronic illnesses and impairments that impede functioning and change them from caregivers to care receivers (Kaiser Family Foundation, 2022) They are also less likely than men to have the immediate support of a spouse and thus more likely to be dependent on formal support services to help them stay in the community.

Medicaid is a major resource for women comprising 69% of all Medicaid recipients (Kaiser Family Foundation, 2022). With the median cost of home care at approximately $3,500 per month and nursing homes at $7,000 per month (Genworth, 2015), few are able to afford these programs. As the ability of older women to remain secure in their own homes is often dependent on the availability of benefits, their rights remain vulnerable.

Lesbian, Gay Bisexual, and Transgender (LGBTQ) Elders

The number of older LGBTQ adults in the United States is estimated at 1.5 to 7 million and this number is expected to double by 2030 (Seegert, 2018). The combination of age and sexual orientation places the human rights of these individuals at particular risk of violation. LGBTQ seniors face higher rates of disability, physical and mental distress, and a lack of access to services (Seegert, 2018).

LGBTQ seniors are more likely to be in poverty than their heterosexual peers with the risk greatest among lesbian couples and transgender individuals (Badgett, Durso & Schneebaum, 2013). LGBTQ seniors also have higher rates of disability, mental distress, and a greater propensity for smoking and excessive drinking than others and are more likely to be socially isolated (Fredriksen-Goldsen et al., 2013). If persons require caregiving, it is the family of choice that tends to fulfill this role, but as these caregivers are not covered by the FMLA (Family and Medical Leave Act), providing such care can be a financial hardship. As marriage equality for gay and lesbian couples was only recently put into effect, a large proportion of LGBT older adults tend not to be legally married. This puts them at additional risk as the rights of their caregiving partners may not be recognized or considered.

Older bisexual adults are more likely to experience greater social isolation and are more prone to depression. Transgender older adults are more likely than their peers to be forced back into the closet or forego needed healthcare. According to the organization Justice in Aging, only 50% of senior-age LGBTQ Americans in long-term care said they were comfortable being out about their orientation (SAGE, 2018). Institutional care poses problems with concerns about discrimination, harassment, and mistreatment by staff (Lambda Legal, 2011). Moreover, the Medicaid spousal impoverishment protections established in 1988 to protect the home and assets of the spouse of a person in a nursing home do not require that states treat same-sex couples in the same way. Consequently, partners may be left financially vulnerable in the community.

Additionally, older LGBTQ adults lack legal protection, which leads to higher rates of discrimination in the work environment, living arrangements, and services. The impact of discrimination against older LGBTQ adults results in an elevated rate of physical and psychological consequences when compared to the general older population (Redcay et al., 2019).

In recognition of the issues and concerns facing this population, the Older Americans Act reauthorized in March 2020 included specific provisions to assure support and services for this vulnerable population. These include requiring that state and local departments of aging conduct outreach to LGBT older people and collect data on their needs and the extent to which they are being met and will be included in all program planning. This recognition both integrates them into the community and recognizes their need for responsive systems and services.

Immigrants

Between the years 1990 and 2010, the number of immigrants in the United States over the age of 65 almost doubled from 2.7 million to nearly 5 million

(Camarota & Ziegler, 20219 The number of working-age (18–64) immigrants increased by 42% between 2000 and 2017, but the number over the age of 64 increased by 108% (Camarota & Ziegler, 2019). This older group composes 16% of all immigrants in the country with 73% naturalized citizens (Camarota & Ziegler, 2019; Migration Policy Institute, 2012).

Compared to their native-born peers, older immigrants are more likely to be living in poverty with half having less than $11,000 in individual income per year (Migration Policy Institute, 2012). Not surprisingly, they depend more on public assistance than those born in the United States with most of this assistance coming from SSI. However, with some exceptions, this assistance, which remains regulated by the states, is only for those who are naturalized citizens or for those who entered the United States before 1996.

Medicare offers benefits only to those who have become citizens and have worked in the United States for at least ten years. Those who have been permanent residents for five years may buy into the program. Medicaid maintains the five-year residency requirement for eligibility although states have the option to offer coverage. The five-year rule also pertains to the Affordable Care Act (ACA) as coverage is limited to older legal residents who have lived in the United States for at least five years. During the Trump administration, individuals seeking to apply for permanent residence would be rejected if they had received any public benefits. This would have placed many older adult immigrants from developing counties at risk. However, as of November 2020, this policy has been stayed by a court ruling (US Citizenship and Immigration Services, 2020).

As well as eligibility restrictions, access to services by older immigrants is often impacted by their limited ability to communicate in English (Leach, 2009). This increases their dependency on their families who themselves may not be knowledgeable about specific programs. Such dependency also can lead to isolation and depression, intensifying needs for mental health care (Wilmouth, 2012). The multitude of factors impacting older immigrants and their accessibility to health care is a flagrant violation of their rights.

Discussion and Implications

Older adults are vulnerable to having their human rights violated as age itself is commonly used as a measure of competency, worthiness, and ability. Stereotypes and biases about older people and their functioning abilities contribute to marginalization and discrimination, which implode fundamental human rights associated with freedom, dignity, participation, health, and security. As long as ageism remains unchallenged, it will continue as a detriment to policies that support and respect the dignity of older adults.

The implications for the profession are vast as social work's commitment to social justice dictates that it advocate for and promote policies that support the most vulnerable in society (CSWE EPAS, 2015; NASW, 2008,

Sec. 6.01). This means moving beyond the needs-based approach, which often provides the basis for social work involvement with older adults, to a rights-based approach that focuses on policies that secure their mandated well-being.

Social workers can also become engaged at the community level with service organizations, older adult coalitions, community resident boards, elected representatives, and research institutions (including educational and healthcare) to address the needs of older adults and highlight the challenges they face. In advocating for policy reform, social workers must use their knowledge and understanding of older adults to influence and educate policy makers to ensure that key policies uphold rather than undermine human rights. They need to advocate for a United Nations Convention on Older People that would give universal recognition to the concerns of this growing population. One way they can strengthen their efforts is by becoming involved in organizations such as NCOA (National Council on the Aging), ASA (American Society of Aging), and AARP (American Association of Retired Persons), which are strong advocacy institutions that work toward policy changes.

Social workers can utilize their specialized training in social policy analysis, advocacy, and community organizing to lead a national movement to raise public awareness and ensure the human rights of all older adults. In essence, they need to:

- (i) identify and engage multiple stakeholders at the local, regional, and national levels to work collaboratively;
- (ii) engage for-profit businesses and non-profit organizations who depend on older adult consumers in supporting (financially and in-kind) a national movement;
- (iii) recruit and train older adults to engage in political action;
- (iv) learn from national movements around the globe that are effectively addressing the rights of older adults;
- (v) advocate with elected representatives across the country to protect the rights of older adults and enhance their well-being;
- (vi) engage media to raise awareness and critical consciousness among the general public;
- (vii) collect and disseminate evidence on the impact of social policies on the lives of older adults; and
- (viii) build a national consensus and action plan to promote the human rights of all older adults.

As human rights advocates, social workers must ensure that policies are fulfilling rights rather than simply addressing needs. A clear example of this is the lack of Medicare coverage for hearing aids and most dental care. While these may easily be perceived as healthcare needs, they are directly connected to human rights as they impact abilities to enjoy full health and actively participate in society.

Utilizing advocacy strategies such as meeting with officials, letters to the editor, testifying at public hearings, and community presentations on human rights and the rights of older adults, social workers can assume leadership roles in promoting rights-based policies. Given their direct involvement with the aging population, they have access to experiences and case studies that can be powerful illustrations of the ways in which policies and services directly impact quality of life, well-being, and rights.

At both the micro and mezzo levels, social workers can help to empower older adults so that their own voices are heard. Encouraging older adults to advocate on issues that impact them through mobilization, organizing, training, and supporting them in their efforts and helping them to perceive needs as rights are important social work roles. Such empowerment increases self-worth and dignity while providing a framework for community participation (Cox, 2014).

However, in order for the profession to take a leadership role with regard to the rights of older adults, it is critical that social workers examine their own attitudes and preconceptions of aging. Years ago, one of the pioneers of gerontological social work wrote that without a decisive commitment to aging, free of biases and stereotypes, the training of gerontological practitioners remained uncertain and problematic (Monk, 1981). Schools of social work have an important role in undermining these biases by helping to ensure that students are offered gerontology courses, exposed to internship opportunities with older adults and that geriatric social work, both clinical and policy practice, is promoted.

By working for social justice and the rights of older adults, social workers can critically impact society in support of changes that affect those they serve and also create a more just society in the process. Yet, working for social justice is not easy. It is a struggle that includes all levels of intervention and depends on the belief that rights can be realized (Wronka, 2008). This struggle is particularly acute as the realization of the rights of older adults impacts both present and future generations.

References

AARP. (2015). *With no COLA increase, AARP urges Congress to pass Medicare Fix*. Retrieved from http://www.aarp.org/about-aarp/press-center/info-10-2015/aarp-urges-congress-to-pass-medicare-fix.html

AARP and NAC. (2015). *Caregiving in the U.S., Annual report*. Washington DC: Author.

American Council on Aging (2021). *How to receive financial compensation via Medicaid to provide care for a loved one*. Retrieved from https://www.medicaidplanningassistance.org/getting-paid-as-caregiver/

Aviv, R. (2017). How the elderly lose their rights. *The New Yorker*, October 19.

Bachelet, M. (2021). *Statement to the 1[1]h session of the open-ended working group on aging*. Retrieved from https://www.ohchr.org/EN/NewsEvents/Pages/DisplayNews.aspx?NewsID=26955&LangID=E

Badgett, M, Durson, L., & Schneebaum, M. (2013). *New patterns of poverty in the lesbian, gay, and bisexual community*. Los Angeles, CA: UCLA: The Williams Institute.

Belleville, B. (2018). *Should you stop working: Guidance for people living with early stage dementia*. Retrieved from https://daanow.org/should-you-stop-working-guidance-for-people-living-with-early-stage-dementia/

Camarota, S., & Ziegler, K. (2019). *Immigrants are coming to America at older ages*. Retrieved from https://cis.org/Report/Immigrants-Are-Coming-America-Older-Ages

Centers for Disease Control (2021). *Older Adults: At greater risk of requiring hospitalization or dying if diagnosed with COVID-19*. Retrieved from https://www.cdc.gov/coronavirus/2019-ncov/need-extra-precautions/older-adults.html

Commission on Long Term Care (2013). *Report to congress*. Retrieved from http://www.medicareadvocacy.org/wp-content/uploads/2014/01/Commission-on-Long-Term-Care-Final-Report-9-18-13-00042470.pdf

Costa-Font, J. (2020). *The Covid-19 crisis reveals how much we value old age*. Retrieved from https://blogs.lse.ac.uk/businessreview/2020/04/15/the-covid-19-crisis-reveals-how-much-we-value-old-age/

Council on Social Work Education (2015). *Educational Policy and Accreditation Standards for Baccalaureate and Master's social work programs*. Washington, DC: Author.

Cox, C. (2014). Personal and community empowerment for grandparent caregivers. *Journal of Family Social Work*, 17.162–174.

Cox, C., & Pardasani, M. (2013). Alzheimer's in the workplace: A challenge for social work. *Journal of Gerontological Social Work*, 56, 643–656.

Cubanski, J., Casillas, G & Damico, A. (2015). *Poverty among seniors: An updated analysis of national and state level poverty rates under the official and supplemental poverty measures*. Kaiser Family Foundation, Issue Brief Retrieved from http://kff.org/report-section/poverty-among-seniors-issue-brief/

Doron, I., & Apter, I. (2010). The debate around the need for a new convention on the rights of older persons", *The Gerontologist, 50*, 5686–593.

Fredriksen-Goldsen, K., Kim, K. Barkan, S., Murcao, A., & Hoy-Ellis, C. (2013). Health disparities among lesbian, gay, and bisexual older adults. *American Journal of Public Health, 103*, 1802–1809.

Dragset, J., Eide, G., & Ranhoff, A. (2013). Anxiety and depression among nursing home residents without cognitive impairment. *Scandinavian Journal of Caring Sciences, 27*, 872.881.

Fulmer, T., Koller, C., & Rowe, J. (2020). R*eimagining Nursing Homes in the Wake of COVID-19*. Retrieved from https://nam.edu/reimagining-nursing-homes-in-the-wake-of-covid-19/

GAO. (2012). *Retirement Security: Women still face challenges, report to the chairman, special committee on aging*. Washington, DC: U.S. Senate

Genworth (2015). *Insights from Genworth's cost of care survey, the cost of long term care*, Retrieved from https://pro.genworth.com/riiproweb/productinfo/pdf/162731.pdf

HelpAge International (2010). *Strengthening older people's rights: Towards a UN convention*. Retrieved from http://www.helpage.org/what-we-do/rights/strengthening-older-peoples-rights-towards-a-convention/

Hurme, S., & Robinson, D. (2021). *What's Working i Guardianship Monitoring: Challenges and Best Practices*, Retrieved from http://law.syr.edu/uploads/docs/academics/Hurme-Robinson.pdf

Human Rights Watch (2020). *Human Rights Dimensions of COVID-19 Response*. Retrieved from https://www.hrw.org/news/2020/03/19/human-rights-dimensions-covid-19-response

Ife, J (2012). *Human rights and social work: Towards rights based practice* (3rd ed.). New York, NY: Cambridge University Press.

International Federation of Social Workers. (2012). *Ageing and older adults*. Retrieved from http://ifsw.org/policies/ageing-and-older-adults/

Kaiser Family Foundation, Medicare's Role for Older Women (May 2013). Retrieved from kff.org/womens-health-policy/factsheet/medicares-role-for-older-women/

Kaiser Family Foundation (KFF) (2020). *Federal and State Share of Medicaid Spending*. Retrieved from https://www.kff.org/medicaid/state-indicator/federalstate-share-of-spending/?currentTimeframe=0&sortModel=%7B%22colId%22:%22Location%22,%22sort%22:%22asc%22%7D

Kaiser Family Foundation (2022). *Medicaid coverage for women*. Retrieved from https://www.kff.org/womens-health-policy/issue-brief/medicaid-coverage-for-women/

Lamda Legal. (2011). *LGBT Seniors raise serious fears about long term care*. Retrieved from www.lamdalegal.org/dc_20110405_lgbt-elders-raise-serious

Leach, M. (2009). America's older immigrants: A profile. *Generations, 32*(4), 343–349.

Medicare. (2015). *When Medicare pays for home health care*. Retrieved from http://www.medicareinteractive.org/page2.php?topic=counselor&page=script&script_id=66

Megret, F. (2011). The human rights of older persons: A growing challenge, *Human Rights Law Review, 11*, 37–66.

Migration Policy Institute. (2012). *Pyramids of U.S. immigrant and native born populations, 1970-present*. Retrieved from http://www.migrationpolicy.org/programs/data-hub/ud-immigration-trends#agesex

Monk, A. (1981). Social work with the aged: Principles of practice. *Social Work, 27*, 65–78.

Moye, J., & Naik, A. (2011). Preserving rights for individuals facing guardianship. *Journal of the American Medical Association, 305*, 936–937.

National Association of Social Workers (2008). *Code of ethics*. Washington, DC: Author.

National Association of Social Workers (2014). *Aging*. Retrieved from https://www.socialworkers.org/pressroom/features/issue/aging.asp

National Council on Aging. (NCOA) (2016). *Economic security for seniors facts*. Washington DC: Author.

Office of the High Commissioner—Human Rights (2021). *Open-ended working group on ageing for the purpose of strengthening the protection of the human rights of older persons*. Retrieved from https://www.ohchr.org/_layouts/15/WopiFrame.aspx?sourcedoc=/Documents/Issues/SForum/SForum2014/Statements/Lane.ppt&action=default&DefaultItemOpen=1

Ottenstein, R., & Jacobson, J. (2006). Gaining a seat at the table. *Journal of Employee Assistance, 36*, 13–15.

Paradise J. (2015). *Medicaid moving forward*, March 9. Retrieved from http://kff.org/health-reform/issue-brief/medicaid-moving-forward/

Reamer, F. (2005). The challenge of paternalism in social work. *Social Work Today*. Retrieved from http://www.socialworktoday.com/news/eoe_0105.shtml

Redclay, A., McMahon, S., Hollinger, V., Mabry-Court, H., & Cook, T. (2019). Policy recommendations to improve the quality of life for LGBT older adults. *Journal of Human Rights and Social Work, 4*, 267–274.

SAGE. (2018). *LGBTQ seniors face unique challenges*. Retrieved from https://www.sageusa.org/news-posts/lgbtq-seniors-face-unique-challenges/

Seegert, L. (2018). *National study finds LGBT seniors face tougher old age*. Retrieved from https://healthjournalism.org/blog/2018/07/national-study-finds-lgbt-seniors-face-tougher-old-age/

Smith Fitzpatrick, C. (2014). *Age discrimination* (AARP Office of Policy Integration). Washington, DC: AARP.

SSA. (2014). *Social security: Basic facts*. Retrieved from http://www.ssa.gov/news/press/basicfact.html_http://www.ssa.gov/news/press/basicfact.html

SSA. (2015). *SSI federal payment amounts for 2015*. Retrieved from http://www.ssa.gov/OACT/COLA/SSI.html

United Nations. (2002). *Political declaration and Madrid international plan of action on ageing* (Second World Assembly on Ageing). New York, NY: United Nations

United Nations. (2013). *World population aging*. New York: Author.

United Nations (1991). *United Nations principles for older persons*. Geneva, Author.

United Nations (2019). *World population ageing*. Retrieved from https://www.un.org/en/development/desa/population/publications/pdf/ageing/WorldPopulationAgeing2019-Highlights.pdf

United Nations, DESA, (2020). *COVID-19 and older persons: A defining moment for an informed inclusive, and targeted response*. Retrieved from https://www.un.org/development/desa/ageing/news/2020/05/covid19/

von Schader, S., & Nazaro, Z. (2015). Employer characteristics associated with discrimination charges under the Americans with Disabilities Act. *Journal of Disability Policy Studies, 26*, 153–163.

U.S. Citizenship and Immigration Services (2020). *Public charge fact sheet*. Retrieved from https://www.uscis.gov/archive/public-charge-fact-sheet

U.S. Equal Employment Opportunity Commission (2018). *The State of Age Discrimination and Older Workers in the U.S. 50 years after the Age Discrimination in Employment ACT (ADEA)* Retrieved from https://www.eeoc.gov/reports/state-age-discrimination-and-older-workers-us-50-years-after-age-discrimination-employment

Waid, M. (2016). *Social Security: A key retirement income source for older minorities*. Washington, DC: AARP Public Policy Institute

Wilmoth, J. (2012). A Demographic profile of older immigrants. *Public Policy & Aging Report, 22*(2), 8–11.

Women's National Law Center (2019). *Women and social security*. Retrieved from https://nwlc.org/resource/women-and-social-security/

Wright, Jennifer L. (2014). Making mediation work in guardianship proceedings: protecting and enhancing the voice, rights, and well-being of elders. *Legal Studies Research Paper*, 14–27. Retrieved from http://ssrn.com/abstract=2477111

Wronka, J. (2008). *Human rights and social justice*. Thousand Oaks, CA: Sage.

10 Gender Identity and Sexual Orientation

Equally Free to Be LGBTQIA+: This Is Who I Am, and We Are!

Tina Maschi, Sarah Malis, Padma Christie, Dean Adams, Rina Goldstein, and Adriana Maya Kaye

Overview of Chapter

This chapter paints a global portrait of gender and sexuality, especially as it relates to rights and needs of the LGBTQIA+ community (Q community) people. It is purposely written from the "insider" and "outsider" perspectives by authors with diverse Q backgrounds and both the lived experiences as well as the knowledge found in the associated scholarship, literature, and media sources. Our collaboration consists of social workers and educators at different stages of personal and professional development from master's or PhD level students and/or faculty members. This chapter is organized as follows: we first introduce the Q population and the key terms and definitions of gender identity (e.g., male, female, transgender) and sexual orientation (e.g., lesbian, gay, transexual). We also explore the important notions of acceptance and the coming out process regarding this community. Next, we provide an overview of the evolution of the Q community, followed by an outline of the core human rights issues outlined by the United Nations affecting this population, such as safety, security, and well-being to address oppression, discrimination, and victimization and criminalization. Directly following, we provide a theoretical and empirically informed analysis based on existing and emerging gender and empowerment theories that address the multilevel intersectional factors, such as intrapersonal, interpersonal, social, structural, and cultural factors, that influence risk and resilience among Q individuals, families, and communities across the life course. We conclude with a review of select global innovations that speak to the promotion of human rights, resilience, and holistic well-being for the Q community worldwide.

Diversity Abound: Q and the Five *W*'s (Who, What, Where, When, and Why)

One of the most diverse communities in the world is known as the lesbian, gay, bisexual, transgender, questioning, asexual/allies, and intersexual community. People from all different backgrounds, cultures, races, genders,

DOI: 10.4324/9781003111269-13

religions, and other identities are seen in the LGBTQIA+ or (Q) community that appears on a worldwide scale.

For the purposes of this chapter, we will refer to the LGBTQIA+ population as either the Q community or Q people. We chose to use the word "Q" as an intergenerational unifying term. In the late 19th century, the origin of the word "queer" among the Q community was once known as a derogatory term (Barker, 2016). Today's older adult Q people were familiar with, and some adversely affected by, the use of this term. Some of the later generations and the older generations embraced this term as a reclaiming and celebration of their diversity, differences, and unconditional acceptance of who they are, gender and sexual identity and beyond. In order for it to be a short form and unifying term, within and without the LGBTQIA+ community, we have chosen the letter Q to be our symbol. It is quite fitting since Q is the 17th letter of the modern alphabet, and it originally is from African and Asiatic languages. It is also mostly associated with the term "Queen," which has multiple meanings within and without the gay community, including being born of royal bloodline and lineage and feminine power (Merriam-Webster, 2020). The term "queen" can also be connected to the most powerful chess piece that each player can use to move any number of unobstructed squares in any direction along a rank, file, or diagonal, regardless of what is standing in the queen's way.

As for human rights, LGBTQIA+ has been classified as a "vulnerable population." The United Nations (UN) recognizes a list of key terms and definitions to represent the Q community, including GBT/LGBTI, Transgender/Trans, Sexual Orientation, Gender Identity, and Gender Expression, as defined in List 10.1 (UN, 2017). Also found in List 10.1 are our recommendations for the UN and advocates on how to use more affirming language when describing Q community subgroups (e.g., gay, lesbian, transgender, bisexual).

List 10.1 *Gender and Sexual Identities and Orientation: Key Terms and Definitions* (Maschi & Kaye, 2019)

In this next section, we provide the key terms and definitions used by the United Nations for what they refer to as GBT/LGBTI people (UN, 2017). They are reviewed in order, respectively. In italics, we also provide our commentary for those definitions that fell short of queer affirming.

- **GBT/LGBTI:** The United Nations asserts that "LGBTI" stands for "lesbian, gay, bisexual, transgender and intersex." This definition also conveys that different cultures may use a variety of terms to describe the Q community and those who exhibit non-binary gender identities.

- **Transgender/Trans:** The United Nations defines Transgender (or "trans") as an umbrella term used to describe a wide range of identities whose appearance and characteristics are perceived as gender atypical—including transsexual people, cross-dressers (sometimes referred to as "transvestites"), and people who identify as third gender."
    - Our recommendations for this definition include omitting the word "transvestites" due to its derogatory and outdated implications and, instead, replacing it with "trans." Lastly, the term "crossdressers" may or may not fall under the category of transgender due to cisgender populations "crossdressing" as an expression, but not a gender identity.
- **Sexual Orientation:** The United Nations describe sexual orientation as a reference to a person's physical, romantic, and/or emotional attraction toward other people. Everyone has a sexual orientation, which is part of their identity. Gay men and lesbians are attracted to individuals of the same sex as themselves. Heterosexual people are attracted to individuals of a different sex from themselves. Bisexual (sometimes shortened to "bi") people may be attracted to individuals of the same or different sex. Sexual orientation is not related to gender identity and sex characteristics.
    - Our recommendations for this definition would be to add that sexual orientation is a spectrum in which each label may not necessarily be characterized by the full physical, romantic, or emotional attraction of each individual. Sexual orientation is a fluid process where sexual labels are not needed to express levels of physical or emotional attraction individuals feel toward others.
- **Gender Identity:** The United Nations expresses gender identity as a deeply felt and experienced sense of one's own gender. Everyone has a gender identity, which is part of their overall identity. A person's gender identity is typically aligned with the sex assigned to them at birth. Transgender (sometimes shortened to "trans") is an umbrella term used to describe people with a wide range of identities—including transsexual people, cross-dressers (sometimes referred to as "transvestites"), people who identify as third gender, and others whose appearance and characteristics are seen as gender atypical and whose sense of their own gender is different to the sex that they were assigned at birth.

   - Our recommendations for this definition would be to see previous comments about the terms "transvestite" and "cross-dresser" in the "transgender/trans" definition cited earlier. Additionally, we would also emphasize adding nonbinary populations to the "third gender" portion of the definition, as a related gender identity.
- **Gender Expression:** The United Nations defines gender expression as the way in which we express our gender through actions and appearance. Gender expression can be any combination of masculine, feminine, and androgynous.

Additionally, we have collectively made the following recommendations to replace commonly used phrases, which describe a dislike or prejudice toward Q communities. The words "homophobia" or "transphobia" do not describe an individual's fear toward Q-communities or gender-variant populations. Instead, it may represent in exposure, misrepresentation, or discriminatory beliefs, or practices against Q-community members. Some phrases to replace this term could be: *Disorientation, Trans-disorientation*, or *Disinclined Exposure*

We have added additional insight into descriptions of key terms for the Q community:

- **LGBTQIA+—**a common abbreviation to describe the subgroups: Lesbian, Gay, Bisexual, Pansexual, Transgender, Genderqueer, Queer, Intersexed, Agender, Asexual, and Ally community. These subgroups represent the diversity of gender identity/fluidity and/or sexual orientations of the LGBTQIA+ community.
- **Gender Identity:** One's innermost concept of self as male, female, a blend of both or neither—how individuals perceive themselves and what they call themselves. One's gender identity can be the same or different from their sex assigned at birth.
- **Gender Fluidity:** refers to the ability to freely and knowingly become one of many of a limitless number of genders, for any length of time, at any rate of change. *Gender fluidity* recognizes no borders or rules of gender.
- **Sexual Orientation:** "An inherent or immutable enduring *emotional, romantic* or *sexual* attraction" (*e.g., love, affection, appreciation, desire*) to other people (e.g., same sex or gender, opposite sex or gender, both sexes or genders).
- **Sexual Orientation:** An inherent or immutable enduring emotional, romantic, or sexual attraction to other people *(e.g., love, affection, appreciation, desire).*

In regard to the total number of people who identify as Q people, research is limited in accurately producing a percentage of Q people who exist worldwide. This limitation is potentially caused by the homophobic discrimination Q people experience when identifying with a sexual orientation and/or gender outside the heteronormative culture. Therefore, the percentage of Q people in the world might reflect a larger number than expected. According to Jones (2021), the Q community in the United States make up about 5.6% of the population, which is approximately 18 to 19 million individuals. On an international scale, approximately 3.22% of adult women and 3.37% of adult men identify as lesbian, gay, and bisexual (Pachankis & Bränström, 2019). Based on these statistics, the world has an approximately 257 million people who fall outside the heterosexual identity. As research pertaining to the Q community continues, it is no surprise to see the rates of people identifying as something outside cis/heterosexual, which is growing (Varella, 2021). Additionally, countries around the world are increasingly growing with acceptance of people who decide to come out as queer, which demonstrates a positive worldwide shift in perspectives (Poushter & Kent, 2020).

This international Q community is also connected by their differing identities that fall outside the heterosexual orientation and heteronormative identity. Despite the potential complications queer people face for simply being different than the norm, several positive personal conceptualizations are formulated by people who identify within the community. According to Harper and colleagues (2012), both flexibility and connectedness are two protective factors that provide Q people with a sense of comfortability and feelings of belonging. In regard to flexibility, research shows that queer people have the opportunity to explore relationships with people outside the heteronormative gender they are expected to be with. In addition, being in the Q community is "about operating beyond powers and controls that enforce normativity" (Nash, 2013). Q people also have the flexibility to express themselves in ways that go against the traditional way, which increases the level of authenticity one has with their identity (Harper et al., 2012). Lastly, Q community members have an increasing level of connection among each other, which fosters an environment of acceptance and love.

The Global Acceptance and Coming Out Process

The Q community is widely known for their resilience even though they face adverse life experiences, such as micro and macro level discrimination on a national and international scale. The level of acceptance for the Q community has been on an upward trend over the past two decades. According to Poushter and Kent (2020), many countries that were surveyed in 2002 showed a significant increase in acceptance for the Q community when resurveyed in 2019. Countries such as South Africa, South Korea, and India, who originally expressed a lack of acceptance when initially surveyed, are slowly beginning to have a shift in societal perspective of sexual orientations and identities outside the heterosexual norm. Research also shows younger generations, regardless of the country, tend to have higher rates of acceptance for the Q community.

Similarly, the "coming out" rate of Q individuals is also on the rise. For example, in the United States, one in six adults who are in "Generation Z" identify as queer, which is the most ever seen within one single generation (Jones, 2021). According to the Youth Risk Behavior Surveillance Survey (as cited in Giordano, 2020), teenagers in the United States during the year 2009 7.3% identified as a part of the Q community, whereas in the year 2017, the percentage increased to 14.3%. This research also reported individuals who identify as female were twice as likely to identify as queer than their male counterparts.

Q History

Looking back at LGBTQIA+ history can inform how we shape a Q human rights agenda that relates to beliefs, practices, and policies within the Q community and the wider society. Throughout history and throughout cultures, there is evidence that same-sex relationships existed, though sometimes criminalized (Morris, 2019). As early as BCE, homosexuality can be seen in the lyrics of Sappho. There is evidence that in Afghanistan, as well as in Albania, children often lived as those of the opposite sex, and others. The prohibition of homosexuality in the Bible implies that it existed in ancient Israel. In Ancient Greece, homosexuality was alive and well. Across time and cultures, "two-spirited" individuals, "female husbands" and people who lived some of their lives as the opposite sex existed. Via various channels, such as missionaries' documentation, travelers' accords, anthropologists' reports, and diplomats' notes, lifestyles that differed from traditional cis-heteronormative ones became better known to the Western world.

For Q history buffs and gamers, the United Nations offers a virtual and interactive history (from 1799 to 2019) of the Q community's "right to love" (UN, 2019; see the history of the right to love if you are gay at United Nations Website Free and Equal Website). This visual map portrays the histories of global countries' records of treatment with the term they use as "same-sex relations" to represent diverse relationships that have and do exist as noted throughout place and time. The Q map also illustrates countries' progress on policies and practices that have criminalized, decriminalized, or re-criminalized starting from 1799. This visual portrayal of a poignant tale of how colonization has attempted to spread fear-based homophobic legislation to many parts of the world. Viewers also see how time influences the successive waves of legal reforms in one global location, others in proximal or distal locations (UN, 2019).

List 10.2 Articles of the UDHR

(Bold font is positively phrased, Regular font is negatively phrased)

Article 1: Right to Equality
Article 2: Freedom from Discrimination
Article 3: Right to Life, Liberty, Personal Security
Article 4: Freedom from Slavery
Article 5: Freedom from Torture and Degrading Treatment
Article 6: Right to Recognition as a Person before the Law
Article 7: Right to Equality before the Law
Article 8: Right to Remedy by Competent Tribunal
Article 9: Freedom from Arbitrary Arrest and Exile
Article 10: Right to Fair Public Hearing
Article 11: Right to be Considered Innocent until Proven Guilty
Article 12: Freedom from Interference with Privacy, Family, Home & Correspondence
Article 13: Right to Free Movement in and out of the Country
Article 14: Right to Asylum in other Countries from Persecution
Article 15: Right to a Nationality and the Freedom to Change It
Article 16: Right to Marriage and Family
Article 17: Right to Own Property
Article 18: Freedom of Belief and Religion
Article 19: Freedom of Opinion and Information
Article 20: Right of Peaceful Assembly and Association
Article 21: Right to Participate in Government and in Free Elections
Article 22: Right to Social Security
Article 23: Right to Desirable Work and to Join Trade Unions
Article 24: Right to Rest and Leisure
Article 25: Right to Adequate Living Standard
Article 26: Right to Education
Article 27: Right to Participate in the Science, Arts, & Cultural Life of Community
Article 28: Right to a Social Order that Articulates this Document
Article 29: Community Duties Essential to Free and Full Development
Article 30: Freedom from State or Personal Interference in the above Rights

Despite varying degrees of global progress, international efforts to protect the human rights of Q populations are growing in fervor. The Universal Declaration of Human Rights unequivocally declares, "All human beings are born free and equal in dignity and rights," as is seen in List 10.2 (The United Nations, 1948, art. 21.3). During 2020, The European Union has called upon all states to ban this inhuman practice (European Parliament, 2020). Countries such as Albania, Australia, Canada, France, Germany, Malta, Ireland, New Zealand, Spain, and United Kingdom have begun or completed placing a full ban on conversion therapy (Human Rights Watch, 2021). Furthermore, the Security Council Resolution is approaching a 20-year anniversary as being the first resolution dedicated to women, peace, and security (United Nations Peacekeeping, 2020). Within this organization, the Colombian peace processes can serve as an example for future assembly action by being the first committee to include a gender subcommittee along with LGBT organizations working toward validating and protecting sexual orientation and gender identity rights on a global scale (e.g., Bouvier, 2017).

Global History of Q Social Movements

Recounting history, the growth of the Q community social-cultural movements was in response to advance rights and needs to the local and global historical and systemic oppression. For centuries, there was persecution by the religious, medical, and governmental authorities. In many cases, homosexuality was illegal and, in some countries, punishable by death (Adam, 1995; Mendos, 2019). From a clinical perspective, the American Psychiatric Association (APA) once classified identifying as LGBTQ+ as a mental disorder (Bayer, 1987). Subsequently, diversity and difference were essentially an outlier that was dealt with by "outlawing" queerness for centuries (APA, 1974; Gonsioreck., 1991). In many cases, queer people feared expressing their voice or being themselves in trepidation of retaliation. Community organizing was also a risk (Stein, 2012).

It was not until the scientific and political revolutions that organizations and resources for Q populations became available and accessible. The 20th-century progressive era brought on a gay liberation movement alongside the social climate of feminism, new sociological lenses, and anthropologies of diversity in difference (Mendos, 2019). During this time period, diverse groups of courageous, intergenerational queer activists began creating inspiration, forming community supports, developing new human rights frameworks, and sparking the global Q movement. However, throughout 150 years of Q social movements, roughly from the 1870s to today, it has yet to be fully diversified even within itself (Stein, 2012). We must recognize that white, male, and Western ideologies gained leverage against homophobia but did not necessarily represent the intersectional viewpoints around queer individuals that identify with various gender, racial, socioeconomic, and national identities.

The "Q" Quest for Human Rights, Freedom, Equality, Justice, and Well-Being

The Q quest for freedom, equality, justice, and well-being and the global human rights movement tell a very colorful story. According to United Nations (UN) data, including the Sustainable Development Goals (SDGs) data, of 195 countries around the world, the majority (*n* = 125; 64%) have had major advances in equality and well-being of the Q people (Human Rights Commission, 2013). The minority (*n* = 70; 36%) of countries around the world continue to criminalize homosexuality or "same sex related acts" (Advocates for Justice and Rights, 2018). Unevenly enshrined and enforced legislation has been a major roadblock for international countries and states to uphold and protect sexual orientation and gender identity rights. In 2011, the Human Rights Council adopted a resolution expressing significant concern at violence and discrimination against individuals based on their sexual and gender identity/orientation (United Nations, 2011).

The call for action to obtain the goal of equality and well-being for the Q community is widely recognized and accepted, and pursued, especially in the United Nations. For example, United Nations Commissioner, Navi Pillay, Born Free and Equal campaign and associated information and publications has three major strategies (Human Rights Commission, 2013). This campaign is the first of global campaign of its kind sponsored by the United Nations. This global Q initiative (1) identifies the core obligations international states have toward LGBT populations and reports how United Nations mechanisms have applied international law in this context and (2) provides an action plan on how rights-holders can report and seek support in violations of human rights law. This document is the first of its kind and may serve as a guide for future aid, intervention, and protection for LGBT+ right holders. As this initiative evolves, it holds great promise to serve as a guide for future aid, intervention, and protection for LGBT+ right holders. This early rallying call has brought us to our current awareness of the global rights movement of Q people and their allies.

An overview of the history of LGBT Rights at the UN can be found online at: https://historia-europa.ep.eu/sites/default/files/Discover/EducatorsTeachers/ActivitiesForYourClassroom/hr-audio-lgbt-rights-en_0.pdf

"Queering" the UDHR

The Universal Declaration of Human Rights (UDHR) was created as an aspirational document and can serve as a mechanism to advance the liberation, empowerment, and health and well-being of Q people who are identified by the UN as a vulnerable group (United Nations Office on Drugs and Crime, 2009). In our assessment, we felt that 60 years of this aspirational document only partially delivered on this process for Q and other minoritized groups. The UDHR was ratified in 1948 as a response to the various atrocities of World War II, especially of genocides of LGBT people (who wore the pink triangle) and other minoritized peoples, such as people of Jewish descent, and/or with disabilities, and gypsies (Maschi, 2016; Maschi & Leibowitz, 2017; UN, 1948). Q people also have historical trauma associated with the shared cultural background of being placed in Nazi concentration camps (Elman,1996).

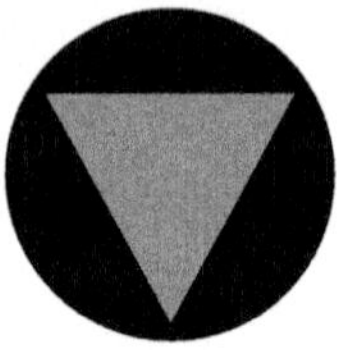

We are remembering the pink triangle (see Picture 10.1) as a pyramid of transformation, returning it from oppression to empowerment. We are placing ourselves at the table when the UDHR is further developed, with our voices present and perspectives honored. In the process of queering this space, we are elevating the UDHR to reflect the affirmative language of queer interpretation in a world where love prevails. We invite readers to join us at the table where we are all united, with our unconditional authentic selves to focus on not what separates us but what brings us together in peace, love, and harmony.

The UDHR serves as the overview document for citizens and countries to create healthy and "justly" societies (Maschi, 2016; Wronka, 2018). Using broad-based and flexible guidelines, the declaration provides some level of diversity and cultural variance in which individuals, groups, and societies can translate these values, principles, and guidelines into laws, policies, and practices. Decision-making is left up to individuals, groups, and societies in how they interpret and adopt these ideals and translate them into tangible forms, such as the development of affirmative Q policies and programs. A diverse, equitable, and inclusive world includes an awareness of the Q community and avenues to ensure that the Q community and their families have representation in leadership positions and design teams to develop and implement solutions, and is of utmost importance (Elman, 1996).

The UDHR is organized within the six major principles of a human rights framework. These six major principles are universality, non-discrimination, the indivisibility and interdependence of political, civil, social, economic, and cultural rights, full participation, accountability, and transparency (see Chapter 2 for more detailed description). These principles are relevant to the Q community and their "rainbow rights" as the Q+ culture pursues liberation, equality, and well-being, especially as it relates to being universally recognized and treated with dignity and respect with access to all rights to participate in politics and their community in the process (Maschi et al., 2015; Maschi, 2016; UN, 2017).

Perhaps the most resonant UDHR rights for the Q community quest for equality is as noted earlier: "All human beings are born free and equal in dignity and rights" and "respect for the inherent dignity and equal and inalienable rights" of all human beings. As echoed in the UN LGBTQ+ campaign, Born Free and Equal, this is clearly a rally call that speaks to and unites the Q and allied cultures (UN, 1948, p. 1; UN, 2019).

Rainbow Reflection Activity: From Facing Down to Facing Up

As we think about how relevant the UDHR has been for the Q community, we reflect on the Holocaust, visualizing the pink triangle worn by Q detainees in the concentration camps. We visualize that the original downward-facing pink triangle symbolized as "less than human" is transformed into an upright resilient pyramid that fosters human potential, expansion, and growth. From this Q empowered space, we are equal participants among the global dignitaries in the crafting of the UDHR. We are present, we speak our truth, and our voices are heard. This process allows us to honor ourselves and release burdens and we reclaim the UDHR with the dance of the light fandango.

We express honor to those who came before us, to ourselves, and all living beings. As we queer this space, we embody the positive so that we best reflect affirmative language that will help create the world that we really want for all living beings.

We are elevating the UDHR to reflect the affirmative language of queer interpretation in a world where love prevails. We invite readers to join us at the table where we are all united, with our unconditional authentic selves to focus on not what separates us but that which brings us together in peace, love, and harmony.

The State of Rainbow Rights

In face of the criminalization of Q people around the world today, and legislation preventing Q community rights, additional safety and security of Q individuals need further efforts to be fully achieved. The good news is that as this growing recognition of the barriers and persistence of human rights violations that impede Q Liberation, there is a wide-scale buy-in and perhaps is universally accepted as part of the United Nations mission. For example, there is increased visibility of Q+ campaigns, such as that one spreadhead by the United Nations Commissioner, Navi Pillay, who created the Born Free and Equal website and reports, and booklets (UN, 2019). This campaign identifies the core obligations international states have toward LGBT populations, as well as how United Nations mechanisms apply international law across diverse global regions and provides an action plan on how rights-holders can report and call upon States to address breaches of international human rights law. This affirmative document is the first of its kind and may serve as a guide for future aid, intervention, and protection for LGBT+ right holders. (For the full version of the document see the chapter appendix for weblinks.)

The very visible attention to Q rights also suggests that the UN's focus moves from a problem/negative focus to a solution/positive focused approach. We underscore the importance of this approach to the Q community, which focuses on resilience and risks with suggested solution-focused movements for remedy. The Born Free and Equal Campaign provides a mechanism of change that promotes global awareness of the struggles but also the resilience in the Q community (Maschi et al., 2020). See the chapter appendix for some suggested readings about this global awareness campaign.

The United Nations Development Program's (UNDP) Human Development Report is as follows. In its "Strategic Plan: 2014–2017," UNDP (2013) defines *inclusion* as "access to opportunities and achievement of outcomes, as captured in human development indices, especially women, female-headed households and youth." Thus, inclusion means that every person has access to opportunities (including the capabilities to do and be as one chooses) and is able to make choices that lead to outcomes consistent with human dignity. While inclusion should be, on one level, universal, UNDP also recognizes that members of certain groups are excluded. These include women, female-headed households, youth, and potentially other groups, such as Q people.

UDHR Values and Principles

The values of the UDHR are particularly to invoke our re-envisioning of the UDHR. We recognize these values in ourselves and others. We recite: I honor and respect the dignity and worth of all persons, the earth, and all living beings. I express compassion, peace, and unconditional love. I recognize the importance of unconditional freedom, care, justice, connection and belonging, service to others, solidarity, and empowerment. These truths belong to everyone, universality, with no exceptions, non-discriminatory, to receive all of the gifts that life can offer for every being to live with purpose, passion, and joy (political, civil, social, economic, and cultural rights, full participation, accountability, and transparency). Please see Chapter 2 for a detailed description of human rights framework (UN, 1948).

Our reframed UDHR preamble reads as follows:

> We the peoples of the united nations determined prepare succeeding generations with the knowledge, values, and skills to promote a common human that is in accordance with nature and natural law. We affirm our faith in fundamental human/natural rights, in the dignity and worth of the person and all living being, in the equal and variant

> rights of gender, sexual, creative expression and unconditional acceptance of the person, group, and culture of nations large and small and to establish conditions under which caring, justice, and respect for the obligations arising from treaties and other sources of international law can be maintained, and to promote social ecological spiritual progress and the high standards of life in larger freedom.

It will also include the following reconstruction of the Preamble to the Charter of the United Nations (UN, 1948):

> To practice tolerance (non-judgment; unconditional acceptance and live together in peace with one another as good neighbors, and to unite our strength to maintain international peace and security, and to ensure, by the acceptance of principles and the institution of methods, that peaceful resolutions will always be sought and armed force shall not be used, save in the common interest, and to employ international machinery and technology for the greatest good of all and for countless generation to come promotion of the ecological, economic, and social advancements and emerging innovation of all people and planet of earth and all its living inhabitants.

Queering the UDHR Articles (Positive *Versus* Negative Declarations)

As shown in List 2, the 30 articles of the UDHR can be categorized as positive and negative affirmative statements. Of the 30 articles, six were phrased negatively using the phrase "freedom from": Discrimination; Slavery; Torture and Degrading Treatment; Arbitrary Arrest and Exile; Interference with Privacy, Family, Home, and Correspondence; and State or Personal Interference in the above Rights. The other 24 articles speak to the right to equality, life, liberty, personal security, recognition before the law, etc.

As noted in the caring justice solution-focused framework, positive phrasing of statements increases chances of obtaining the outcome we want, as opposed to what we do not want, as in the use of negative phrasing (see Tables 10.1, 10.2 and Figure 10.1; Drisko & Maschi, 2016; Maschi & Aday, 2014). To redress the conflicting language, we reorganized the UDHR articles into positive themes, by clustering the rights with major themes written with affirmative language (see List 10.3). We moved from Human Rights to Natural Rights (Humans, the earth, and all living beings in the Universal Environment). As members of a historically marginalized community in which binaries were created, we envision a world in which gender and sexual orientation are united (UN, 2017; UNDESA, 2017).

Table 10.1 From Problem-Focused to Solution-Focused Thinking and Approaches: Decision-Making

Problem Focused **Fear-Based Thinking (Survival Mode, Contraction)**	**Solution Focused** **Creative Thinking (Creative and Expansive)**
Problem-focused Trauma/stressed/crisis Negative/pessimistic/stressed Dualistic/binary thinking Linear thinking only, Deductive thinking predominant Ego-driven and intellectual only focus Self-preservation Self-focused (ego-centric) Self-centered or either-or impulsive fear-based decision-making Closed minded Irrational biased Judgmental Competitive Power over vertical Hierarchy/domination Control-focused Criticizes/discriminates Does not honor diversity and difference Top down partial decision-making Cultural arrogance	Solution-focused and mission-driven Resilient; crisis as opportunity Relaxed, creative, positive, optimistic Unity/collective (I/We) systems thinking Linear and systems thinking Circular/deductive and inductive thinking Heart driven, emotional, compassionate Group-focused Open-minded Collective centered decision-making (for the highest good of all; sustainable) Positive thoughts and emotions Fair and non-judgmental, compassionate caring Horizontal power within/power with model Non-judgmental Collaboration/partnerships Honors diversity and difference Grass roots participation; bottoms up approach] Shared decision-making Cultural humility

Source: *Maschi & Morgen, 2020; Maschi et al., 2020*

Table 10.2 From Problem to Creative Solution Focus—Part 1: Example Identified Issues/Problems

Levels of Assessment and Intervention	*Problem Focus Example*	*Suggested Solutions*
Cultural Level: Transmitted through cultural, community, and mass media systems	Negative media messages about the issue focus (e.g., showing continuous violence on TV; fear-based strategies about the spread of illnesses and no focus on recovery)	Build an affirmative compassionate/caring justice partnership culture using mass media; watch positive programming on TV or no TV; support and frequent alternative mass media programs, including for LGBTQIA+ people

Levels of Assessment and Intervention	*Problem Focus Example*	*Suggested Solutions*
Structural/ Institutional Level: Transmission through social policies and institutions	Reactionary social action; engage policy campaigns that focus on what we don't want; campaigns that use double negatives, such as end community violence, gun violence, or end discrimination, end poverty Collective phraseology-how we discuss and develop goals and indicators of change Economic and business systems—competitive and hierarchal institutions	Contemplative reflexive social action; engage in positive policy campaigns of what we do want; revise campaigns that use double negatives, such as end LGBTQIA+ community violence or gun violence, and positively reframe them to what we do want (e.g., the compassionate and peaceful community campaign; liberation, empowerment, and well-being
Personal Level: Transmitted through everyday relationships	Uses negative phraseology and disrespectful verbal and non-verbal behaviors; describes people derogatorily, disrespectfully, or by a label; does not use humanizing language or engage in abusive behaviors in personal and professional settings	Use new phraseology and respectful verbal and non-verbal behaviors; in personal life—tell loved ones you love them; learn conflict resolution strategies; n practice—call LGBTQIA+ people and allies by their preferred first names as opposed to their diagnoses; if needed, rephrase the description: a person in a recovery program
Internal Level: Impact of other levels on the psychological, emotional, and overall well-being of individuals	Person who engages in self-criticism and internalized oppressive beliefs	Promote self-directed wellness, self-empowerment, peer-led individual and group support, community connections
Research and Evaluation: Exploratory, intervention, participatory research, and diverse perspectives	No research on the topic; research abuses—no participatory research; findings not available for public consumption Rational focused science; lack of diverse perspectives; control of research and funding by outside parties and experts without the lived experience or situation; all stakeholders not involved	Research from diverse perspectives and ways of knowing; use of qualitative, quantitative, mixed methods, participatory, and emerging methods (evaluation of assessment interventions at all levels); engage key stakeholders in research, especially as the researchers and not just the "researched"; grassroots, community-based led research initiatives that engage all key stakeholders in identifying the problem(s) and solutions (Maschi & Youdin, 2012; Maschi, 2016)

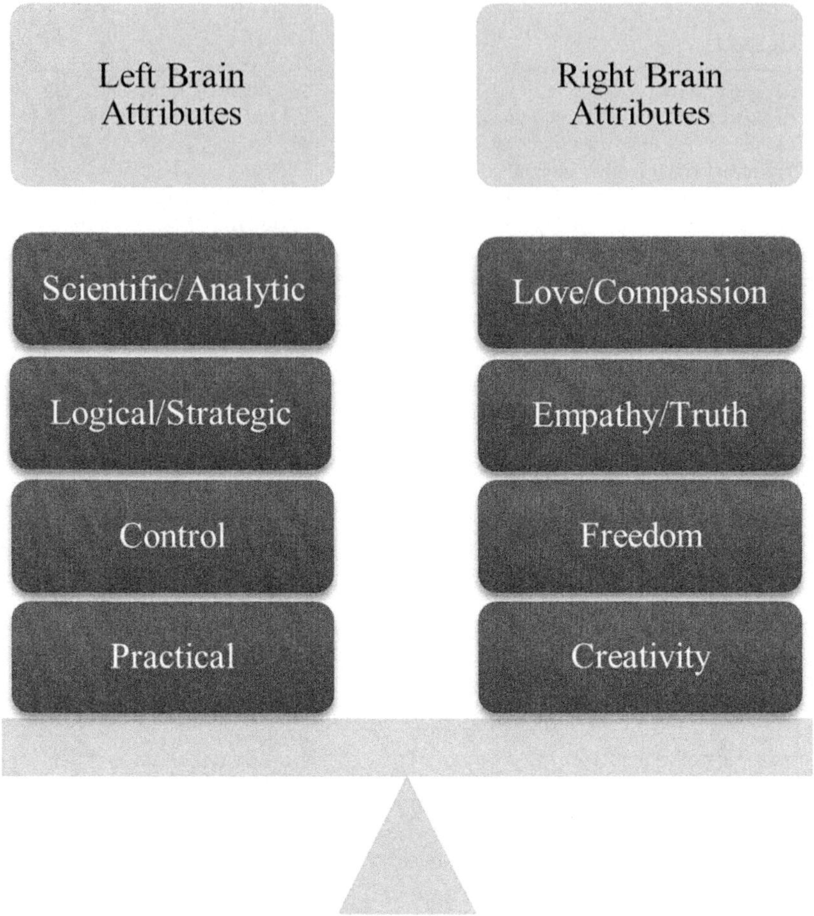

Figure 10.1 Select Left and Right Brain Attributes

List 10.3 UDHR Positive Declarations

(Major affirmative themes of the UDHR for individuals, groups, families, communities, organizations, and societies).

Our queering of the 17 goals in your and my world, found below are abundance, wealth, prosperity abounds, food is plentiful, health is wellbeing, gender is in balance, cleansed love, light, and hot and cold.

I/We express gratitude and appreciation for these universal rights and commitment to uphold these rights for myself and others. These positive truths that I/We have are the:

1. Right to Life, Liberty, Freedom, and Movement
2. Right to Safety, Security, and Protection
3. Right to Unconditional Love, Recognition, and Acceptance
4. Right to Authenticity, Independence, Self Determination
5. Right to Health, Wealth/Prosperity/Abundance, Happiness, and Holistic Well-Being
6. Right to a Vocation (e.g., work), Avocation (to be of service/express universal love)
7. Right to Equality, Justice, Order, Fairness, Truth (Mutual Accountability and Transparency)
8. Right to Innocence (non-judgment, non-guilty)
9. Right to Love, Right Relationships and Mutual Supports with Family, Peers, Affiliates, Neighbors, and Support
10. Right to the Participate in the Arts, Sciences, and the Cultural Life of the Community
11. Right to Beliefs, Conscience, and Spirituality and Contemplative Beingness
12. Right to Diversity and Inclusion, Association, and Belonging
13. Right to Natural Rights and Solidarity Rights

The 17 Sustainable Development Goals (SDGs) to Transform Our World

Also of relevance to the Q community are these equal recognition and inclusions to the promise of the positive results of Sustainable Development Goals (SDGs, see List 10.4). The SDGs are the blueprint to achieve a better and more sustainable future for humans, the earth, and all living beings (UN, 2017; UNDESA, 2017). Building on the achievement of the millennium development goals MDGs (e.g., achieve financial well-being, education, gender equality, health, environmental sustainability, and global partnerships) to address the global challenges we face, including poverty, inequality, climate change, environmental degradation, peace and justice, unduly affects the Q community along with other minoritized communities. Although these SDGs are important, we bold print goals that address the Q communities, especially related to the social determinants of health and justice (access to financial, food security, safety, health, education, gender equality, work, peace, cooperation and partnerships, justice, and strong institutions), as is seen in List 10.4.

List 10.4 UN SDGs

The highlighted goals next pertain to Intersectional Q equality rights regarding access to rights, health, and justice.

Goal 1: no poverty
Goal 2: zero hunger
Goal 3: good health and well-being
Goal 4: quality education
Goal 5: gender equality
Goal 6: clean water and sanitation
Goal 7: affordable and clean energy
Goal 8: decent work and economic growth
Goal 9: industry, innovation and infrastructure
Goal 10: reduced inequality
Goal 11: sustainable cities and communities
Goal 12: responsible consumption and production
Goal 13: climate action
Goal 14: life below water
Goal 15: life on land
Goal 16: peace and justice strong institutions
Goal 17: partnerships to achieve the goal

Theoretical Underpinning for the Next Wave of the LGBTQIA+ Culture: Individual, Relational, Collective Liberation, and Empowerment

Caring Justice Partnership Perspective for Q and Minoritized Groups

The Caring Justice Partnership Perspective (CJPP) is a conceptual/theoretical model that offers a heart-centered philosophy that infuses the core principles of care and justice (e.g, Maschi & Morgen, 2020; Maschi et al., 2020). Given the historic oppression of Q and other minoritized groups, adopting a perspective that is heart and value centered is an imperative. This perspective can be applied as a solution to individual and societal unsolved problems that involve simple problems or even complex problems affecting multiple systems (Maschi et al., 2020). This includes problems such as violence, crime, health, and justice disparities that intersect with the political, social, economic, health systems, local and global systems, especially related to the Q community.

This perspective aligns and compliments feminist and human rights perspectives for promoting awareness, liberation, and empowerment. Given the importance of gender identity, these perspective offers a balanced perspective and recognize the masculine and feminine principles innate in all individuals whether they identify as male, female, transgender, or other. Additionally, it intentionally does so by moving from problem-focused (negative) thinking to solution-focused (positive) thinking to focus on the ideal. For example, Q people seek freedom from gender and sexuality oppression only.

Q people also equally seek freedom from violence, all injustices, and health disparities. It is important for the wider community to expand their thinking that it is not only about gender and sexual rights but about all of the rights guaranteed to all living beings. Once we recognize all aspects of what we do not want for all of us for the simple task of being "human," we can let go of what separates and instead embrace what unites up. It also will be helpful for the Q and heteronormative communities that we all need gender and sexual liberation if we truly want each of us to be our authentic selves, authentic communities, and have rewarding relationships with our families and communities.

For example, what we might visualize is how to achieve peace, justice, and health for all if human and natural rights are valued and practiced. These values and principles include but are not limited to honoring the intrinsic value, dignity, and worth of the person and developing creative, present-oriented, and solution-focused ways to create opportunities for care and justice through ethics, principles, and guidelines that promote peace, health, and well-being of individuals, families, groups, and communities to support the capacity to overcome life adversities and become stronger—not only surviving but also thriving (Maschi & Morgen, 2020).

New Ways of Thinking and Being

Additionally, Caring Justice offers an integrated solution-focused thinking model (Maschi et al., 2020). It draws inspiration from Einstein's quote: "You can't solve the problem with the same level of thinking that created the problem;" Caring justice identifies the problem and moves into solution-focused thinking (see Tables 10.1, 10.2, 10.3, and 10.4) The Caring Justice is a decision-making and action plan. We also provide recommendations for daily affirmative practices of empowerment. It helps to identify fear-based negative thinking and replace it with solution-focused positive thinking for assessment-realizing diverse, equitable, inclusive, peaceful, safe, and healthy individuals, groups, and communities for all Q people.

For example, the dominance of problem-focused thinking that favors the negative, binary or dualistic, hierarchy, competition conflict, and domination will lead to negative processes and outcomes and repetitions of tragedies (Maschi et al., 2020, Maschi et al., 2021). Examples include the repetition and patterning of global pandemics, political violence, mass violence and genocide, global war and conflict, and climate change. In comparison, a solution-focused perspective favors the positive, I/We unity thinking (*interconnectedness*), holistic circular thinking, cooperation, peace and calmness,

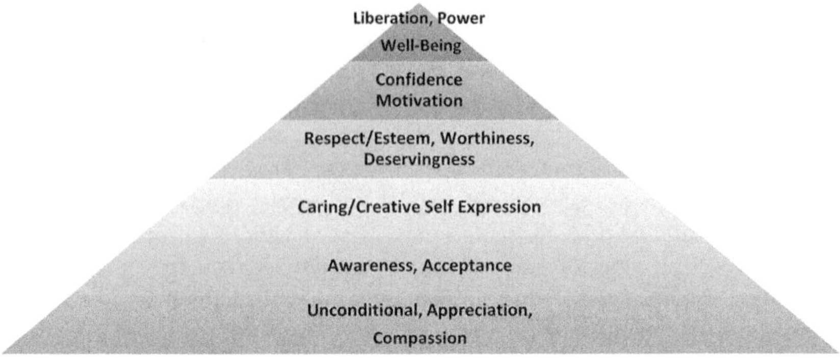

Figure 10.2 Unconditional Self-Love Pyramid

and equality leads to sustainable solutions and intervention designs fueled by peace, understanding, compassion, justice, and equality (see Tables 10.1, 10.2, and 10.3) provides examples of public health and safety problems and outlines differences between a problem-focused and solution-focused perspective and how this impacts the ability to deliver peaceful, healthy, and just outcomes for Q people and their families and communities.

> *This pyramid can be applied to oneself, this model romantic relationships, family, peers, and/or others to map the path to relational power/ empowerment and liberation, local to global communities within the LGBTQIA+ community and the wider world to map the path to community power/ empowerment and liberation.*
>
> (Maschi & Kaye, 2019)

The Caring Justice perspective unconditionally addresses "inner love, justice, and peace," and right and left-brain integration for all genders (see Figures 10.1, 10.2, 10.3, and 10.4; Maschi & Morgen, 2020). Persons and inner and external environments embody aspects of "caring" or "compassion" and are expressive/feminine and nurturing principles as well as instrumental/ masculine aspects (e.g., protection, balance and truth, order, rationality, structure, and rule of law), the system is in balance and leans toward equality. Additionally, the Caring Justice approach is solution-focused, and strengths-resilience based. It reflects the balance and integration of the right (feminine) and left (masculine) sides of the brain that inform different ways of thinking, feeling, and behaving (Maschi & Morgen, 2020). The CJPP posits that finding peace within can occur when individuals take responsibility for healing their inner wounded masculine and feminine selves and get back into a state of unconditional love (for self and others) and balance. As individuals become integrated and whole again, we can begin to cocreate loving-kindness relationships, communities, and the global natural world that flourish. In the next section, we provide some select exemplars of how individuals have created organizations that embody caring justice.

The core concepts and drivers embodied in the Caring Justice perspective are "care" and "justice" (Maschi & Morgen, 2020). These are two fundamental aspects for the health functioning of a complex system, such as the human body as well as a local to global community. In order to survive and thrive, care (e.g., emotional and instrumental care) and justice (e.g., balance homeostasis) are necessary. In the Caring Justice perspective, "caring" refers to emotional and behavioral aspects that include unconditional love, empathy, compassion, authenticity, treating others with dignity and respect, acknowledgment of the worthiness and wellness of self and others, prudent optimism, and unity in the form of inner and outer relational interconnections, and being of service to others. The core aspect of justice is represented by ideals of truth, rationality, balance, order, harmony, morality, and equity/equality. In the model, the critical drive is the presence of care that reaches a level of unconditionality in the form of unconditional love that supersedes sympathy and empathy.

Caring Justice Practice Innovation: Unconditional Living and Empowerment

A Caring Justice process of empowerment maps that pathways to dismantle, release, and/or transform internalized (e.g., homophobia, xenophobia) and externalized oppression (e.g., marginalization, discrimination, victimization, and criminalization; (see List 10.5; Maschi & Kaye, 2019). Another concept that draws upon liberation and empowerment theories is the "Unconditionally Me" mindset (Maschi & Kaye, 2019).

Figure 10.3 illustrates the pathways in which individuals, groups, and/or communities use a conscious practice of unconditional living to boost confidence and motivation that fosters liberation, empowerment, and well-being for minoritized groups, such as the Q community, people of color, and women experience. Through this unconditional conscious practice, the promotion of personal, relational, and mass liberation, empowerment,

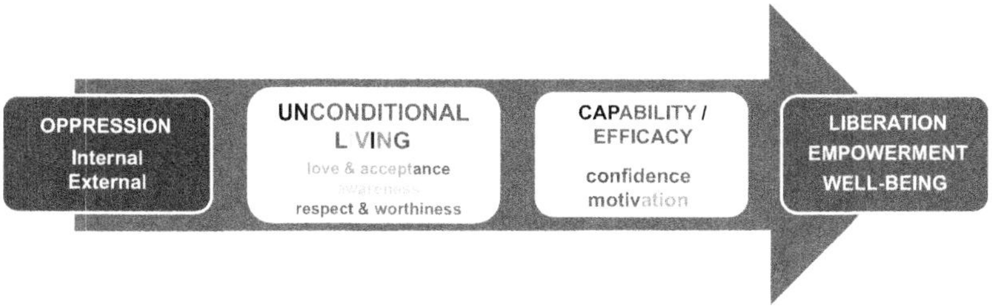

Figure 10.3 From Oppression to Liberation, Unconditionally Me

and well-being for oppressed individuals and groups, such as LGBTQIA+ and their families and communities, can be advanced locally and globally. According to Maschi and Kaye (2019), this model illustrates the pathways to dismantle, release, and transform internalized otherness (e.g., homophobia) and externalized oppression (e.g., marginalization, discrimination, and victimization). Using the aforementioned unconditional living framework can help boost collective consciousness, confidence, and motivation that fosters liberation, empowerment, and well-being.

Using the "Unconditionally Me" mindset can support LGBTQ+ and other oppressed populations to reach their full potential, which includes unconditional love toward oneself and others. We can refer to a definition of unconditional love, which posits that this declaration of self-love transcends all behavior, is selfless, and is in no way reliant upon any form of reciprocation. Through this holistic unconditional love framework, the promotion of personal, relational, and mass liberation for oppressed individuals and groups (e.g., LGBTQ+ populations) can be used to empower other oppressed groups, from a local and global lens. See List 10.5 for the key terms and conceptual definitions of the model.

List 10.5 Unconditional Empowerment Conceptual Theoretical Terms

Definitions taken from Maschi and Kaye (2019).

- **Love** as the base essence of our being that is devoid of all false pride and fear. It is *Great Love*, love also as appreciation. Love as the source of everything, love as absolute love and unity. Love and appreciation as a daily practice that includes compassion and kindness in action for self, others, and the world (universal love).
- **Compassion as Love:** The meaning of compassion often refers to the ability to recognize the suffering of self and others and then take action to help. Compassion is a tangible expression of love and kindness for those suffering.
- **Conditional Love** is an attachment to and feeling for someone that depends on them behaving in a certain way. It is the old way of love thinking, feeling, and doing. At its heart is the premise that the person giving the love (partner, parent, child, spouse, concept, belief) does so because they get something back in return—namely a response from the person receiving the love (the beloved) that meets their, often unrealistic, expectations.
- **Unconditional Love** exists in the absence of any benefit for the lover (e.g., partner, parent, child, spouse, concept, belief). **This is**

of love thinking, feeling, and doing. It transcends all behavior and is in no way reliant upon any form of reciprocation. It is completely and utterly **selfless**. It cannot be given in as much as it flows without effort from one's heart rather than coming consciously from one's mind. There is nothing that can stand in the way of unconditional love. At its heart is the premise that the person giving the love (partner, parent, child, spouse, concept, belief) does so because they get something back in return—namely a response from the person receiving the love (the beloved) that meets their, often unrealistic, expectations.

- **Efficacy/Capability** refers to the confidence, competence, and capability to produce a desired or an intended result. Key drivers are individual and/or group confidence and motivation to achieve an intended outcome.
- **Self-Liberation** refers to a personal act or process of freeing oneself from internal or external controls. The freedom to be one's "true" self "unconditionally" and pursue personal growth, purpose, passion, and joy.
- **Collective Liberation** refers to a group act or process of freeing themselves from internal or external controls. The freedom to be one's "true" culture "unconditionally" and pursue personal growth and purpose, passion, and joy.
- **Force (False-Power)**

  A disconnected self fueled by underlying fear as a weakness and quick to panic and overwhelmed.

  Accustomed to dualistic thinking and hierarchical relationships (externally focused power, power over).

  Assertion of false power and false control of others and the community/environment.

  Limited inner and outer awareness, integrity, understanding, and compassion.

  Fueled by underlying fear as a weakness and quick to panic and overwhelmed.

  Accustomed to dualistic thinking and hierarchical relationships (externally focused power, power over).

  Assertion of false power and false control of others and the community/environment.

  - Limited inner and outer awareness, integrity, understanding, and compassion.

- **True Power as Empowerment**

  - A unified self-fueled by an internal inner awareness, strength, and resilience.

Accustomed to vertical egalitarian relationships (power with) with others and the community/environment.
Emanates, inner and outer awareness, integrity, understanding, and compassion.
Fueled by an internal inner awareness, strength, and resilience.
Accustomed to vertical egalitarian relationships (power with) with others and the community/environment.

- Emanates, inner and outer awareness, integrity, understanding, and compassion.

Related Resources

For those interested in using the Unconditionally Me intervention in personal life practice, please contact *justicecaring@gmail.com* or *drtinamaschi59@gmail.com*

For readers who want to dig deeper into Q-specific issues highlighted by the UN, see the Born Free and Equal resource on the United Nations Website (*www.ohchr.org/documents/publications/bornfreeandequallowres.pdf*). The UN also has Fact sheets regarding human rights and challenges facing lesbian, gay, bi, trans and intersex (LGBTI) people and the actions that can be taken to tackle violence and discrimination and protect the rights of LGBTI people everywhere (*www.unfe.org/learn-more/*). They highlight the following issues:

1. LGBT Rights: Frequently Asked Questions
2. International Human Rights Law
3. Equality and Non-Discrimination
4. Criminalization
5. Violence
6. Refuge and Asylum
7. Intersex
8. Bullying and Violence in School
9. Transgender
10. Bivisibility
11. Youth Homelessness

References

Adam, B. D. (1995). *The rise of a gay and lesbian movement.* Farmington Hills, MI: Twayne.
Advocates for Justice and Rights (2018). *Sexual orientation and gender identity,* May 5, 2021. Retrieved from https://www.icj.org/themes/sexual-orientation-and-gender-identity/

American Psychological Association (1974). *Standards for educational and psychological tests.* Washington, DC: Author.

Barker, M. J. (2016). *Queer: A graphic history*. Icon Books.

Bayer, R. (1987). *Homosexuality and American psychiatry: The politics of diagnosis* (2nd ed.). Princeton, NJ: Princeton University Press.

Bouvier, V. M. (2017). Gender and role of women in Colombia's peace process. *UN Women*. Retrieved from https://www.unwomen.org/en/digital-library/publications/2017/2/gender-and-the-role-of-women-in-colombias-peace-process#view

Drisko, J., & Maschi, T. (2016). *Content analysis: Pocket guide to social work research*. New York: Oxford University Press.

Elman, R. Amy (1996). Triangles and tribulations. *Journal of Homosexuality, 30*, 1–11.

European Parliament (2020, September 17). *Determination of a clear risk of a serious breach by Poland of the rule of law*. Retrieved from www.europarl.europa.eu/doceo/document/TA-9-2020-0225_EN.html

Giordano, R. (2020, February 10). *More high school students than ever are coming out, but their despair remains acute*. Retrieved from https://www.inquirer.com/health/gay-lesbian-teenagers-doubled-suicide-rates-20200210.html

Gonsiorek, J. C. (1991). The empirical basis for the demise of the illness model of homosexuality. In J. Gonsiorek and J. Weinrich (Eds.), *Homosexuality: Research implications for public policy* (pp. 115–136). Thousand Oaks, CA: Sage.

Harper, G. W., Brodsky, A., & Bruce, D. (2012). What's good about being gay? Perspectives from youth. *Journal of LGBT Youth, 9*(1), 22–41. https://doi.org/10.1080/19361653.2012.628230

HRC (n.d.). *Sexual Orientation and Gender Identity Definitions*. Human Rights Campaign. Retrieved from https://www.hrc.org/resources/sexual-orientation-and-gender-identity-terminology-and-definitions

Human Rights Commission (2013). *Born free & equal: Human rights, sexual orientation, sex and gender*. Auckland: Human Rights Commission.

Human Rights Watch (2021, February 24). *Global trends in LGBT rights during the Covid-19 Pandemic*. Retrieved from https://www.hrw.org/news/2021/02/24/global-trends-lgbt-rights-during-covid-19-pandemic

Jones, J. M. (2021, April 3). *LGBT Identification rises to 5.6% in latest U.S. estimate*. Retrieved from https://www.gallup.com/home.aspx

Maschi, T. (2016). *Applying a human rights approach to social work research and evaluation: A rights research manifesto*. New York: Springer Publishing.

Maschi, T., & Aday, R. (2014). The social determinants of health and justice and the aging in prison crisis: A call to action. *International Journal of Social Work, 1*(1), 1–15.

Maschi, T., & Leibowitz, G. (2017). *Forensic social work: A psychosocial legal approach across diverse populations and settings* (2nd ed.). New York: Springer Publishing.

Maschi, T., & Morgen, K. (2020). *Aging behind prison walls: Trauma and resilience*. New York, NY: Columbia University Press.

Maschi, T., Morgen, K., Bullock, K., Kaye, A., & Hintenach, A. M. (2021). Aging in prison and the social mirror: Reflections and insights on care and justice. *Journal of Elder Policy, 1*(2). doi: 10.18278/jep.1.2.6 https://www.ipsonet.org/publications/open-access/journal-of-elder-policy/jep-volume-1-number-2-winter-2020-2021

Maschi, T., & Kaye, A. (2019). *Unconditionally LGBTQIA+: Moving from victimization and criminalization to liberation* [PowerPoint slides] New York, NY: Fordham University

Maschi, T., & Youdin, R. (2012). *Social worker as researcher: Integrating research with advocacy*. Boston, MA: Pearson Publishing.

Maschi, T., Kaye, A., & Rios, J. (2020). Co-constructing community with 2020 vision of care and justice. National Association of Social Work Specialty Practice. *Sections: Mental Health Newsletter*, pp. 5–9.

Maschi, T., Viola, D., & Koskinen, L. (2015). Trauma, stress, and coping among older adults in prison: Towards a human rights and intergenerational family justice action agenda. Traumatology. Advance online publication. http://dx.doi.org/10.1037/trm0000021

Mendos, Lucas Ramón (2019). *State-sponsored homophobia 2019 (PDF)*. Geneva: ILGA, p. 429. Retrieved from https://ilga.org/downloads/ILGA_State_Sponsored_Homophobia_2019.pdf

Merriam Webster (2020). *Queen definition*. Retrieved from https://www.merriam-webster.com/dictionary/queen

Morris, B. J. (2019). *History of lesbian, gay, bisexual and transgender social movements*. Washington, DC: American Psychological Association.

Nash, C. (2013). Queering neighbourhoods: Politics and practice in Toronto. *ACME: An International Journal for Critical Geographies, 12*(2), 193–219. Retrieved from https://www.acme-journal.org/index.php/acme/article/view/960

Pachankis, J. E., & Bränström, R. (2019). How many sexual minorities are hidden? Projecting the size of the global closet with implications for policy and public health. *PLOS ONE, 14*(6). https://doi.org/10.1371/journal.pone.0218084

Poushter, J., & Kent, N. (2020, October 27). Views of homosexuality around the world. *Pew Research Center's Global Attitudes Project*. Retrieved from https://www.pewresearch.org/global/2020/06/25/global-divide-on-homosexuality-persists/

Stein, M. (2012). *Rethinking the gay and lesbian movement*. New York: Routledge.

The United Nations (1948). *Universal declaration of human rights*. Retrieved from http://www.un.org/en/documents/udhr/

UNDP (2013). *2013 human development report 2013*. New York: UNDP.

United Nations (2011). *A history of LGBT rights at the UN*. Retrieved from https://historia-europa.ep.eu/sites/default/files/Discover/EducatorsTeachers/ActivitiesForYourClassroom/hr-audio-lgbt-rights-en_0.pdf.

United Nations (2017, October 11). UN free & equal | definitions. *UN Free & Equal*. Retrieved from https://www.unfe.org/definitions/

United Nations (2019, February 5). *UN Free & Equal | THE HISTORY OF THE RIGHT TO LOVE (IF YOU'RE GAY)*. *UN Free & Equal*. Retrieved from https://www.unfe.org/the-history-of-the-right-to-love-if-youre-gay/

United Nations, Department of Economic and Social Affairs (UNDESA, 2017, October 11). *Sustainable Development Goals: The 17 Goals*. Retrieved from https://sdgs.un.org/goals

United Nations Office on Drugs and Crime (2009). *Handbook for prisoners with special needs*. Retrieved from www.unhcr.org/refworld/docid/4a0969d42.html

United Nations Peacekeeping (2020). *20 years of women, peace and security*. Retrieved from https://peacekeeping.un.org/en/20-years-of-women-peace-and-security

Varrella, S. (2021). U.S. homosexuality—statistics & facts. *Statista*. Retrieved from https://www.statista.com/topics/1249/homosexuality/

Wronka, J. (2018). *Human rights and social justice: Social action and service for the helping and health professions*. Thousand Oaks, CA: Sage Publication.

Appendix

Weblinks

Disabilities vision weblink. https://www.un.org/development/desa/disabilities/envision2030.html.

UN LGBT adaptations: https://www.ohchr.org/en/issues/discrimination/pages/lgbtunresolutions.aspx.

Resolutions that the UN has instated to protect gay people can be found here: https://www.hrc.org/news/ten-ways-the-united-nations-has-protected-lgbtq-human-rights

Unitarian Universalist Office of the UN's LGBTQ/SOGI Human Rights Program overview, see *www.uua.org/lgbtq/witness/international*. Here is the International Commission of Jurists' overview of LGBT rights violations around the world and efforts made to diminish them: *www.icj.org/themes/sexual-orientation-and-gender-identity/*. For a general overview of the LGBTQ rights at the United Nations: *https://en.wikipedia.org/wiki/LGBT_rights_at_the_United_Nations*.

11 Disability, Social Justice and Human Rights

The Experience of the United Kingdom

Peter Simcock and Caroline Lee

Introduction

As central to its purpose, its mission and its role, social justice has been a core social work value throughout the history of the profession (Reamer, 2006; Hodgson & Watts, 2017; Poston-Aizik et al., 2019). Social work educators are required to include content on social justice in their course curricula and the concept 'permeates social work definitions and codes of ethics across the world' (Martinez-Herrero, 2017: 16). Many have argued that its focus on social justice is what distinguishes social work from other helping professions (Kwong Kam, 2014; Mehrotra et al., 2019). Despite this long-standing commitment to social justice, an increase in professionalisation and bureaucratic practice has seen social work scholars lament the profession's move away from promoting social justice as its main goal (Kwong Kam, 2014; Postan-Aizik et al., 2019). In a world of increasing social injustice, there are therefore calls for social work education and practice to reclaim their focus on social justice as a central principle and value (Mehrotra et al., 2019; Watson, 2019).

The International Federation of Social Work (IFSW) and the International Association of Schools of Social Work (IASSW) (2018) make it clear that social workers' responsibility to promote social justice relates not only to society overall but also 'to the people with whom they work'. Many of those using social work services are disabled, and as the world's largest and fastest-growing minority population (Series, 2020), it is probable that irrespective of setting, practitioners will work with disabled people. However, just as social work practice with disabled people has been neglected in the academic and professional literature (Simcock & Castle, 2016), disability has been somewhat marginalised by social activists, and the disability perspective on social justice overlooked by policymakers (Mladenov, 2016; Singh 2020). For example, disability is notable by its absence in the Canadian campaigning tool to promote social justice known as the Leap Manifesto. Furthermore, despite evidence of human rights violations across the globe, Series (2020) highlights the omission of disabled people from the minorities listed as being at risk of discrimination in Article 2 of the Universal

DOI: 10.4324/9781003111269-14

Declaration of Human Rights (UDHR) and Article 14 of the European Convention on Human Rights (ECHR). Disabled people's particular needs were also omitted from the original version of the United Nations' Millennium Development Goals (Mittler, 2016). It is therefore unsurprising that there are calls for further work on social justice in the disability research and practice arenas (Perrin, 2019).

In this chapter, we explore what social justice means in the context of disability, before considering two particular social justice concerns facing disabled people: the disproportionate impact of the Covid-19 pandemic and the phenomena of hate and mate crime. Though there are various social work approaches to the promotion of social justice (Watts & Hodgson, 2019), we then offer three suggestions for practice in disability settings: adopting a critical perspective to practice, a focus on human rights and being an ally to the Disability Rights Movement. Notwithstanding the variable disability terminology used in academic, legal and political spheres (Iriate et al., 2016), throughout the chapter we predominantly refer to 'disabled people', rather than 'people with disabilities', as this is the preferred term of the United Kingdom (UK) Disability Movement and reflects our understanding of disability as socially imposed.

What Do We Mean by Social Justice in the Context of Disability?

If social workers working with disabled people are to promote social justice, they need to have an understanding of what it means. This is complicated by the lack of a single definition and the many different interpretations and understandings of the notion (Krol, 2019; Postan-Aizik et al., 2019). Nevertheless, its foundations are found in the concepts of human rights, fairness, equality and dignity (Watts & Hodgson, 2019). When considering social justice in the context of disability, it is helpful to reflect upon the observation of Goodley and colleagues (2019: 987) that 'disability is place of oppression but also possibility'. Not only is an understanding of social justice insufficient if it neglects disabled people (Kittay, 2019), a disability perspective on the concept is vital for the realisation of social justice for *everyone* (Mladenov, 2016; Singh, 2020). Such argument was maintained by the UK Disability Rights Commission, which predicted a failure in the country's public policy goals of economic prosperity, full employment, better health, and a reduction in child poverty and crime levels, if disabled people's experiences were ignored.

Though a very diverse population, various shared experiences of disabled people are considered social justice concerns, such that Goodley et al. (2019: 979) contend that 'disabled people find themselves in dangerously precarious situations all over the world'. Such situations include:

Poverty: an association between disability and poverty is well established (Thomas-Skaf & Jenney, 2020). The majority of disabled people live in poverty in developing nations (Iriate et al. 2016). Nonetheless, higher rates of poverty are also recorded among disabled people in the developed world, including the UK (Ghosh et al., 2016), where the prevalence of disability is also observed to increase in economically deprived areas (Odell, 2016). Notwithstanding disabled people's increased likelihood of experiencing poverty, cuts to welfare benefits as part of the UK's austerity policies have largely targeted this population (Watson, 2019).

Employment: related to higher rates of poverty are the high levels of disabled people's exclusion from the labour market (Iriate et al., 2016). While disabled people are less likely to be in paid employment (United Nations, 2020), a UK-based longitudinal study also found a correlation between the onset of impairment and a decline in employment (Ghosh et al., 2016); similarly, undesired early retirement has been observed among those acquiring impairment (Arndt & Parker, 2016; Simcock, 2020a).

Access to Health, Social Care and Education: globally, disabled people are reported to have limited access to, and substantially poorer outcomes from, education, health and social care services (Iriate et al., 2016; United Nations, 2020). This includes the exclusion of disabled children from mainstream schools, bullying at school and the experience of discrimination at universities, and failure to meet disabled people's social care needs as a result of reductions in welfare services (World Health Organisation and The World Bank, 2011; Ghosh et al. 2016).

Violence, Abuse, Neglect and Discrimination: in her theorising on social justice, Iris Marion Young (see Chapter One) notes violence as one of the five faces of oppression. Watts and Hodgson (2019) highlight that disabled people are considerably more likely than non-disabled people to experience violence; this includes institutional violence, abuse, neglect, discrimination and other forms of ill-treatment (Malinga & Gumbo, 2016; Jenkins, 2018; Thomas-Skaf & Jenney, 2020). Drawing on research from both the United Kingdom and the United States, Odell (2016) concludes that disabled children are more at risk of abuse than non-disabled children. Although there are multiple contributory factors for such increased risk (Gilligan, 2016), social workers have been observed to tolerate neglect of disabled children, owing to assumptions made about the difficulties parents may have caring for their child (Thomas-Skaf & Jenney, 2020).

In addition to the situations described earlier, social workers should explore social injustice through an intersectional lens. The experiences of disabled people of colour, disabled people from sexual minorities, Indigenous disabled people and older disabled people have been described using terms such as 'multiple marginalisation' and 'double burden' (Ghosh et al., 2016; Conover & Israel, 2019; Perrin, 2019). The UN Special Rapporteur on the Rights of Persons with Disabilities (2017: 11) draws particular attention to the 'systematic and multiple discrimination' faced by disabled women and girls, something observed in both the developed and developing world, and throughout the life course (Ghosh et al., 2016).

As described in Chapter 1, the work of Amartya Sen and John Rawls on theories of social justice is particularly relevant to social work. Such theorising can also inform our understanding of social justice in the context of disability. For example, Sen (1999) illustrated his human capabilities approach to social justice by highlighting the association between poverty and disability described earlier. He contends that disability may not only impact on an individual's ability to earn but that disabled people may require additional income in order to achieve the same capabilities (Ghosh et al., 2016); put simply, 'a disabled person can do fewer things with the same resources, than a non-disabled person' (Martinez-Herrero, 2017: 34). Drawing on Rawls' distributive perspective, social justice can only be achieved where a fair share of resources and the benefits of social co-operation are made available. However, disabled people often lack access to necessary resources. For example, Thomas-Skaf and Jenney (2020) report on disabled children's lack of access to therapeutic services and unequal access to adequate support is similarly noted (Mladenov, 2016). Nevertheless, other theorists have argued that redistribution alone is insufficient if social justice is to be attained for *all* people (Kwong Kam, 2014; Krol, 2019). In particular, Kittay (2019) critiques a Rawlsian perspective on social justice in the context of disability, in relation to fair terms of social co-operation. She highlights the limitations of arguing that enabling disabled people to engage in work is justification for additional resources, because for some disabled people, no amount of support can facilitate this (*ibid.*). She therefore contends that to render a theory of social justice inclusive of disabled people, it must be founded on the notion of the inevitable interdependence of all people.

Social workers in disability settings and scholars undertaking disability research are also influenced by Nancy Fraser's theorising on social justice, albeit that thus far, this has only focused on gender, class, race and sexuality (Mladenov, 2016; Krol, 2019). Disabled people's experiences have been understood using Fraser's model of social justice in a number of ways. For example, Shrewsbury (2015) drew upon the model to examine the under-representation of disabled students accessing the legal, medical and teaching professions, and Danermark and Gellerstedt (2004) used it to make sense of disabled people's exclusion from modern society.

The usefulness of Fraser's social justice model in a disability context is evident because of its concern with parity of participation (Mladenov, 2016; Krol, 2019). Full and meaningful participation has been the focus of disability campaigning and the work of the Disability Rights Movement since the 1970s, and in 1981 was adopted as the theme of the International Year of Disabled Persons (Malinga & Gumbo, 2016; Mladenov, 2016). Barriers to full and effective participation are also explicit in the very definition of disability contained in the UN Convention on the Rights of Persons with Disabilities (CRPD). Acknowledging that participation demands access to necessary resources, redistribution is one element of Fraser's 'tripartite model of social justice' (Mladenov, 2016). Such redistribution must involve enhanced access to appropriate support (*ibid.*), such that disabled people's participation in society and the enjoyment of their human rights is achieved (UN Special Rapporteur on the Rights of Persons with Disabilities, 2017). Nonetheless, as the name of the model suggests, Fraser maintains that redistribution alone is insufficient, and must be combined with cultural recognition and political representation, for social justice to be realised (Krol, 2019). Applying the second of these elements to the experience of disabled people, Krol (2019) refers to the pervasive devaluing of disabled lives, and misrecognition of disabled people's worth. Such misrecognition is often centred on the stigmatisation of dependence, applicable to disabled people in receipt of care and support services, and propagated through a 'welfare dependency' narrative, evident in conservative media and political discourse (Mladenov, 2016). Using the example of disabled university students' exclusion from social interaction with peers, Krol (2019) illustrates their misrepresentation in higher education, the third element of Fraser's model. This is a social injustice, as their opportunity to participate fully is denied (Mladenov, 2016). Keeping in mind that the promotion of social justice necessitates redistribution, recognition and representation, we now turn to consider two social justice concerns facing disabled people in particular: the disproportionate impact of the Covid-19 pandemic, and the phenomena of hate and mate crime.

Disabled People and the Covid-19 Pandemic

On 11th March 2020, the World Health Organisation declared that the Covid-19 outbreak, initially reported in Wuhan, China, in December 2019, had been characterised as a pandemic. Although the Covid-19 coronavirus has impacted upon all our lives, certain groups have been disproportionately affected, including disabled people (Lee & Miller, 2020; Smith, 2020). The UN Office of the High Commissioner for Human Rights (OCHR) made particular reference to the number of Covid-19 related deaths among the disabled population. In the UK, while not published until June 2020, official statistics revealing the number of disabled people who had died of the virus were alarming. These figures suggest a two to three times higher death rate for disabled people than the general population; for individuals with a learning disability (intellectual impairment), the death rate is six times higher than the general population (Office for National Statistics (ONS), 2020).

The health needs of disabled people may differ from their non-disabled peers (Jenkins, 2018) and the presence of underlying health conditions, associated with some impairments, is known to increase the risk of negative outcomes of Covid-19 infection (Rotenburg, 2021). Nevertheless, Rotenburg (2021) maintains that health inequalities have exacerbated such risk, a position confirmed by the ONS, which observes a statistically significant increased risk of death from Covid-19 for disabled people, even when taking factors such as underlying health conditions and living in a care home into account. Abbasi (2021) uses Engel's phrase 'social murder' to describe the failure of the UK

Government to pay sufficient attention to these inequalities and the ways in which they have intensified the effects of the pandemic. In a very literal sense, the disproportionate impact of Covid-19 on disabled people illustrates Lundy's (2011: 38) claim that 'social injustice is killing people'.

Criticising the lack of action taken by various nations to protect disabled people during the pandemic, the OCHR published specific guidance in April 2020, making recommendations to alleviate the disproportionate impact. This guidance does highlight instances of good practice. For example, it refers to the Bioethics Committee of the San Marino Republic Covid-19 triage guidance, which explicitly prohibits disability discrimination, and the accessible Covid-19 related public health information available on the New Zealand and Mexican government websites.

In the UK, the political rhetoric and response to the pandemic have been described as 'disablist and worrying' (Hoskin & Finch, 2020). In June 2020, the Disability Law and Policy Project (2020), published *An Affront to Dignity, Inclusion and Equality*, which documents the ways government Covid-19 policy-making is contrary to provisions protecting disabled people found in both national and international equality and human rights legal provisions. In the same month, research published by the user-led disability organisation Inclusion London (2020), *Abandoned, Forgotten and Ignored*, presents disabled people's experiences during the pandemic, which are characterised by discrimination, disadvantage and a feeling that government has either overlooked their needs or treated disabled people as an afterthought. By March 2021, disabled people's organisations had developed a list of 24 ways in which disabled people's rights had been breached during the pandemic; this list illustrated the 'profound injustice done to disabled people by the UK government' (Pring, 2021). Disabled people's rights have been affected in the following ways:

Restrictions to health, care and education based rights: the Coronavirus Act 2020, emergency legislation introduced during the pandemic, saw a downgrading of the statutory duties on local authorities in England in relation to disabled people's rights to social care and special educational needs provision. Illustrating its impact, Inclusion London (2020) describe local authorities across the country adopting different approaches to the provision of social care, such that many disabled people lost essential care and support services. Furthermore, survey findings from a Research Institute for Disabled Consumers study (2020) reveal that 50% (n = 421) of respondents were no longer receiving health or personal care home visits, despite having identified care and support needs. Similarly, over 3000 families of disabled children reported having essential care services stopped (Disabled Children's Partnership, 2020). In addition to the Coronavirus Act, the UK Government introduced lockdown guidance that discriminated against disabled people who needed to exercise outdoors more than once a day, and NHS England visitor guidance prevented personal assistants from accompanying disabled people with communication and high support needs when attending hospital (Simcock, 2020b).

Problems with Personal Protective Equipment (PPE): disabled people describe difficulties accessing PPE, while some direct payment recipients tell of insufficient monies to source such equipment, leaving them either to place themselves and their personal assistants at increased risk of infection or to cancel required support and rely on family and friends (Hoskin and Finch, 2020; Inclusion London, 2020). Deaf, deafblind and hearing impaired people have felt overlooked because of the push for universal mask wearing, owing to the substantial impact this has on communication and interpersonal interaction (Saunders et al., 2020; Simcock, 2020b).

Non-accessible or late information: a lack of timely, accessible public health information has also contributed to inequalities for disabled people. This has included delays in providing Covid-19 related guidance to direct payment users and disabled people living in supporting living accommodation (Inclusion London, 2020; Rook Sweeney, 2020), and a failure to provide British Sign Language interpreters at televised government briefings (Inclusion London, 2020). Particularly concerning is the failure of the Health and Social Care Secretary to produce guidelines prohibiting disability discrimination in relation to rights to life-sustaining treatment in the event of contracting Covid-19 (Inclusion London, 2020). This has resulted in psychological distress for many disabled people, who fear that they will be denied necessary health care (Hoskin & Finch, 2020) and sent a message that misrecognised the value of disabled lives (Singh, 2020). This is not a situation unique to England: Singh (2020) highlights allegations of medical rationing based on disability discrimination within the United States, and Rotenburg (2021) contends that across the world, limited consideration has been given to the prioritisation of disabled people for the Covid-19 vaccine.

Such injustices, often a direct result of government policy (Morris, 2021), have left disabled people feeling that they are 'expendable in the fight against Covid' (Hoskin & Finch, 2020), and there have been calls from disabled people's organisations, academics and Members of Parliament for an independent, public inquiry into the disproportionate number of deaths of disabled people (Abbasi, 2021). Nevertheless, these injustices are not new: the pandemic has revealed and intensified existing and long-standing inequalities experienced by disabled people (Hoskin & Finch, 2020), including those related to access to health and social care (Rotenburg, 2021).

Disabled People and Phenomena of Hate and Mate Crime

UK legislation defines disability hate crime as

> A criminal offence motivated by hatred or prejudice towards a person because of their actual or perceived disability. It is also a criminal offence in which immediately before, after or during the offence the

perpetrator demonstrates hostility towards a person because of their disability.

(Section 146 of the Criminal Justice Act 2003)

In the UK there has been evidence of a rise, year on year, in reported incidences of hate crime specifically affecting disabled people. The disability rights charity United Response cite police figures for 2019–2020 which record 7,333 disability hate crimes reported across England and Wales—an increase of 12% from the previous year (United Response, 2020).

The phenomenon of hate crime directed against learning disabled people (intellectual disability) in particular illustrates the broader impact of social and economic inequalities (Sin, 2016; Healy, 2020). Underpinned by UK government austerity policies, the cuts to government funding for social care have reduced the opportunities for people to live independently with dignity and to participate socially (Malli et al., 2018; Ryan, 2019). The erosion of social care and the welfare benefits safety net for all in society appears to have contributed to an increase in hate crime against disabled people (Disability Rights UK, 2012; Quarmby, 2015). Ryan (2019: 47) contends that the UK right-wing media have fuelled disablist rhetoric, citing among others an article published in the Daily Express newspaper arguing for a 'crack down' on 'sick note culture'.

In addition to the inequalities made evident by the Covid-19 pandemic discussed earlier, hostility and discrimination towards disabled people have also been compounded by the continued public health crisis. Research in the UK suggests that disabled adults have been targeted in public for not wearing face masks (Scope, 2020). A joint survey conducted by UK charities Disability Horizons and Leonard Cheshire reports on an increase of verbal and physical abuse to which disabled people have been subjected during the pandemic, citing examples of people being spat at in public, receiving online abuse for accepting food parcels, and accusations of being 'less deserving' of the Covid vaccine (Pring, 2020a). Value assumptions regarding the lives of disabled people are also evident at a systematic level within the health care system. A UK-based study found that learning disabled people had been automatically placed on an unlawful order of Do Not Resuscitate in hospital without prior consultation (Care Quality Commission, 2020).

The personal impact of this form of hostility is difficult to quantify. However, previous studies have pointed towards the significant impact on well-being that directly experiencing hate crime brings (Mencap 2000; Richardson et al., 2016). Hate crime victims are more than twice as likely to experience fear, difficulty sleeping, anxiety or panic attacks or depression compared with victims of overall crime (Office for National Statistics (ONS), 2019).

In 2017, the British Crown Prosecution Service (CPS) made a statement which sought to clarify the difference between a disability hate crime and crimes committed against disabled people. Crimes committed against disabled people are defined as

> Any crime in which disability is a factor, including the impact on the victim and where the perpetrator's perception that the victim was disabled was a determining factor in his or her decision to offend against the specific victim. Some crimes are committed because the offender perceives the disabled person to be vulnerable and not because the offender dislikes or hates the person or disabled people.

Examples of types of crimes committed against disabled people are

> 'Mate crime' or 'befriending crime': the victim is groomed or befriended and subjected to financial or sexual exploitation; or made to commit minor criminal offences such as shoplifting; or the victim's accommodation is taken over to commit further offences, such as taking/selling drugs, handling stolen goods, encouraging under-age drinking and sexual behaviour.
>
> (CPS, 2017)

The usefulness of this distinction is debateable and raises questions about whether or not disabled people are automatically considered as vulnerable to crime owing merely to their impairment. Such questions have practical importance, as the ways in which both disability and vulnerability are understood by social workers directly influences practice (Fawcett, 2009), as considered later in this chapter.

Although in the UK there is no legal definition of the term 'Mate Crime', the term was coined to describe the sorts of coercive and abusive behaviours specifically experienced by people with a learning disability by so-called friends (ARC, 2013). Voluntary sector services in the UK continue to document the high levels of discrimination and harassment that many people with a learning disability (including people on the autistic spectrum) experience daily (Mencap, 2000; Chaplin & Mukhopadhyay, 2018). The increased prevalence of mate crime affecting people on the autistic spectrum in particular has also been identified (ONS, 2018). A regional UK study conducted by Charity *Autism Together* found that 80% of respondents had experienced bullying or exploitation from someone they considered a friend (Vasey, 2017).

The UK has witnessed high-profile cases at the 'extreme end' of mate crime, which has resulted in the violent deaths of learning disabled people. Steven Hoskin, Gemma Hayter and Keith Philpott are especially notable in that their abusers were regarded as friends (Equality and Human Rights Commission, 2011).

The Murder of Steven Hoskin

In 2008, the Joint Committee on Human Rights produced a report entitled *A Life Like Any Other?*, following an enquiry into the extent to which the human rights of adults with learning disabilities were being upheld. In this report, they cite the case of Steven Hoskin, the details of which were summarised in the press:

> In a particularly disturbing murder case involving a man with profound learning difficulties, a teenage girl and two men tortured 38-year-old Steven Hoskin before forcing him to his death from a 100ft viaduct in St Austell, Cornwall . . . Yesterday, they were jailed for murder and manslaughter. As well as drugging him with 70 paracetamol tablets, burning him with cigarettes and forcing him to walk around on a dog lead, the offenders made Mr Hoskin confess to being a paedophile before killing him.
>
> (Guardian, Society, 31 July 2007)

The serious case review (a local authority commissioned inquiry following the death of an adult with care and support needs) into Steven's death was published later that year (Flynn, 2007). This review highlighted over 40 missed opportunities to intervene by a number of external agencies involved in Steven's life, notably police, social care, housing and ambulance services, pointing to a systemic failure on behalf of agencies to work together. Steven's death was not recognised or investigated as a disability hate crime. Nonetheless, due to his perceived level of vulnerability, it arguably falls into the category of a crime against a disabled person or mate crime (CPS, 2017).

The review's recommendations led to an eventual change in English legislation, placing adult safeguarding (adult protection) on a statutory footing, including the introduction of Multi Agency Safeguarding Adults Boards (Care Act, 2014). This legislation provides a rights-based framework for social work practice with adults in England and a more proactive approach to safeguarding adults. A rights-based approach for learning disabled people is also underpinned by UK social policy (see, for example, *Valuing People*, 2000 and *Valuing People Now*, 2009). This policy is founded on the concepts of normalisation and inclusion in society, challenging traditional assumptions of vulnerability and risk (Wolfensberger et al., 1972; Wolfensberger, 1983; O'Brien, 2006). Nevertheless, without a wider political commitment, which advocates for a joined-up approach to supporting disabled people to access housing, paid employment and public services, there is a risk that this becomes meaningless rhetoric.

Promoting Social Justice in Social Work Practice With Disabled People

Martinez-Herrero (2017) asserts that social work interventions will be ineffective unless informed by a social justice perspective. Consequently, social workers need to move beyond an understanding of social justice and develop an ability to put the principle into practice (Banks, 2006). In the context of increased social welfare privatisation, cuts to social services' budgets, constraining institutional policies, and an emphasis on individual approaches such as care management, to do so is particularly challenging (Ahmed, 2011; Kwong Kam, 2014; Postin-Aizik et al., 2019). In the second part of this chapter, we now suggest three practice approaches that support the promotion of social justice in the context of work with disabled people, starting with the importance of adopting a critical perspective.

Adopting a Critical Perspective to Practice

Critical thinking, critical reflection and critical judgment are essential social work tools for promoting social justice (Morgan, 2015; Mehrotra et al., 2019). Watts and Hodgson (2019) maintain that a lack of criticality in practice contributes to stereotypical and prejudicial views about those whom social workers support. In the context of work with disabled people, practitioners' understandings of disability influence their interventions (Odell, 2016). Perrin (2019) therefore encourages further research into diverse ways of knowing and understanding the phenomenon. Marginalising or ignoring these diverse understandings contributes to social injustice (Smith, 2010).

Notwithstanding the many ways in which a social model of disability has influenced national and international policy and practice, the medical model retains dominance, even in social work education and practice (Perrin, 2019; Thomas-Skaf & Jenney, 2020). Consequently, disabled people are perceived as 'defective folk' (Conway, 2018: 2), in need of professional intervention, charity or pity (Goodley et al., 2019). Koubel (2016) warns that social workers' interventions will be adversely affected if such a model is central to their understanding of disability, arguing that it results in infantilisation and a neglect of disabled people's strengths. This is echoed by Andrews et al. (2019), who refer to the way in which euphemistic language, such as 'differently abled' or 'special' denies both the structural oppression encountered by disabled people and also their potential. The impact of a deficit-based understanding is observed in the medical rationing policies during the Covid-19 pandemic, described earlier. As Ryan (2020) notes, the notion that an 'early death is somehow natural for disabled people is still worryingly prevalent'.

Associated with a deficit-based understanding of disability, and of particular concern to many disabled people, is their categorisation as 'the vulnerable' or even 'the *most* vulnerable' (Koubel, 2016; Stewart & MacIntyre, 2018; Ryan, 2019), a term used frequently during the Covid-19 pandemic and applied to disabled victims of hate crime (Mathews, 2018; Shannon, 2020). The perception of disabled lives as vulnerable lives has resulted in the disempowerment, dehumanising and 'othering' of disabled people and the denial of their human rights (Simcock, 2020a). Overlooking the heterogeneity of disabled people (Jenkins, 2018) and the fluid nature of vulnerability (Stewart and MacIntyre, 2018; Simcock, 2020a), perceiving people as *inherently* vulnerable owing to impairment is especially problematic. It results in failure to address the relational, situational and structural factors that construct their vulnerability, such as economic deprivation, unequal access to health and social care, and the abusive actions of others (Koubel, 2016; Inclusion London, 2020; Simcock, 2020a; Morris, 2021). In the context of hate crime, the vulnerability label may result in victim blaming (Mathews, 2018; Thomas-Skaf & Jenney, 2020) and sanction paternalistic intervention, resulting in over protection rather than access to justice (Simcock, 2020a).

The social justice-orientated social worker needs to adopt a critical perspective on the difficulties disabled people face and challenge dominant yet oppressive understandings of disability (Goodley et al., 2019; Hoskin & Finch, 2020). A starting point is to think critically about the way in which oneself understands disability. For example, when reading this chapter, did you position disabled people as service users only and never as social workers themselves? Mehrotra et al. (2019) observe how disabled people are presented as service users and never as social workers or social work students throughout social work course syllabi. Thomas-Skaf & Jenney (2020) recommend that social workers develop their knowledge by drawing upon the insights of Critical Disability Studies scholarship, a body of work rich in counter-narratives that challenge dominant understandings of disability (Goodley et al., 2019). As there is evidence of internalised disability discrimination among disabled people (Foster-Pratt et al., 2019), it is also essential for social workers to challenge negative self-perception informed by pervasive deficit-based understandings and to influence the attitudes of family members and other professionals (Gilligan, 2016; Freidman, 2019).

Social workers should also be informed by a social construction model of vulnerability (Kwong Kam, 2014; Koubel, 2016). There have been calls to pay more attention to the particular risks disabled people are vulnerable to, rather than the mere identification of the population as a vulnerable group (Simcock, 2020a). Nonetheless, Simcock (2020a) recommends that social workers explore not only what disabled people feel vulnerable about and to, but also the situations *when* they feel vulnerable, paying particular attention to situational, structural and pathological factors that construct such vulnerability. Adopting a social construction model of vulnerability also requires social workers to avoid stigmatising disabled people's dependence (Mladenov, 2016). Reflecting the theorising of Kittay, described earlier in this chapter, this involves acknowledging the universality of interdependence (Singh, 2020). Furthermore, it necessitates social work practice focused on the identification, recognition and promotion of disabled people's rights, on an equal footing with the non-disabled majority, and a move away from paternalistic and overly protective intervention (Koubel, 2016; Potten, 2016).

A final way in which social workers can challenge deficit models of disability is to utilise strengths-based approaches to practice, recognising and reinforcing disabled people's agency, resilience, and resources (Kwong Kam,

2014; Stanley, 2016). Smith (2010) argues that this goes beyond the identification of personal strengths, talents and skills that disabled people may have *despite* their impairments, and exploration of the ways in which particular conditions themselves are conceptualised as strengths. For example, participants in Simcock's (2020a) study on deafblindness describe their dual sensory loss as a 'gift', offering opportunities and insights that would have otherwise been missed. A strengths-based approach recognises the value and personhood of disabled people. In the words of Woodward (2020), 'We aren't simply disabled or vulnerable, we are also the policy makers, journalists, entrepreneurs and everything else you can imagine'. We now turn to consider how a focus on human rights assists social workers to promote social justice, paying particular attention to the UN Convention on the Rights of Persons with Disabilities, a legal instrument that eschews the 'language of vulnerability' (Series, 2020: 81).

A Focus on Human Rights

Like social justice, the promotion of human rights is considered fundamental to social work, as reflected in the IFSW definition. Social justice and human rights are not only conceptualised as interconnected (Martinez-Herrero, 2017), but the securing of human rights is seen as a mechanism for attaining social justice (Hodgson & Watts, 2017) and a socially just society perceived as one in which human rights are respected (Martinez-Herrero, 2017). Conway (2018) contends that disability needs better inclusion in human rights policy-making and public discourse, a position with which Krol (2019) agrees by highlighting a failure to secure disabled people's human rights as itself a disabling barrier.

Social workers may engage in a range of human rights-based practice, including advocacy and activism (Watts & Hodgson, 2019). However, as human rights are 'not just abstract concepts [but] are defined and protected by law' (Martinez-Herrero, 2017: 20), it is vital that social workers have a sound knowledge of human rights legal instruments and how they relate to disabled people's lives (Ahmed, 2011). There is a range of such legal provisions, many of which emerged over the latter half of the 20th century as a result of the campaigning activities of the disability movement, such as the Americans with Disabilities Act 1990 (Series, 2020). On a national level, other important instruments include the *Additional Protocol to the American Convention on Human Rights in the Area of Economic, Social and Cultural Rights*, the *African Charter on Human and People's Rights* and the *Incheon Strategy to 'Make the Right Real' for persons with disabilities in Asia and the Pacific (2013–22)*.

At an international level, of considerable importance to the lives of disabled people is the *UN Convention on the Rights of Persons with Disabilities* (CRPD). This convention is described as the 'highest international standard to promote and protect the rights' of disabled people (UN Special Rapporteur on the Rights of Persons with Disabilities, 2017: 8) and a 'landmark achievement for inclusive law-making [and] disability advocacy' (Series, 2020: 80). Adopted by the UN in December 2006, the CRPD came into force in 2008 and was signed by 158 countries within its first eight years. It was developed by disabled people and is informed by a human rights model of disability, valuing disabled lives as part of human diversity (Krol, 2019). The CRPD places a range of obligations on states, including a requirement to ensure national legislation and policy are compatible with the convention, and responsibility to guarantee disabled people's access to wide-ranging support services. Although no country has yet achieved full compliance, for nations who have signed and ratified the CRPD, it is binding in international law (Series, 2020). Its enforceability in domestic law varies among signatory states, depending on whether they are monist (international conventions become domestic law if ratified) or dualist (ratified international conventions are only domestic law if parliament passes legislation to this effect) (Series, 2020). Nevertheless, even in states where the convention is not directly binding in domestic law, there is evidence that its provisions are informing the decision-making of higher domestic courts (see, for example, the UK Court of Appeal case *Burnip v Birmingham City Council and Another* [2012]). Furthermore, Mittler (2016) observes that even those states that have signed but not ratified the CRPD, for example the United States, have committed to respect the general obligations it imposes.

The purpose of the CRPD is described In Article 1:

> to promote, protect and ensure the full and equal enjoyment of all human rights and fundamental freedoms by all persons with disabilities, and to promote respect for their inherent dignity.

The remaining 49 Articles cover substantive civil, political, economic, social and cultural rights, both positive and negative, and provisions for their implementation and monitoring. Series (2020) refutes the notion that the CRPD establishes no new rights, highlighting multiple novel provisions that speak directly to the experiences of disabled people, such as the right to independent living (Article 19). Indeed, the CRPD contains rights of particular relevance to the injustices faced by disabled people described in this chapter. For example, during humanitarian emergencies, such as the Covid-19 pandemic, Article 11 requires governments to take all necessary steps to ensure the protection and safety of disabled people. Article 16, the right to freedom from exploitation, violence and abuse, and Article 13, the right to access to justice are especially important to those experiencing disability hate crime. The latter is fundamental to the enjoyment of all human rights, yet several barriers impact on disabled people's equitable access to justice (Ruck Keene, 2020). The UN Special Rapporteur on the Rights of Persons with Disabilities, the Committee on the Rights of Persons with Disabilities and the Special Envoy of the secretary-general on disability and accessibility have therefore collectively produced specific guidelines on access to justice for disabled people. Ruck Keene (2020) believes that these guidelines have transformative potential in relation to securing disabled people's substantive rights. Notwithstanding the importance of the CRPD, Mittler (2016) observes limited understanding of its potential among welfare organisations. Consequently, it is incumbent upon social workers to raise awareness of the convention and the rights contained within it.

Although some legal provisions promote human rights, Krol (2019) refers to the role law and policy can have in maintaining social injustices faced by disabled people. For example, Steele (2020) examines the ways in which UK criminal law has contributed to the sustained oppression of disabled people, particularly that related to court diversion practices. Therefore, in order to promote human rights, social workers should support people to challenge existing discriminatory and oppressive law and policy, and lobby against any suggested legal changes that would have such effect (Watts and Hodgson, 2019). In the UK, such action has seen successful challenge to the discriminatory regulations relating to the prohibition of more than one episode of outdoor activity during the lockdown and the NHS England visitor policy preventing disabled people from being accompanied by a personal assistant if admitted to hospital, described earlier in this chapter.

Despite such positive outcomes, by itself, critical knowledge of the law is insufficient for the promotion of disabled people's human rights (Ife, 2010; Series, 2020). Hodgson and Watts (2017) emphasise the values element of human rights-based practice, which involves relationship-based practice focused on the 'human' in human rights discourse (Martinez-Herrero, 2017). In their exploration of social work in adult protection settings, Spreadbury & Hubbard, (2020) describe this practice as informed by a human rights *perspective* rather than a human rights legal framework. This requires more than just legal knowledge, but an ability to recognise human rights abuses, work to empower disabled people to secure their rights, and ensuring professional decision-making is informed by human rights principles (Martinez-Herrero, 2017; Spreadbury & Hubbard, 2020). The importance of such an approach is highlighted by Potten (2016), who describes the potential escalation of minor infringements of rights to systematic abuse. Adopting a human rights perspective necessitates social work involvement in advocacy, policy development, political lobbying and social action such as engagement in public demonstrations (Payne, 2020).

Being an Ally to the Disability Rights Movement

Describing it as essential to anti-oppressive practice, Kwong Kam (2014: 736) asserts that 'being an ally is key to advancing social justice'. Considered practice at the macro level, owing to its focus on the interests of particular groups (Payne, 2020), social workers have allied themselves to rights movements, such as the Civil Rights movement in the United States and anti-apartheid movement in South Africa, throughout history (Martinez-Herrero, 2017). In the context of disability, Foster-Pratt et al. (2019) contend that being an ally to the disability community is essential to the promotion of social justice, and such allyhood is recommended by both the World Health Organisation (WHO & World Bank, 2011) and UN Special Rapporteur on the Rights of Persons with Disabilities (2017). Moreover, collaboration between states and disabled people's organisations is mandated by the CRDP (Article 4(3)). Commenting on addressing inequalities faced by disabled people exposed by the Covid-19 pandemic, Liz Sayce, former chief executive of Disability Rights UK, emphasised, 'We cannot go it alone. We need allies and there are lots of potential allies on this agenda' (cited in Pring, 2020b).

Being an ally requires social workers to consider approaches focused on wider social change rather than methods of intervention aimed at supporting individuals (Watts & Hodgson, 2019). It involves forming alliances with disabled people's organisations and self-advocacy groups at a local, national and global level (Goodley et al., 2019) and forming egalitarian relationships with disabled people (Kwong Kam, 2014). Kwong Kam (2014) maintains that being an ally means working *with* people and not *for* them and that such an approach necessitates the sharing of power and recognition of service-user expertise.

The particular expertise of user-led disabled people's organisations has been highlighted (Morgan, 2015) and, like other social movements (Mehrotra, 2019), the potential for the disability movement and disability activists to effect social change should not be underestimated. Indeed, Iriate et al. (2016: 6) describe worldwide disability movements as 'major drivers of change'. For example, the work of the disability movement was pivotal to the emergence of user-led organisations and rights-based legislation such as the Rehabilitation Act in the US and the Disability Discrimination Act in the UK (Morgan, 2015; Conway, 2018). In the context of social care, one of the most significant changes brought about as a direct result of the campaigning of disabled people's organisations was the availability of direct payments as a means of meeting care and support needs (Morgan, 2015). Activism on a smaller scale is also achieving change, such as the campaigning work of a disabled students' collective aimed at tackling discrimination experienced on campus at their UK-based university (Aylen, 2020).

Being an ally may involve collaborative community organising and development, group work, cultural projects, evaluation work, advocacy, and training and skills development (Watts & Hodgson, 2019; Payne, 2020). Social workers should draw on their networking and relationship-based skills to facilitate collaboration (Watson, 2019), bringing together disabled people and their organisations to address the concerns that matter to them (Thomas-Skaf & Jenney, 2020). Kwong Kam (2014) suggests that as an ally, social workers can assist organisations to identify and articulate disabled people's needs; this in turn supports disabled people to inform the policies that affect them, essential to participation and thus social justice (Mladenov, 2016). Such work has been effective in addressing some of the injustices exacerbated by the Covid-19 pandemic described earlier. For example, a collaboration of disabled people's organisations and their allies presented a statement to NHS England, along with a list of guiding principles, in relation to fears that they will be denied life-sustaining treatment. This resulted in confirmation from NHS England that the NHS must safeguard disabled people's rights. Additionally, a number of local authorities in England decided not to adopt the option of downgrading their social care duties, made available by the Coronavirus Act 2020, following campaigning by disabled people's organisations and their allies (Hoskin & Finch, 2020).

The responsibility to promote social justice via effective social change may leave individual social workers feeling overwhelmed; being an ally to the disability movement offers the solidarity needed (Watson, 2019). Nonetheless, Goodley et al. (2019) argue that learning about disability necessitates embracing the expertise of disabled people. As such, allyhood with the disability movement not only provides such solidarity but also offers social workers the opportunity to explore their own biases, often influenced by ableism and a dominant medical model of disability (Foster-Pratt et al., 2019), and to explore how their professional knowledge and skills can best serve disabled people (Morgan, 2015). As Malinga and Gumbo (2016: 64) assert,

> [t]he struggle for disabled people is not a struggle for [non-disabled] people who can jump in and out of policy making: it is a struggle for disabled people, and all they need is support for the cause.

Conclusion

Despite the view expressed by some within the disability movement that social work no longer has a role with disabled people, we maintain that practice framed within a social justice perspective has a positive contribution to make. It is a complex, yet highly rewarding area of practice. Nevertheless, just as social work in disability settings is often overlooked in the academic and professional literature, so too has disability been marginalised by social activists, and the disability perspective on social justice ignored by policymakers. Though a very diverse population, various shared experiences of disabled people are considered social justice concerns. This chapter has explored some of these concerns and contends that adopting a critical perspective, focusing on human rights, and being an ally to the Disability Rights Movement, enables social workers to put the social justice principle into practice.

Suggested Further Reading

Mladenov, T. (2016). Disability and social justice. *Disability and Society, 31*(9): 1226–1241
Ryan, F. (2019). *Crippled: Austerity and the demonization of disabled people.* London: Verso
Series, L. (2020). 'Disability and human rights. In N. Watson and S. Vehmas (Eds.), *Routledge handbook of disability studies* (2nd ed.). London: Routledge
Simcock, P., & Castle, R. (2016). *Social work and disability.* Bristol: Polity Press.

References

Abbasi, K. (2021). 'Covid-19: Social murder, they wrote—elected, unaccountable, and unrepentant' *British Medical Journal* [online]. Retrieved from http://dx.doi.org/10.1136/bmj.n314

Ahmed, M. (2011). *Social work reform: Promoting rights, justice and economic well-being* [online]. Retrieved from www.communitycare.co.uk/2011/03/10/social-work-reform-promoting-rights-justice-and-economic-well-being/

Americans with Disabilities Act 1990, Retrieved from https://www.eeoc.gov/americans-disabilities-act-1990-original-text

Andrews, E. E., Forber-Pratt, A. J., Mona, L. R., Lund, E. M., Pilarski, C. R., & Balter, R. (2019) #SaytheWord: A disability culture commentary on the erasure of 'disability'. *Rehabilitation Psychology, 64*(2), 111–118.

ARC (2013). *Safety net project* [online]; Retrieved from http://arcuk.org.uk/realchangechallenges/real-change-challenge-mate-crime/

Arndt, K., & Parker, A. (2016). 'Perceptions of Social Networks by Adults who are Deafblind'. *American Annals of the Deaf, 161*(3), 369–383.

Aylen, S. (2020). *Support and action the Exeter University Disability Campaign 2020 to stop discrimination.* [online]. Retrieved from www.change.org/p/university-of-exeter-support-and-action-the-exeter-university-disability-campaign-2020-to-stop-discrimination?utm_content=cl_sharecopy_23876293_en-GB%3A1&recruiter=545676431&utm_source=share_petition&utm_medium=copylink&utm_campaign=share_petition

Banks, S. (2006). *Ethics and values in social work* (3rd ed.) London: Palgrave.

Care Act (2014, Retrieved from https://www.legislation.gov.uk/ukpga/2014/23/enacted

Care Quality Commission (2020). *Reviewing the use of do not resuscitate decisions during COVID-19* [online]. Retrieved from www.cqc.org.uk/news/stories/reviewing-use-do-not-resuscitate-decisions-during-covid-19.

Chaplin, E., & Mukhopadhyay, S. (2018). 'Autism spectrum disorder and hate crime.' *Advances in Autism, 4*(1), 30–36.

Conover, K. J., & Israel, T. (2019). 'Microaggressions and social support among sexual minorities with physical disabilities' *Rehabilitation Psychology, 64*(2), 167–178.

Conway, M. (2018). 'What about disability and social justice?' *Review of Disability Studies: An International Journal, 13*(1), 1–3.

Crown Prosecution Service (CPS) (2017). *Disability hate crime public statement;* [online]; Retrieved from www.cps.gov.uk/sites/default/files/documents/publications/disability-hate-crime-public%2520statement-2017.pdf.

Danermark, B., & Gellerstedt, L. C. (2004). 'Social justice: Redistribution and recognition—a non-reductionist perspective on disability'. *Disability & Society, 19*(4), 339–353.

Disability Law and Policy Project. (2020). *An affront to dignity, inclusion and equality* [online]; Retrieved from www.law.ox.ac.uk/news/2020-07-02-affront-dignity-inclusion-and-equality-coronavirus-and-impact-law-policy-practice

Disability Rights UK. (2012). *Press portrayal of disabled people: A rise in hostility fuelled by austerity?* Retrieved from www.disabilityrightsuk.org/how-we-can-help/independent-living/stop-disability-hate-crime#sthash.zdeR1qPW.dpuf.

Disabled Children's Partnership. (2020). *Left in Lockdown—Parent carers' experiences of lockdown* Retrieved from https://disabledchildrenspartnership.org.uk/wp-content/uploads/2020/06/LeftInLockdown-Parent-carers'-experiences-of-lockdown-June-2020.pdf.

Equality and Human Rights Commission (2011). *Hidden in plan sight. Inquiry into disability-related harassment.* Retrieved from https://www.equalityhumanrights.com/sites/default/files/ehrc_hidden_in_plain_sight_3.pdf

Fawcett, B. (2009). Vulnerability: Questioning the certainties in social work and health. *International Social Work, 52*(4), 473–484.

Flynn, M. (2007). *The murder of Steven Hoskin; serious case review—executive summary.* Cornwall Adult Protection Committee, Cornwall [online]; Retrieved from www.scie-socialcareonline.org.uk/the-murder-of-steven-hoskin-a-serious-case-review-executive-summary/r/a11G00000017tmDIAQ.

Foster-Pratt, A. J., Mueller, C. O., & Andrews, E. E. (2019). 'Disability, identity and allyship in rehabilitation psychology: Sit, stand, sign and show up'. *Rehabilitation Psychology, 64*(2), 119–129.

Friedman, C. (2019). 'Family members of people with disabilities' explicit and implicit disability attitudes'. *Rehabilitation Psychology, 64*(2), 203–211.

Ghosh, S., Dababnah, S., Parish, S. L., & Igdalsky, L. (2016). 'Disability, social exclusion and poverty'. In EG. Iriate, R. McConkey and R. Gilligan (Eds.), *Disability and human rights.* London: Palgrave.

Gilligan, R. (2016). 'Children's rights and disability'. In EG. Iriate, R. McConkey and R. Gilligan (Eds.), *Disability and Human Rights.* London: Palgrave.

Goodley, D., Lawthorn, R., Liddiard, K., & Runswick, K. (2019). 'Provocations for critical disability studies'. *Disability & Society, 34*(6), 972–997.

Healy, J. (2020). 'It spreads like a creeping disease': Experiences of victims of disability hate crimes. *Austerity Britain, Disability and Society, 35*(2), 176–200.

Hodgson, D., & Watts, L. (2017). *Key concepts & theory in social work.* London: Palgrave.

Hoskin, J., & Finch, J. (2020). 'Covid 19, disability and the new eugenics: Implications for social work policy and practice.' *Social Work 2020 under Covid-19 Magazine 4th Ed.* [online]; Retrieved from https://sw2020covid19.group.shef.ac.uk/2020/06/02/covid-19-disability-and-the-new-eugenics-implications-for-social-work-policy-and-practice/.

Ife, J. (2010). 'Human rights and social justice. In M. Gray and S. A. Webb (Eds.), *Ethics and value perspectives in social work*'. London: Palgrave.

Inclusion London. (2020). *Abandoned, Forgotten and ignored. The impact of the coronavirus pandemic on disabled people.* London: Inclusion London.

International Federation of Social Work & International Association of Schools of Social Work (2018). *Global social work statement of ethical principles* [online]; Retrieved from www.ifsw.org/global-social-work-statement-of-ethical-principles/

Iriarte, E. G., McConkey, R., & Gilligan, R. (2016). 'Disability and human rights: Global perspectives'. In E. G. Iriate, R. McConkey and R. Gilligan (Eds.), *Disability and human rights.* London: Palgrave.

Jenkins, R. (2018). 'Safeguarding adults with learning disabilities'. In G. MacIntyre, A. Stewart, and P. McCusker (Eds.), *Safeguarding adults: Key themes and issues.* London: Palgrave.

Kittay, E. F. (2019). *Love's labor: Essays on women, equality and dependency.* London: Routledge.

Koubel, G. (2016). 'Constructing safeguarding'. In G. Koubel (Ed.), *Safeguarding adults and children.* London: Palgrave.

Krol, C. (2019). *A human rights and social justice perspective of disability and participation in higher education* [unpublished thesis]. Western Sydney University.

Kwong Kam, P. (2014). 'Back to the 'social' of social work: Reviving the social work profession's contribution to the promotion of social justice'. *International Social Work, 57*(6), 723–740.

Lee, H., & Miller, V. J. (2020). 'The disproportionate impact of Covid-19 on minority groups: a social justice concern'. *Journal of Gerontological Social Work.* Retrieved from https://doi.org/10.1080/01634372.2020.1777241

Lundy, C. (2011). *Social work, social justice and human rights: A structural approach to practice* (2nd ed.). Toronto: University of Toronto Press.

Malli, M., Sams, L., Forrester-Jones, R., Murphy, G., & Henwood, M. (2018). 'Austerity and the lives of people with learning disabilities. A thematic synthesis of current literature' *Disability and Society, 33*(9), 1412–1435.

Malinga, J. T., & Gumbo, T. (2016). 'Advocacy and lobbying: The road map from charity to human rights'. In E. G. Iriate, R. McConkey and R. Gilligan (Eds.), *Disability and human rights.* London: Palgrave.

Martinez-Herrero, M. I. (2017). *Human rights and social justice in social work education: A critical realist comparative study of England and Spain* [unpublished thesis]. Durham University.

Mathews, I. (2018). 'Representations of vulnerability, innocence and evil in the murder of a disabled people'. *Disability & Society, 33*(10), 1620–1638.

Mehrotra, G., Hudson, K. D., & Self, J. M. (2019). 'A critical examination of key assumptions underlying diversity and social justice courses in social work'. *Journal of Progressive Human Services, 30*(2), 127–147.

Mencap. (2000). *Living in fear. The need to combat bullying of people with a learning disability.* London: Mencap.

Mladenov, T. (2016). 'Disability and social justice'. *Disability and Society, 31*(9), 1226–1241.

Mittler, P. (2016). 'The UN convention on the rights of persons with disabilities: Implementing a paradigm shift'. In EG. Iriate, R. McConkey and R. Gilligan (Eds.), *Disability and human rights.* London: Palgrave.

Morgan, H. (2015). 'Working with disabled people'. In M. Webber (Ed.), *Applying research evidence in social work practice.* London: Palgrave.

Morris, J. (2021). *Why have so many disabled people died of Covid-19?* [online]; Retrieved from https://jennymorrisnet.blogspot.com/2021/03/why-have-so-many-disabled-people-died.html.

O'Brien, J. (2006). *Reflecting on social roles: Identifying opportunities to support personal freedom & social integration* [online]; Retrieved from https://cincibility.files.wordpress.com/2013/03/social-role-inventory.pdf.

Odell, T. (2016). 'Safeguarding children with disabilities'. In G. Koubel (Ed.), *Safeguarding adults and children.* London: Palgrave.

Office for National Statistics (2019). *Hate crime England and Wales, 2018–2019* [online]; Retrieved from www.gov.uk/government/statistics/hate-crime-england-and-wales-2018-to-2019.

Office for National Statistics (2020). *Coronavirus (COVID-19) related deaths by disability status, England and Wales: 2 March to 14 July 2020* [online]; Retrieved from www.ons.gov.uk/peoplepopulationandcommunity/birthsdeathsandmarriages/deaths/articles/coronaviruscovid19relateddeathsbydisabilitystatusenglandandwales/2marchto14july2020.

Payne, M. (2020). *How to use social work theory in practice: An essential guide*. Bristol: Policy Press.

Perrin, P. B. (2019). 'Diversity and social justice in disability: The heart and soul of rehabilitation psychology'. *Rehabilitation Psychology, 64*(2), 105–110.

Poston-Aizik, D., Shdaimah, C. S., & Strier, R. (2019). 'Positioning social justice: Reclaiming social work's organising value'. *British Journal of Social Work*. [online]; Retrieved from doi: 10.1093/bjsw/bcz111

Potten, J. (2016). 'Safeguarding in learning disability practice: Rights, risk, vulnerability and empowerment'. In G. Koubel (Ed.), *Safeguarding adults and children*. London: Palgrave.

Pring, J. (2020a) Coronavirus: Fears over 'face covering hate crime' as new laws go live [online]; available at: www.disabilitynewsservice.com/coronavirus-fears-over-face-covering-hate-crime-as-new-laws-go-live/ (Accessed: 24/04/2021).

Pring, J. (2020b) *Coronavirus: Peer calls for an end to use of 'vulnerable' to describe disabled people* [online]; Retrieved from www.disabilitynewsservice.com/coronavirus-peer-calls-for-an-end-to-use-of-vulnerable-to-describe-disabled-people/

Pring, J. (2021). *Government's 'shocking' pandemic rights list of shame* [online]; Retrieved from www.disabilitynewsservice.com/governments-shocking-pandemic-rights-list-of-shame/.

Quarmby, K. (2015). *To combat disability hate crime, we must understand why people commit it.* [online]; Retrieved from www.theguardian.com/society/2015/jul/22/combatdisability-hate-crime-understand-people-commit

Reamer, F. G. (2006) 'Keeping social justice in social work'. *Social Work Today,* 1–2.

Research Institute for Disabled Consumers (2020). *RIDC Covid-19 Survey* [online]; Retrieved from www.ridc.org.uk/sites/default/files/uploads/Research%20Reports/Covid19_030420/RiDC_Covid19_FullResults_030402020.pdf.

Richardson, L., Beadle-Brown, J., Bradshaw, J., Guest, C., Malovic, A., & Himmerich, J. (2016). "I felt that I deserved it"—experiences and implications of disability hate crime", *Tizard Learning Disability Review, 21*(2), 80–88.

Rook Sweeney. (2020). *Challenge to lack of COVID-19 guidance for people in supported living.* [online]; Retrieved from https://rookirwinsweeney.co.uk/challenge-to-lack-of-covid-19-guidance-for-people-in-supported-living/.

Rotenburg, S. (2021). *We need equitable access to the Covid-19 vaccine for disabled people* [online]; Retrieved from https://blogs.bmj.com/bmj/2021/02/02/sara-rotenberg-we-need-equitable-access-to-the-covid-19-vaccine-for-disabled-people/

Ruck Keene, A. (2020). *Mental capacity report: Practice and procedure* (Issue 107). London: Essex Chambers.

Ryan, F. (2019). *Crippled: Austerity and the demonization of disabled people*. London: Verso.

Ryan, F. (2020). *Coronavirus has made it even easier to forget about disabled people* [online]; Retrieved from www.theguardian.com/commentisfree/2020/apr/29/

coronavirus-disabled-people-inequality-pandemic?fbclid=IwAR39l1pG4rhPDhr2sb7k1bx0O8H5Cqs42SzS-aojDJyE98v-Kl95Am4c4X0.

Saunders, G. H., Jackson, I. R., & Visram, A. S. (2020). 'Impacts of face coverings on communication: An indirect impact of COVID-19'. *International Journal of Audiology*. [online]; Retrieved from https://doi.org/10.1080/14992027.2020.1851401

Scope. (2020). *My disabled friends are being met with aggression because they cannot wear a mask* Retrieved from www.scope.org.uk/news-and-stories/disabled-people-and-wearing-masks/.

Sen, A. (1999). *Development as freedom*. New York, NY: Knopf.

Series, L. (2020). 'Disability and Human Rights'. In N. Watson and S. Vehmas (Eds.), *Routledge handbook of disability studies* (2nd ed.). London: Routledge

Shannon, B. (2020). '*The virus and 'the vulnerable': Have labels cost lives?* [online]; Retrieved from https://rewritingsocialcare.blog/2020/07/24/vulnerable/

Shrewsbury, D. (2015). 'Disability and Participation in the Professions: Examples from higher and medical education'. *Disability & Society, 30*(1), 87–100.

Simcock, P. (2020a) *The lived experience of vulnerability among adults ageing with deafblindness: An interpretative phenomenological analysis* [unpublished thesis]. King's College London.

Simcock, P. (2020b) 'When physical distancing means losing touch: Covid-19 and deafblind people'. *Social Work 2020 under Covid-19 Magazine 4th Ed.* [online]; Retrieved from https://sw2020covid19.group.shef.ac.uk/2020/06/02/when-physical-distancing-means-losing-touch-covid-19-and-deafblind-people/.

Simcock, P., & Castle, R. (2016). *Social work and disability*. Bristol: Polity Press.

Sin, C. H. (2016). 'Commentary on " 'I felt I deserved it'—experiences and implications of disability hate crime'. *Tizard Learning Disability Review, 21*(2), 89–94.

Singh, S. (2020). 'Disability Ethics in the Coronavirus crisis'. *Journal of Family Medicine and Primary Care, 9*(2), 2167–2171.

Smith. S. R. (2010). 'Social Justice and Disability: competing interpretations of the medical and social models'. In K. Kristiansen, S. Vehmas and T. Shakespeare (Eds.), *Arguing about disability: Philosophical perspectives*. Abingdon: Routledge

Spreadbury, K., & Hubbard, R. (2020). *The adult safeguarding practice handbook*. Bristol: Policy Press.

Stanley, T. (2016). 'A practice framework to support the Care Act 2014'. *The Journal of Adult Protection, 18*(1), 53–64.

Steele, L. (2020). *Disability, criminal justice and law. Reconsidering court diversion*. London: Routledge.

Stewart, A., & MacIntyre, G. (2018). 'Safeguarding adults: Key issues and concepts'. In G. MacIntyre, A. Stewart, and P. McCusker (Eds.), *Safeguarding adults: Key themes and issues*. London: Palgrave.

Thomas-Skaf, B. A., & Jenney, A. (2020). 'Bringing social justice into focus: Trauma-Informed work with children with disabilities'. *Child Care in Practice*. [online]; Retrieved from https://doi.org/10.1080/13575279.2020.1765146

United Nations. (2020). *Policy brief: A disability-inclusive response to Covid-19*. Geneva: United Nations.

United Response (2020). *Disability hate crime* [online]; Retrieved from www.unitedresponse.org.uk/get-involved/campaign/disability-hate-crime/

UN Special Rapporteur on the Rights of Persons with Disabilities. (2017). *Support services to ensure the inclusion of persons with disabilities*. Geneva: United Nations.

Vasey, S. (2017). 'Mate crime: how to spot it, stop it and prevent it'. *Learning Disability Practice, 20*(1), 11–11.

Watson, P. (2019). 'Key themes for safeguarding practice: Challenges and priorities'. In C. Chisnell and C. Kelly (Eds.), *Safeguarding in social practice: A lifespan approach* (2nd ed.). London: Sage.

Watts, L., & Hodgson, D. (2019). *Social justice theory and practice for social work. Critical and philosophical perspectives*. Singapore: Springer.

Wolfensberger, W. (1983). Social role valorization: A proposed new term for the principle of normalization. *Mental Retardation, 21*(6), 234.

Wolfensberger, W. P., Nirje, B., & Olshansky, S, et al. (1972). *The principle of normalization in human services*. Toronto: National Institute on Mental Retardation.

Woodward, O. (2020). *Coronavirus: The shielders turning the word 'vulnerable' on its head* [online]; Retrieved from www.bbc.co.uk/news/disability-53351241.

World Health Organisation and World Bank (2011). *World report on disability 2011*. [online]; Retrieved from www.who.int/teams/noncommunicable-diseases/sensory-functions-disability-and-rehabilitation/world-report-on-disability.

12 The Human Rights of "Prisoners"

It Is about People and Community, Not Prisons

Tina Maschi, Keith Morgen, and A. Maya Kaye

Introduction

As we begin to discuss prisoners as a vulnerable population as classified by the United Nations, we ask readers to pause and reflect on this shared narrative of risk and resilience from a 56-year-old woman in an American prison who has served five years.

> *Prison is a hard place. Pure Hell! As long as you are in khaki, you are considered non-human. I miss my family and want to go home so bad. I don't feel there is enough mental health available on a regular basis or the comfortable feeling of just expressing yourself without the fear of being put in lockdown. The elder suffer the most because there isn't much for them, us. The medical here makes no sense. Until you have an ailment, you are put off and time holds you back. I have the starts of osteoporosis and seeing how some people young and old are treated makes me suffer and deal with it. I look at it that I will deal with it when I get home. In the meantime I hurt and deal with it. Prayer and God is what gets me through every day, moment, second I am here. Overall, it's horrible and wouldn't wish this on my worst enemy.*

This quote is just one example of the challenges experienced by vulnerable groups across the world. The crimes against humanity and the imprisonment of vulnerable groups have been historically intertwined with the United Nations and its mission to promote the Earth and individuals' human rights and "leave no one behind." As societies responded to bring forth a kinder and gentler world, the drafting and ratification of the Universal Declaration of Human Rights (UDHR, 1948) was a significant turning point in the aftermath of the atrocities and genocide of children, the Jewish population, people with disabilities, and migrants (UN, 1948).

The Universal Declaration of Human Rights has the potential to inspire and pave the way for the attainment of political, civil, social, economic, and cultural rights for humanity, the Earth, and all living beings, including the primarily overlooked group of individuals at risk of incarceration, incarcerated and formerly incarcerated people. Since the UDHR, more than

DOI: 10.4324/9781003111269-15

seventy human rights treaties have been adopted, which are now in force permanently at global and regional levels. The UDHR preamble underlines the norm of "respect for the intrinsic dignity, and equal and inalienable rights" of all human beings (UN, 1948, p. 1).

Of the 30 UDHR articles, several specifically speak to those at risk of incarceration and incarcerated of all races, ethnicities, and ages. For example, Article 25 notes, "Everyone has the right to a standard of living that is sufficient for health and wellbeing" (UN, 1948, p. 5). These provisions are applicable both before, during, and after prison terms and include accommodation, medical, mental, and social care, as well as the right to protection in the event of unemployment, illness, disability, or old age (UN, 1948). Article 3 provides that "everyone shall have the right to life, liberty, and protection of person" (UN, 1948, p. 3), and Article 5 provides that "no one shall be subjected to torture or cruel, inhuman or degrading treatment or punishment" (UN, 1948, p. 3). These two articles are critical, given the growing understanding of the histories of trauma and oppression based on societal statuses, racial/ethnic minorities, class, gender, disability, and immigration.

The UDHR also serves as a broad blueprint for the design and implementation of international policies and legal standards that protect people in prison and the subgroups of vulnerable individuals from victimization, neglect, mistreatment, and substandard health care. For example, Article 22 of the UDHR underlines that "everyone has the right to social security," which many countries describe as social protections and "holistic" wellbeing (UN, 1948, p. 5). Social protection is consistent with the principle of human agency and the right of every person to have the best opportunity to achieve social, economic, and cultural wellbeing in their country, including those individuals and groups living in poverty and prison (UN, 1948).

Furthermore, two UN treaties, the International Covenant on Civil and Political Rights (ICCPR; UN, 1966a) and the International Covenant on Economic, Social and Cultural Rights (ICESC; UN, 1966b), clarify the right to services, particularly for incarcerated individuals. For example, article 10 of the ICCPR defines prison rehabilitation as a central factor. It notes that the "penitentiary system shall comprise the care of prisoners and their reformation and social rehabilitation shall be the central goal" (UN, 1966a, p. 3). Article 12 of the ICESC acknowledges "the right of all to enjoy the highest attainable level of physical and mental health" (UN, 1966b, p. 4). Such rights involve continuous improvement of environmental conditions, prevention, treatment and control of disease transmission, and appropriate medical services (UN, 1966b). Adopting foreign policies based on these provisions will help promote incarcerated individuals' wellbeing during their lifetime.

This chapter will overview the central issues of a vulnerable group that relate to people in prison. We offer a summary of the current global prison portrait, explore some of the United Nations' key areas to address the prison crisis such as (1) incarcerated individuals with special needs (e.g., foreign people, Indigenous people, drug users, women, children, people of color, people with disabilities, older adults, LGBTI people); (2) sentencing policies and alternatives to imprisonment; and (3) access to justice and legal aid. Next, we highlight select incarceration and post-incarceration issues such as trauma, discrimination, and access to health and mental health treatments. We also review the United Nations standards and norms on the treatment of incarcerated people as well as the UN Sustainable Development Goals (SDGs) and promising international practices. Finally, we offer an overview of social work practice recommendations when working with this vulnerable group of people in prison.

Review of the Literature: Global Prison Portrait

Historically, social work has been resistant to prepare social workers with the knowledge, values, and skills to practice in the criminal justice system. However, over the past decade (2010–2020+), a growing awareness of and response to policing, courts, and imprisonment as a mechanism of oppression has ignited essential debates regarding the levels of social work, police, and community engagement (Maschi et al. (2019); Robbins et al., 2015). Individuals with intersecting identities based on race, class, gender and sexual identity, immigration, mental health, or disability status, and geographic location have been unduly affected and are at the highest risk of criminal justice involvement. For example, the "get tough on crime" era of the 1970s with punitive policies, such as "Truth in Sentencing" and "Three Strikes You Are Out," led to the rise of the prison population in the United States (Maschi et al., 2021). The 2020 pandemic has brought to the surface the cracks in prisons' health, education, economic, social, and political systems. When it comes to the loopholes related to mass incarceration, even though global crime rates have been declining, the prison population rate has increased worldwide.

For example, a 2019 report by the Penal Reform International [PRI] estimates more than 10 million men, women, and children are in prison worldwide—an increase of 20% between 2002 and 2015. The number of women and girls in prison worldwide increased by 53% between 2000 and 2017. Most of the people imprisoned around the world come from marginalized backgrounds. In the context of counter-terrorism operations, children around the world are either detained or living in prisons. Sadly, inadequate prison conditions and institutionalization have compromised children's cognitive development and increased post-traumatic stress and suicide rates (PRI, 2019).

The increasing number of incarcerated women, often harshly sentenced for morality crimes and drug offenses, also reveals the challenges of prisons that cater to a predominantly male population. Such ill-equipped institutions lack gender-specific care and inadequate to non-existent rehabilitation opportunities, leading to increased risk of ill-health, reinforced discrimination, and higher risk of reoffending. Even though the death penalty has decreased globally, life sentence usage has increased by 84% between 2000 and 2018, leading to overcrowded, unsanitary, and violent prison conditions (PRI, 2019).

These substandard prison conditions coupled with cruel correctional practices (e.g., solitary confinement, torture), shortage of staff, and budget cuts, are shown to impede rehabilitation and harm incarcerated individuals' health and mental health, resulting in severe violations of human rights (PRI, 2019). Racial disparities are also well documented in the African American population in the United States. According to the Sentencing Project (2013), one out of every ten Black males in their 30s is in prison or jail on any given day. Black men have a one-in-three chance of being imprisoned in their lifetime, compared to one in seventeen for white men. The incarceration rate for Black men is 6.7 times that of white men (Guerino et al., 2011).

The United States still maintains its position as the country with the world's highest national imprisonment rate (675 incarcerated individuals per 100,000 of the national population). The following countries with the largest prison populations are El Salvador (597 per 100,000) and Turkmenistan (552 per 100,000). Since the 11th World Prison Population List was published in 2015, significant changes in individual countries have occurred. For example, between 2015 and 2018, there was a significant increase in the imprisonment rate in Cambodia (68% increase in prisoners per 100,000 of the national population), Nicaragua (61%), Egypt (53%), and the Philippines (48%). There have also been significant decreases in the past three years in Mexico (23%) and Romania (22%) (PRI, 2019).

Prison Populations

Next, we are briefly reviewing the current situation of vulnerable populations such as women, children and youth, older people, and lesbian, gay, bisexual, transgender, and intersex (LGBTI).

Women

Although women and girls are considered a minority in the global prison population (6.9%), they are rapidly increasing, compared to male incarcerated individuals. For example, from 2000 to 2017, women and girls in prison increased by 50% globally, compared to 20% of males. The causes of imprisonment reported are non-violent offenses, low-level drug trafficking offenses, and morality offenses such as failed virginity tests and suspected abortion. For example, in 2014 in Brazil, 63% of women in prison had minor drug-related crimes compared to a quarter of men. Owing to the double inequality of gender and race—which is also associated with low socioeconomic status and education—women from Indigenous and ethnic minorities face significant disadvantages in the criminal justice system. In Canada, Australia, and New Zealand, the rate of criminalization and incarceration of Indigenous women is especially troubling (PRI, 2019).

Children and Youth

Another global trend related to ageism and racial and other minority discrimination is the imprisonment of children and youth. As a result of social discrimination, children and youth minorities are more likely to be arrested, prosecuted, and imprisoned for longer terms than members of the majority population in a significant number of countries. (ACLU, 2012). For example, in a 2018 report by the Juvenile Justice Advocates International, out of 118 countries surveyed, 26% did not have pre-trial detention limit for children, 43% had pre-trial detention limit that applies only to children, and 31% had pre-trial detention limit that apply to both adults and children (Juvenile Justice Advocates International [JJAI], 2018). In the United States, about 48,000 juveniles are incarcerated in facilities away from home on any given day because of juvenile justice or criminal justice involvement. The vast majority are kept in repressive, correctional-style prisons, and thousands are held without being trialed (Sawyer, 2019).

Older People

The global aging prison population crisis has been affected by punitive criminal justice policies. People aged 55 and older, for example, will account for a third of the prison population in the United States by 2030 (Maschi & Kaye, 2019). Since the 1970s and 1980s, the United States has been at the forefront of the most recent tough-on-crime criminal justice reforms (Maschi, Viola, & Sun, 2013). Unfortunately, other countries have since followed suit, setting in motion an upward trend of mass imprisonment of many convicted people destined to grow old, if not die, in overcrowded prisons (Kinsella, 2004). More recently, countries have started to move away from unnecessarily punitive measures that impact elderly adults in prison and toward a more compassionate approach. Currently, correctional systems around the world are dealing with the growing surge of older adults in need of comprehensive treatment and community reintegration programming, including end-of-life care, even though they were not equipped to take on the position of long-term care facilities (Aday, 2006; Stone et al., 2011).

Lesbian, Gay, Bisexual, Transgender, and Intersex (LGBTI)

Over the last few years, progress has been made in the rights of lesbians, gays, bisexuals, transgender people, and intersex (LGBTI) people—but only in certain parts of the world. For example, in 2018, the Association for the

Prevention of Torture [APT] developed a guide for monitoring bodies that provide an overview of how authorities should identify patterns of abuse against LGBTI people and proposes measures to prevent ill-treatment and torture (Association for the Prevention of Torture [APT], 2018). Notably, the Supreme Court of India unanimously decided to decriminalize same-sex marriages in 2018, and Angola followed suit in early 2019. In other parts of the world, the "don't tell, don't ask" prison policies require that incarcerated LGBTI people make themselves invisible. Such policies are alarming because they deny their human dignity and encourage authorities to disregard and neglect their responsibilities to respect and fulfill these rights (PRI, 2019).

The Rights-Limitations of Justice-Involved Individuals Around the Globe

Historically, a common thread in the use of incarceration that outpaces global population growth is that incarcerated people overwhelmingly come from disadvantaged and oppressed communities across the world. A substantial number of people run afoul of the law for reasons related to poverty. They lack the financial means to pay adequate legal representation or monetary bail once they enter the system, so they are more likely to obtain prison sentences than non-custodial alternatives. The consequence is a cycle of deprivation from which people struggle to break free. This pattern continues over generations, as research shows that children of incarcerated individuals are more likely to become involved in the criminal justice system themselves (Burton, 2006; PRI, 2019).

Prison Overcrowding

Overcrowding in prisons continues to be a global problem, owing in part to the widespread use of pre-trial detention. According to the Institute for Criminal Policy and Research (ICPR), the number of inmates in 121 countries exceeds the official prison capacity. Nonetheless, this is likely underestimating the actual situation, not least because individual inmates or portions of prisons can be overcrowded even though the entire prison system is not. Overcrowding has a significant effect on the lives of incarcerated individuals, resulting in unsanitary and violent environments that are detrimental to their physical, mental health, and recovery. Staff employed in overcrowded prisons are also at risk, as they are more likely to face possible abuse, the risk of contracting infectious diseases, as well as increased stress and mental health problems. When prisons are overcrowded, prison administration and services are spread so thin that they can only provide the bare necessities to those in their care (PRI, 2019).

Overcrowding strategies are outlined in detail in a variety of international and regional guidelines and resources. Overall, they include enhancing crime prevention programs, expanding the use of alternatives to pre-and post-trial incarceration, updating sentence lengths, restricting the use of recall of inmates on parole or probation, and maintaining consistency in sentencing practices. Amnesties and pardons are still seen as a temporary solution to overcrowding and other more politicized causes. Since overcrowding in prisons is a significant factor impacting both inmates' and staff's physical and mental health, states should improve crime reduction, decriminalize minor crimes, review sentencing proportionality, and broaden the use of alternatives to imprisonment (PRI, 2012; UNODC, 2013, PRI, 2019).

Closing Space for Civil Society Organizations

Under the criminal justice and prison systems, civil society organizations play a crucial role. They act as regulatory bodies, exposing human rights abuses and corruption. Some of the essential functions of civil society organizations are to:

a) provide legal assistance to incarcerated individuals,
b) track conditions and care within prisons through formal and informal mechanisms,
c) link incarcerated people with their families and communities,
d) help prison staff and advocate for transparency and accountability,
e) share information, knowledge, and skills to build consensus on evidence-based law and policy, and
f) offer services that are essential for incarcerated individuals' rehabilitation and reintegration into society on release.

Civil societies organizations are especially important because they bridge the divide between communities and prisons, bringing a sense of normalcy to environments that are often far from ordinary. To work effectively, civil society organizations need a conducive atmosphere to function (e.g., operating in a favorable economic, political, social, cultural, and legal climate that enables people to participate in civil society) (PRI, 2019).

Over the last ten years, there has been a disturbing trend toward limiting civil society's operating space. According to data from the International Center for Not-for-Profit Law, between 2004 and 2010, more than 50 countries considered or adopted laws limiting civil society (Rutzen, 2015). Given the increased international emphasis on counterterrorism, civil society actors who participate in politically sensitive or human-rights-related activities are mainly targeted. As a result of such restrictions, civil society organizations are hindered in obtaining funding and communicating with governments (PRI, 2019). For example, the UN Special Rapporteur on the rights to freedom of peaceful assembly and association describes how having a complex legal environment "has the effect of destabilizing and threatening associations by creating doubt and raising the administrative burden of continuing their activities, thus instilling fear of action among their members" (United Nations Human Rights, 2018).

Even though the effect of closing civil society organizations varies from country to country and sector to sector, because of their human rights orientation, organizations focused on criminal justice and prison reform are often affected the most. While in some cases this has resulted in assaults, threats, criminal prosecution, and coercion, in other cases, organizations have closed, relocated, or adapted to their new environment in some ways. Unfortunately, the effects of restricting the space of civil society organizations are felt more acutely in countries with substandard prison systems that rely on civil society organizations for material support for incarcerated individuals. Another potentially problematic issue is that such civil society organizations may internalize a form of self-censorship and shift their focus from more sensitive matters (e.g., revealing the use of torture in detention facilities) to less sensitive ones, it becomes more tangible (e.g., provision of services to people leaving prison) (PRI, 2019). Civil society organizations fighting for criminal justice and prison reform must operate in a safe environment free of threats and arbitrary restrictions. States should provide a secure and enabling atmosphere for civil society based on international human rights law and backed by a transparent national legal system (PRI, 2019).

Sentencing Policies and Alternatives to Imprisonment

Pre-Trial Detention

Pre-trial incarceration should be a last resort, used only when warranted and following the right to liberty and the presumption of innocence. Even though it can only be used under very restricted circumstances, around 30% of detainees worldwide have not been sentenced. In some countries, more than 60% of those incarcerated are in pre-trial custody. On any given day in 2016, when the most recent figures were released, nearly 3 million people were kept in pre-trial detention and other forms of remand incarceration worldwide. Since it does not include detention in police custody, this number is likely to be underestimated. Poor adherence to time limits, lack of access to legal representation, and inability to pay monetary bail are two common causes of prolonged pre-trial detention, both related to poverty. For example, according to a 2018 report by Kenya's Office of the Director of Public Prosecutions, nine out of ten pre-trial inmates were given bail or bond. Still, they could not afford the terms, and about the same proportion had no legal representation (PRI, 2019).

The consequences of pre-trial detention can be devastating. Individuals who are put in pre-trial detention are abruptly separated from their families and social relations. Pre-trial detainees are often held in worse conditions than convicted individuals and are more likely to be tortured. Adults and children held in pre-trial detention increase the risk of coercion, false confessions, unfair plea bargains, increased corruption, physical and mental violence, prison overcrowding, long-term social and developmental effects, and increased recidivism. Pre-trial detention that is unreasonable or prolonged may also harm public perceptions of the justice system (PRI, 2019).

As part of the PRI recommendations, non-custodial interventions should be used more often, and states should implement efficient mechanisms to ensure that people in prison are held for no longer than is explicitly instructed by law. For example, in New Zealand, the number of people held in pre-trial custody was decreased in a relatively short period in 2018. The decrease was associated with efficiencies of the system, such as having bail counselors in prisons, and providing bail support services at court hearings, including linking new remand individuals with electronic monitoring (PRI, 2019).

Evidence-Based Sentencing

Globally, a dynamic combination of objectives affects sentencing decisions. These priorities include recovery, social security, and deterrence, in addition to punishment. The severity and duration of penalties for similar offenses significantly vary worldwide, which means that these goals are perceived somewhat differently. There is some evidence that prison sentences are lengthening in many jurisdictions, especially for serious offenses. Harsher sentencing procedures are determined by a progressively punitive atmosphere of political and media discourse about punishment, policy changes, new sentencing guidelines, new sentencing precedents, and assumptions about new or different offending trends (PRI, 2019).

Many countries have developed sentencing guidelines and/or formed an advisory sentencing council or commission to aid in sentencing decisions. For example, in some jurisdictions, there has been a movement toward more evidence-based sentencing strategies, which seek to enhance sentencing decisions by providing courts with an objective evaluation of the static and complex variables that affect the probability of reoffending. A risk "score" is usually given to an incarcerated person to guide diversion interventions. For example, a non-custodial sentence can be given to a low-risk criminal behavior, whereas those at a higher risk of criminal behaviors are more likely to be incarcerated. The point is that these risk assessment tools can reliably, impartially, and critically forecast the risk of reoffending (PRI, 2019).

Death Penalty

While there has been some progress toward the global abolition of the death penalty (e.g., 109 of 193 UN States Members have repealed the death penalty for all offenses), there have been reports of a resumption of incarcerated individual's executions in Thailand (June 2018), Japan (July 2018), Taiwan

(August 2018), Iraq (May 2018). In 2018, conditions on death row in the US state of Virginia were so bad that a federal district court granted an injunction to resolve the situation after a complaint was filed challenging the conditions. The claimants, who were all on death row, argued that their conditions were unconstitutional as they were subjected to cruel and unusual punishment such as no contact visits; no congregate meals; no congregate leisure, worship, educational, or social programming; only three showers a week; and only five hours of outdoor recreation per week in separate, isolated cages (PRI, 2019).

According to available data, there are approximately 500 women on death row around the world. Most of these women have been sentenced to death for the murder of a close family member, primarily because of a history of gender-based abuse. The second-most common category of crimes for which women are sentenced to death is drug-related offenses, especially in the Middle East and Asia. Although there is little research on the living conditions of women on death row, most of the states that maintain the death penalty have detention conditions that fall well short of minimum requirements (PRI, 2019).

Life Sentencing

As a result of the global movement toward abolition and limits on the death penalty, many states have adopted life imprisonment as their most severe punishment. For example, formal sentences of life imprisonment are in practice in 183 out of 126 countries. There has also been an increase in *de facto* life sentences worldwide (e.g., Mexican federal system fixed-term sentences of up to 140 years). In the United States, the number of prisoners serving life without parole has increased significantly, accounting for half of all people serving full life. When it comes to vulnerable populations such as youth, even though the Washington State Supreme Court (2018) ruled that life without parole sentences for youth is unconstitutional, many states still allow these sentences for crimes committed by youths under the age of 18 (PRI, 2019).

Alternatives to Imprisonment

The UN Standard Minimum Rules for Non-Custodial Measures (the Tokyo Rules) encourage states to use alternative measures to incarceration more generally, considering each country's political, economic, social, and cultural circumstances, as well as the criminal justice system's goals and objectives. Incarcerated individuals can escape the harmful effects of incarceration by using alternative measures. Alternative measures are still in progress in many parts of the world, and greater coordination and cooperation are required to ensure their effectiveness (PRI, 2019). Non-custodial sanctions should be used more often, particularly for minor and non-violent crimes, to encourage offenders to keep their employment, help their families, compensate victims, and hold society accountable. Instead of extending the net of criminal justice oversight, non-custodial penalties should fix the root causes of crime, be gender-sensitive, and substitute prison (PRI, 2019).

Access to Justice and Legal Aid

Access to justice is a fundamental principle of the rule of law. It is particularly relevant to understanding communities and citizen's pathways to and through prison. It also helps create an opening to access justice instead of focusing on the barriers affecting only the "vulnerable." As Article 7 of the UDHR states, all people, regardless of diversity and difference, have equal protections. Historically, people who become involved in the criminal justice system consists of those individuals and group that represent vulnerable groups, such as racial/ethnic minority men and women and youth (especially African Americans and Latinos in the United States), persons with immigration and mental health histories.

Many of these people experienced societal oppression before prison (Maschi & Morgen, 2021). In several instances, most were unable to voice their concerns, exercise their rights, challenge discrimination, or keep decision-makers accountable without access to justice. The High-Level Meeting on the Rule of Law's Declaration highlights everyone's right to equal access to justice, including representatives of disadvantaged groups. It reaffirms Member States' commitment to providing equitable, open, reliable, non-discriminatory, and accountable services that facilitate access to justice for all (Universal Human Rights Instruments, 2021; Nations Office on Drugs and Crime [UNODC], 2013).

The work of the United Nations in seeking solutions in the field of the rule of law includes initiatives that help Member States' efforts to ensure access to justice. Justice should be delivered in a fair and non-discriminatory manner. In the Declaration of the High-Level Meeting on the Rule of Law, member States stressed the judicial system's independence and impartiality, and dignity as an essential condition for upholding the rule of law and ensuring no discrimination in the administration of justice. The UN system collaborates with national partners to create national action strategies and programs for justice reform and service delivery to improve access to justice. The United Nations entities support the Member States in strengthening justice in areas including monitoring and evaluation; empowering the poor and marginalized to seek responses and remedies for injustice; improving legal security, legal awareness, and legal aid; civil society and parliamentary oversight; addressing challenges in the justice sector such as police brutality, inhumane prison conditions; civil society and parliamentary oversight (Access to Justice, 2021).

As legal aid services are an essential part of any strategy to improve access to justice, one of the most critical barriers to it is the cost of legal advice and representation. With that in mind, the Declaration of the High-level Meeting on the Rule of Law committed the Member States to take all necessary steps to provide fair, transparent, adequate, non-discriminatory, and accountable services that promote access to justice for all. In an attempt to establish minimum standards for the right to legal assistance in the criminal justice systems, in December 2012, the General Assembly unanimously adopted the "UN Principles and Guidelines on Access to Legal Aid in Criminal Justice Systems"—the first international instrument on the right to legal aid providing practical guidance on how to ensure access to effective criminal legal services (Universal Human Rights Instruments, 2021; UNODC, 2013).

Guided Discovery: Discrimination, Health, and Mental Health Access

Incarcerated people are a vulnerable and underserved group with specific health needs that go unmet all too often. In general, their health and mental health are lower than those of their community counterparts worldwide. Developmental and learning disabilities, attention deficit disorders, anxiety disorders, arthritis, cancer, heart or lung disease, and cognitive disability or dementia are examples of physical or mental health problems that incarcerated people may face. For example, about 96% of incarcerated adolescents and adults have experienced trauma and have signs or illnesses related to post-traumatic stress (Maschi et al., 2011). Additionally, 40 to 70% of incarcerated individuals in US prisons and abroad have drug abuse issues, and suicidality rates are significantly higher. Compared to the general population, incarcerated adults are seven times more likely to commit suicide than community-dwelling people; incarcerated youth are 18 times more likely to commit suicide than non-incarcerated youth (World Health Organization, 2014).

Inadequate nutrition, overcrowding, and infectious diseases such as tuberculosis are up to 84 times higher in prison than in the general population. Tobacco use is another primary health concern among the incarcerated. According to global figures, incarcerated people smoke at a rate of 28% (WHO, 2014). Special needs groups within the prison population have their health rights violated, including women, children, individuals with mental health problems, and those who use drugs. Providing treatment in a prison environment has proven to be a difficult task. It involves a "whole-of-government" policy in which prison healthcare is incorporated into broader public health and social care systems and meets community-level expectations. Besides, there must be continuity of treatment between the community and the prison. Since most incarcerated individuals will be released back into society, ensuring adequate medical care improves the incarcerated' wellbeing and the general public's health. The greater their wellbeing needs are fulfilled, the more likely they are to play a meaningful role in society (PRI, 2019).

To that extent, it is essential to understand the criminal justice system and the legal paths to incarceration. It is also crucial to consider how the criminal justice system interacts with community health care systems and whether they are part of a host justice system. When it comes to the criminal justice system, the police are the first people a young person or adult who is accused of committing a crime meets. If anyone is arrested, they can be held in custody or jail before they appear in court. If found guilty in court, the judge can order release, probation, participation in an alternative to incarceration program, or placement in a secure juvenile or adult correctional facility, such as a federal or state prison. After serving their sentence, the individual is released on parole or under the supervision of community corrections. However, in some cases, the person completes their maximum sentence and is released to the community with no parole reporting requirement (Maschi & Morgen, 2021).

As for health care services, community-based healthcare facilities, emergency departments, inpatient services, and outpatient clinical services are all part of the continuum of care over the life course of humans. Thus, they should be readily available to incarcerated and formerly incarcerated people as well. Nonetheless, discrimination based on race, class, gender, sexual identity, mental wellbeing, and immigration status is overrepresented in the criminal justice system. Still, people with these characteristics have less access to community health care. As a result, it is critical to address health and justice inequalities in any criminal justice system discussion, particularly related to intersectionality. While racism is a global social problem, racial disparities in the general population of the United States are well-known and well-documented. Minorities have less access to services, lower-quality care, and worse health outcomes than whites (Adler & Newman, 2002; Adler & Rehkopf, 2008; Groman & Ginsburg, 2004; Smedley et al., 2003, PRI, 2019).

In terms of racial/ethnic, class, and age group comparisons, a significant proportion of both the young and the elderly in incarceration have encountered accumulated disadvantages throughout their lives. Homelessness, poverty and financial problems, low educational attainment, lack of family support and family problems, lack of access to care, and trauma, violence, abuse, and other stressful life events (i.e., becoming a victim and witness of violence and living in a poverty-stricken neighborhood) before incarceration are all social determinants of health and criminal justice involvement (Sampson & Lauritsen, 1997; World Health Organization, 2014). Voting rights can be denied to formerly incarcerated people with felony convictions, particularly in terms of participatory or political wellbeing (ACLU, 2010). Obtaining required social welfare services, such as housing and health care, can be difficult, particularly for veterans (ACLU, 2010, 2012).

United Nations Policies: Incarcerated People

The United Nations Office on Drugs and Crimes (UNODC) is ideally positioned within the United Nations framework to assist Member States in resolving the prison crisis by promoting human rights-compliant penal reform measures. The Office assists in implementing international crime prevention and criminal justice principles and norms and serves as the secretariat for intergovernmental mechanisms to draft or update those standards (Universal Human Rights Instruments, 2021).

The following are the United Nations standards and norms on the treatment of incarcerated people:

- United Nations Standard Minimum Rules for the Treatment of Prisoners (the Nelson Mandela Rules)
- Basic Principles for the Treatment of Prisoners (1990)
- Body of Principles for the Protection of All Persons under Any Form of Detention or Imprisonment (1988)

Alternatives to imprisonment

- United Nations Standard Minimum Rules for Non-custodial Measures—"the Tokyo Rules" (1990)
- Basic Principles on the Use of Restorative Justice Programmes in Criminal Matters (2000)

Women offenders and prisoners

- United Nations Rules for the Treatment of Women Prisoners and Non-custodial Measures for Women Offenders— "the Bangkok Rules" (2010)
- Updated Model Strategies and Practical Measures on the Elimination of Violence against Women in the Field of Crime Prevention and Criminal Justice (2010)

Incarcerated Children

- United Nations Standard Minimum Rules for the Administration of Juvenile Justice (1985)
- United Nations Rules for the Protection of Juveniles Deprived of their Liberty (1990)
- United Nations Model Strategies and Practical Measures on the Elimination of Violence against Children in the Field of Crime Prevention and Criminal Justice (2014)

Foreign prisoners

- Model Agreement on the Transfer of Foreign Prisoners and Recommendations on the Treatment of Foreign Prisoners (1985)

Access to legal aid

- United Nations Principles and Guidelines on Access to Legal Aid in Criminal Justice Systems (2012)

Crime prevention

- United Nations Guidelines for the Prevention of Crime (2002)
- United Nations Guidelines for Cooperation and Technical Assistance in the Field of Urban Crime Prevention (1995)
- United Nations Guidelines for the Prevention of Juvenile Delinquency—Riyadh Guidelines (1990)

The Nelson Mandela Rules of 2015

The 2015 Nelson Mandela Rules are an updated edition of the original 1955 Standard Minimum Rules for Prisoners' Care (or Standard Minimum Rules-SMRs). In 2015, the General Assembly of the United Nations unanimously adopted Mandela's Rules of Practice, which set basic requirements for effective prison management (Penal Reform International, [PRI], 2016). Following are five fundamental concepts that can direct the practice of social work that are consistent with the ethical mandates of the professions while performing correctional health care: (1) incarcerated persons shall be treated as human beings with respect for their inherent dignity and value; (2) they shall be treated following their needs, without discrimination; (3) torture or other ill-treatment shall be prohibited; (4) prison shall aim to protect society and reduce reoffending; and (5) the safety of prisoners, staff, service providers and visitors shall be a central concern (Penal Reform International [PRI], 2016).

The Mandela Rules further specify the responsibilities of prison health workers, including social workers. Prison health personnel should be separate from prison officials and security staff and be employed by health care providers (as opposed to corrections). Prison health workers also have the absolute responsibility to provide humane treatment to their patients and never be involved in the protection or punishment of incarcerated people. Clarifying roles and obligations may help direct social workers to resolve ethical dilemmas, such as denial of care by the institution to an inmate, which may lead to a dual conflict of allegiance between serving the patient or the institution. The Mandela Rules also provide access to physical and mental health services. According to the Rules of Practice, states must offer health services at the same standard of care as in the community when people are stripped of their liberty. Besides, inmate health care should be in close coordination with community health programs to ensure continuity of care between prison and the community (Rules 24–29, 31).

The position of health practitioners in prison must be distinct from that of the prison administration. The same ethical and technical requirements apply to inmate health employees as to those outside the prison. Their function in prisons is to assess, support, and manage their prison patients' physical and mental health. This includes prevention and care for infectious diseases, drug abuse, mental wellbeing, and dental care. Health care professionals must not be involved in prison administration matters, such as disciplinary actions, and their professional decisions must not be overruled or ignored by non-medical prison staff. Prison health workers are obliged to disclose any evidence of torture or other inhumane treatment (Rules 25, 30–34).

These principles and guidelines will help social workers contend with ethical dilemmas, such as dual allegiance conflicts. They may include documenting abuses and offering psychiatric care and advocacy in the event of torture and cruel, inhuman, and unusual punishment, physical or sexual harassment by an inmate by a correctional officer, or institutional negligence in the event of prolonged solitary confinement and resulting physical and mental degradation of an imprisoned person (PRI, 2016).

UN Sustainable Development Goals

The role of the UN Sustainable Development Goals is essential to understand the experiences of vulnerable groups in prisons, especially given the ongoing high rates of violence, crime, and corruption worldwide. Most if not all individuals in prison have experienced being both a victim and perpetrator of a crime and, in many cases, wrongful convictions, primarily due to racial profiling (Alexander, 2016). The 17 Sustainable Development Goals (SDGs) adopted by all the United Nations Member States in 2015 are part of the 2030 Agenda for Sustainable Development. In general, it commits to "leave no one behind," including people in prison. It shares a blueprint for peace and prosperity for people and the world in the present and future.

The SDGs are an urgent call to action for all countries—developed and emerging—to work together in a global partnership. They understand that eradicating poverty and other forms of deprivation must be combined with efforts to improve health and education, minimize inequality, and boost economic development—all while combating climate change and protecting our oceans and forests (UN-Sustainable Development Goals [SDGs], 2021). While the Sustainable Development Goals are not legally binding, each UN member state is "required to take responsibility and create a national structure" for achieving all the goals, which includes voluntary national reviews (VNRs) (Penal Reform International [PRI], 2017). These social and environmental conditions especially pertain to prisons known mainly for the substandard conditions that perpetuate poor health and high risk of early mortality and lifetime poverty, and lack of access to full participation in their communities.

As part of the broader community-based criminal justice trajectory (police, pre-detention trial, detention, jail placement, probation/community supervision, corrections-prison secure care, parole/prison release/reentry), opinions vary on the role of prisons. Some argue they are discriminatory and institutions of oppression and should be abolished. On the opposite spectrum, some say that prisons play a critical role in ensuring society's safety on those deemed too dangerous to be in the community and put public safety at risk. Public views vary on the continuum of whether prisons should be humane versus inhumane. For the SDGs, the rule of law should create a stable and inclusive society by ensuring appropriate and rights-based enforcement of the rule of law (PRI, 2017).

When it comes to prison reform, its critical elements are highlighted in the SDGs goals and targets, such as to provide basic healthcare and sanitation to incarcerated individuals *(goals 3 and 6)*, to address the needs of vulnerable populations such as women and girls *(goals 5 and 10)*, and to introduce successful education and recovery programs *(goals 4 and 8)*. Prisons should be able to work at their optimum and produce positive results for the broader community if they are reformed through the lens of sustainable development and inclusive society (PRI, 2017). With that said, incarcerated individuals must be included in the commitment to "leave no one behind" in countries' efforts to implement the SDGs. More specifically, the UN has offered support to countries in the prevention and elimination of violence against children and women in the field of crime prevention and criminal justice, protection of victims and witnesses, crime prevention, judiciary reform, prosecution services, access to legal aid, prison reform and alternatives to imprisonment, and police reform (UNODC-Access to justice, 2021).

International Promising Practices and Initiatives

Different international promising programs, practices, and initiatives have continued to emerge over the past two decades across the world. These responses are designed to foster the health and wellbeing of justice-involved individuals of all ages and backgrounds in communities, prisons, and post-community reintegration. Promising age-sensitive practices often include comprehensive case management services for medical, mental health, substance abuse, family, social services, housing, education or vocational training, spiritual counseling, exercise and creative arts programs, employment, and retirement counseling. Program-specific aspects include age and cognitive capacity, sensitive environmental modifications (e.g., segregated units), interdisciplinary staff and volunteers trained in intersectional identities, specific correctional care, specialized case coordination, family and inmate peer support and volunteering, mentoring, and self-help advocacy group efforts. Additionally, many programs that serve justice-involved people worldwide include restorative justice interventions across various communities and criminal justice settings (Maschi & Kaye, 2019).

The work developed by the United Nations on prison reform leads to the prevention of torture, cruel or degrading treatment, and the preservation of the rights of those deprived of their liberty, emphasizing gender-based and other forms of discrimination. Key areas to address the prison crisis are (1) incarcerated individuals with special needs (e.g., foreign people, Indigenous people, drug users, women, children, people of color, people with disabilities, older adults, LGBTI people); (2) sentencing policies and alternatives to imprisonment; (3) access to justice and legal aid; and (4) social reintegration and recidivism prevention. The UNODC offers policy guidance and capacity-building to minimize the overuse of incarceration and increase the use of alternatives to imprisonment. Such strategies enhance prison management to ensure safe and humane prison conditions, including meeting the special-needs groups of incarcerated individuals and assisting them in their social reintegration (UNODC-Access to Justice, 2021).

For example, The UN Rules for the Treatment of Women Prisoners and Non-Custodial Measures for Women Offenders (the Bangkok Rules) have been enforced through various progressive initiatives. In Brazil, if pregnant women and mothers of children under the age of 12 are convicted of non-violent offenses, the Brazilian Federal Supreme Court has agreed that they will be put under house arrest rather than held in pre-trial custody. In the United States, the Equality for Incarcerated Women Act was passed in Florida, ensuring that women have free and unrestricted access to hygiene products and banning male workers from conducting strip and cavity searches on women (PRI, 2019).

Social Work Practice Recommendations

When it comes to the role of social workers in the criminal justice system, given their expertise to work with people and communities, they can help address the health, social, structural, and legal needs of justice-involved individuals. Given the complexity of micro, mezzo, macro levels, social workers may draw from specialist advanced generalist skills (The Advanced Generalist Public Health Model) and sometimes referred to as forensic social work.

Given the growing practice arena at the intersection of social work, public health, and criminal justice, social workers must be prepared to serve in correctional settings and advocate for better healthcare conditions in the criminal justice system. As policies seek to minimize incarceration and improve prison conditions, social workers are invited to engage in various roles such as the change advocate, the researcher, and the program developer and evaluator (IPRT, 2016). The Nelson Mandela Rules corroborate such high demand as it highlights the need for specialists such as social workers and interprofessional partners in correctional environments to assist in improving the wellbeing of incarcerated people (rules 74 and 78; IPRT, 2016).

The social work profession and the public also have a growing concern with correctional wellbeing and mental health care. As prisons are integrated into the community and only separated by barbwire fences, imprisoned minors, teenagers, and older adults will return to their communities after serving their sentences. As a result, the welfare of all citizens should be of great concern to the broader society, even though they are incarcerated. Furthermore, having everyone in the community in good health prevents financial burden. For example, maintaining one's wellbeing while incarcerated improves overall populations' health, decreases health and justice inequalities, lowers overall healthcare costs and recidivism, increases public safety, and reduces the overall size of prison populations (ACLU, 2012).

When it comes to the scope of forensic social work, to represent justice-involved individuals, social workers must be prepared to discuss and address their clients' physical and mental health needs as well as social and legal problems most effectively. Social workers, frequently in partnerships with counselors and medical practitioners, play an essential role in integrating health and justice, whether dealing with justice at the macro, mezzo, or micro-level. For example, a hospital social worker may render services to incarcerated and formerly incarcerated patients.

A prison social worker can also work in a regional medical unit within a prison and provide discharge preparation services for soon-to-be-released individuals with chronic and terminal illnesses. As for correctional environments, such as jails, the course of health and mental health treatment is most frequently rooted in the prison system, from clinics and primary care to end-of-life hospital care. Social workers in community corrections also offer direct care or treatment, such as therapy and case management services, connecting previously incarcerated people to community health, mental health, and drug addiction facilities, such as public health homes. Regardless of the job settings of social workers, it is likely that some of their clients will have a history of criminal justice, thus the need for social workers to develop generalist and advanced skills in practice, policy, and advocacy.

Summary and Reflection

This chapter summarizes human rights in prisons and other criminal justice settings, emphasizing social work and psychosocial treatment in collaboration with allied practitioners. Health and justice inequalities exist in both the United States and overseas, with the criminal justice system functioning as the *de facto* health and mental health care system. Social workers and other related practitioners who work in the system may be most successful in correctional environments if they are skilled in generalist and advanced treatment that combines science, practice, policy, and advocacy. Adopting empirically validated and evidence-based practices can help to improve health and wellbeing while also breaking the cycle of recidivism for our society's most vulnerable individuals and groups. When working in a team-based manner inside and through care systems, social workers, psychologists, and other allied professionals can make a massive difference in improving care.

We conclude this chapter with a quote from a 55-year-old man in prison and the impact on staff who work in such facilities, such as social workers, psychologists, and correctional officers. We ask that you explore the decision-making and choices of the officers on duty to handle a dying person in prison and his family members. After reading, please reflect upon what accounts for the thoughts, feelings, and behaviors of the staff and its impact on this family.

Quote From a 55-Year-Old Man in Prison Who Work in a Prison Infirmary

The apathy of the guards toward dying inmates was unconscionable. We had one inmate about 30 years old, whose wife and two small children were given permission for a special visit because he was near death. As shift change approached, a nurse entered the room and the family had to stand outside of the door. A female guard yelled to the nurse, "Isn't he dead yet? I don't want to have to stay late to do the paperwork." The two little girls were sobbing in no time. We also had an inmate turn 100 years old there. He was completely bed-ridden. He passed away eventually. I was left wondering how society was being served by that. In the six months that I worked there, six to seven inmates passed away. Hepatitis and diabetes cases abounded, with many amputations.

References

Access to Justice. (2021). Retrieved from https://www.unodc.org/unodc/en/Human-rights/access-to-justice.html

Aday, R. H. (2006). Aging Prisoners' Concerns toward Dying in Prison. *OMEGA—Journal of Death and Dying, 52*(3), 199–216. https://doi.org/10.2190/chtd-yl7t-r1rr-lhmn

Adler, N. E., & Newman K. (2002). Socioeconomic disparities in health: Pathways and policies. *Health Affairs (Millwood), 21*, 60–76.

Adler, N. E., & Rehkopf, D. H. (2008). U.S. disparities in health: Descriptions, causes, and mechanisms. *Annual Review of Public Health, 29*, 235–252.

Alexander, M. (2016). *New Jim Crow: Mass incarceration in the age of colorblindness*. New Press.

American Civil Liberties Union [ACLU]. (2010). Voting with a criminal offense history. Retrieved from http://www.aclu.org/racial-justice-voting-rights/voting-criminal-record-executive-summary

American Civil Liberties Union [ACLU]. (2012). *At America's expense: The mass incarceration of the elderly*. Retrieved from https://www.aclu.org/criminal-law-reform/report-americas-expense-mass-incarceration-elderly

Association for the Prevention of Torture [APT]. (2018). *Towards the effective protection of LGBTI persons deprived of liberty: A monitoring guide*. Geneva. Retrieved from https://atlas-of-torture.org/api/files/1556025997707ajsxnh2aod4.pdf

Burton, M. (2006). *Address to 'child and youth offenders. What works*. Retrieved from https://www.beehive.govt.nz/speech/address-child-and-youth-offenders-what-works

Groman, R., & Ginsburg J. (2004). Racial and ethnic disparities in health care: A position paper of the American College of Physicians. *Annals of Internal Medicine, 141*(3), 226–232.

Guerino, P., Harrison, P., & Sabol, W. (2011), U.S. Department of Justice, Bureau of Justice Statistics, *Prisoners in 2010*. Retrieved from http://bjs.ojp.usdoj.gov/content/pub/pdf/p10.pdf (accessed 6 January 2013).

Irish Penal Reform. (2016). *IPRT Annual Review 2016–2017*. Retrieved from www.iprt.ie. www.iprt.ie/what-we-do/iprt-annual-review-2016-2017/

Juvenile Justice Advocates International. (2018). *Children in pretrial detention: Promoting stronger international time limits*. Cambridge, MN: Juvenile Justice Advocate International. Retrieved from www.jjadvocates.org/wp-content/uploads/2020/02/JJAI-Children-in-Pretrial-Detention.pdf

Kinsella, C. (2004). *Correctional health care costs*. Lexington, KY: The Council of State Governments. Retrieved from www.csg.org/knowledgecenter/docs/TA0401CorrHealth.pdf.

Maschi, T., & Kaye, A. (2019). Incarcerated older adults. Retrieved from www.giaging.org/issues/incarcerated-older-adults/

Maschi, T., & Morgen, K. (2021). *Aging behind prison walls studies in trauma and resilience*. New York, NY: New York Columbia University Press.

Maschi, T., Morgen, K., Hintenach, A., & Kaye, A. (2021). Aging in prison and correction policy in global perspectives. *Oxford Research Encyclopedia of Criminology and Criminal Justice*.

Maschi, T., Morgen, K., Zgoba, K., Courtney, D., & Ristow, J. (2011). Trauma, stressful life events, and post-traumatic stress symptoms: Do subjective experiences matter? *Gerontologist, 51*, 675–686.

Maschi, T., Rees, J., Leibowitz, G., & Bryant, M. (2019). Educating for rights and justice: A content analysis of forensic social work syllabi. A content analysis of forensic social work syllabi. *Social Work Education, 38*, 177–197.

Maschi, T., Viola, D., & Sun, F. (2013). The high cost of the international aging prisoner crisis: wellbeing as the common denominator for action. *The Gerontologist, 53*(4), 543–554.f

Penal Reform International [PRI]. (2016). *Global prison trends 2016*. London: Penal Reform International. Retrieved from https://www.penalreform.org/resource/global-prison-trends-2016-2/

Penal Reform International [PRI]. (2017). *The sustainable development goals and the criminal justice system*. London: Penal Reform International. Retrieved from https://cdn.penalreform.org/wp-content/uploads/2017/05/Global_Prison_Trends-2017-Full-Report-1.pdf

Penal Reform International [PRI]. (2019). *Global prison trends 2019*. London: Penal Reform International. Retrieved from https://cdn.penalreform.org/wp-content/uploads/2019/05/PRI-Global-prison-trends-report-2019_WEB.pdf

Robbins, S. P., Vaughan-Eden, V., & Maschi, T. (2015). From the editor—it's not CSI: The importance of forensics for social work education. *Journal of Social Work Education, 51*(3), 421–424.

Rutzen, D. (2015). Civil society under assault. *Journal Of Democracy, 26*(4), 28–39. doi: 10.1353/jod.2015.0071

Sampson, R. J., & Lauristen, J. H., 1997. A life-course theory of cumulative disadvantage and the stability of delinquency. In T. Thornberry (Ed.), *Advances in criminological theory and delinquency: Vol. 7*. New Brunswick, NJ: Transaction Publishers, 1–29.

Sawyer, W. (2019). *Youth confinement: The whole pie 2019*. Northampton, MA: Prison Policy Institute. Retrieved from https://www.prisonpolicy.org/reports/youth2019.html

Sentencing Project (2013). *Racial disparity*. The Sentencing project web site. Retrieved from http://www.sentencingproject.org/template/page.cfm?id=122

Smedley, B., Stith, A., & Nelson, A. (2003). *Unequal treatment: Confronting racial and ethnic disparities in health care*. Washington, DC: The National Academies Press.

Stone, K., Papadopoulos, I., & Kelly, D. (2011). Establishing hospice care for prison populations: An integrative review assessing the UK and USA perspective. *Palliative Medicine, 26*(8), 969–978. https://doi.org/10.1177/0269216311424219

Sustainable Development Goals. (SDGs). (2021). Retrieved from https://sdgs.un.org/goals

United Nations [UN]. (1990). *Basic principles for the treatment of prisoners.* Retrieved from https://www.ohchr.org/EN/ProfessionalInterest/Pages/BasicPrinciplesTreatmentOfPrisoners.aspx

United Nations (1948), *The universal declaration of human right.* Retrieved from www.un.org/en/documents/udhr/.

United Nations. (1966a). *International covenant on economic, social, and cultural rights.* Retrieved from http://www2.ohchr.org/english/law/cescr.htm.

United Nations. (1966b). *International covenant on political and civil rights.* Retrieved from http://www.ohchr.org/EN/ProfessionalInterest/Pages/CCPR.aspx.

United Nations [UN]. (1985). *International transfer of sentenced persons.* United Nations: Office on Drugs and Crime. Retrieved from https://www.unodc.org/unodc/en/organized-crime/transfer-of-sentenced-persons.html

United Nations [UN]. (1988). *Protection of all persons under any form of detention or imprisonment.* Retrieved from https://www.ohchr.org/EN/ProfessionalInterest/Pages/DetentionOrImprisonment.aspx

United Nations [UN]. (1990). *Rules for the protection of juveniles deprived of their liberty.* Retrieved from https://www.ohchr.org/EN/ProfessionalInterest/Pages/JuvenilesDeprivedOfLiberty.aspx

United Nations[UN]. (1990). *United Nations Guidelines for the Prevention of Juvenile Delinquency.* Retrieved from https://www.ohchr.org/documents/professionalinterest/tokyorules.pdf

United Nations [UN]. (1990). *United Nations standard minimum rules for non-custodial measures (The Tokyo Rules).* Retrieved from https://www.ohchr.org/documents/professionalinterest/tokyorules.pdf

United Nations [UN]. (2002). *ECOSOC Resolution 2002/13 Action to promote effective crime prevention.* Retrieved from https://www.unodc.org/documents/justice-and-prison-reform/crimeprevention/resolution_2002-13.pdf

United Nations [UN]. (2013). *United Nations principles and guidelines on access to legal aid in criminal justice systems.* Retrieved from https://www.unodc.org/documents/justice-and-prison-reform/UN_principles_and_guidlines_on_access_to_legal_aid.pdf

United Nations [UN]. (2015). *Rules for the treatment of women prisoners and non-custodial measures for women offenders with their commentary.* Retrieved from https://www.unodc.org/documents/justice-and-prison-reform/Bangkok_Rules_ENG_22032015.pdf

United Nations Human Rights. (2018). *Special Rapporteur on the rights to freedom of peaceful assembly and of association.* Geneva: United Nations Human Rights. Retrieved from https://www.ohchr.org/en/issues/assemblyassociation/pages/srfreedomassemblyassociationindex.aspx

United Nations Office on Drugs and Crime (UNODC). (2013). *Handbook on strategies to reduce overcrowding in prisons.* Vienna: United Nations. Retrieved from https://www.unodc.org/e4j/data/_university_uni_/handbook_on_strategies_to_reduce_overcrowding_in_prisons.html?lng=en

United Nations Office on Drugs and Crime [UNODC]. (2013). *United Nations principles and guidelines on access to legal aid in criminal justice systems.* New York: United Nations.

Retrieved from https://www.unodc.org/documents/justice-and-prison-reform/UN_principles_and_guidlines_on_access_to_legal_aid.pdf

United Nations Office on Drugs and Crime [UNODC]. (2009), *Handbook for prisoners with special needs*. Retrieved from www.unhcr.org/refworld/docid/4a0969d42.html.

Universal Human Rights Instruments. (2021). Retrieved from https://www.ohchr.org/en/professionalinterest/pages/universalhumanrightsinstruments.aspx

World Health Organization [WHO] (2014). *Prisons and Health*. Retrieved from http://www.euro.who.int/__data/assets/pdf_file/0005/249188/Prisons-and-Health.pdf?ua=1

13 Women's and Girls' Rights Are Human Rights

Smita Ekka Dewan, Sandra G. Turner, Rina Goldstein, and Tina Maschi

Chapter Overview

This chapter provides an overview of human rights of women and girls. It presents the key concepts related to human rights and their applicability and implications for women and girls across the world. A brief overview of international laws and conventions created to protect the human rights of women and children is provided. We use four theories, that is. feminist theory, oppression theory, empowerment theory, and the caring justice framework to explain the various factors that influence the well-being of women and girls. Following this, we examine eight key social issues that highlight the vulnerability of women and girls to the violation of human rights.

Introduction

Gender plays an important role in all aspects of human life, and its implications can be seen in all social, political, economic, and cultural indicators of well-being. As a result of gender inequalities, women and girls have very different outcomes than men and boys for every social problem that affects individuals, families, and communities. At every stage of their life span, women and girls also experience multiple barriers and violations of their human rights. In this chapter, we examine these inequalities using a human rights framework.

Key Concepts

Gender

Gender is a hierarchical concept and refers to the socially constructed roles, behaviors, and norms attributed to being a woman, girl, man, or boy (World Health Organization [WHO], 2019). Variations of gender are defined by culture, societies, and across times, and are subject to change. Although different than sex, gender is intrinsically related. Sex is defined by physiological and biological markers, such as hormones, chromosomes, and reproductive organs associated with women, men, and intersex individuals. Gender

DOI: 10.4324/9781003111269-16

identity, however, refers to the individual, internal experience of a person's instinctive feelings regarding their gender. It may not correspond to their sex designated at birth or physiological sex attributes. Gender is the social expression of sex or gender identity. Gender concepts relate to interpersonal norms between those of the same or different genders.

Intersectionality

Gender hierarchy creates inequality and discrimination. These occur socially and economically and are compounded with factors such as ethnicity, disability, age, sexual orientation, socioeconomic status, and geographic location, and can cause an exacerbation of gender-based discrimination, often referred to as intersectionality (WHO, 2019). The intersectionality framework has been consistently used to highlight how multiple identities and their interconnectedness influence the experiences of oppression. The "interlocking systems of oppression" (Crenshaw, 1991) are most clearly at play when the human rights of women and girls are examined. According to Hamilton et al. (2009), viewing oppression from a holistic lens of intersectionality enhances the understanding of the depth and complexity of oppression and social suffering. Intersectionality acknowledges the multiplicity and complexity of the experiences of women and girls and asserts that oppression and discrimination is result of an intersection of race, gender, sexual orientation, gender identity, economic class, and disability, among others. Specific foci within an intersectionality framework are biological, psychological, social, political, history, and cultural influences. Social systems are interrelated, and power differentials abound and should be viewed as such when assessing for intersectionality among individuals, families, communities, and social systems.

Equality and Equity

Equality and non-discrimination are the core principles in many human rights laws. The International Labour Organization ([ILO], 2016) cites various targets within the Sustainable Development Goals (SDGs) that relate to gender inequality, such as equal access to education (SDG 4), overall gender equality (SDG 5), decent work for all (SDG 8), equal pay (SDG 8), and equal opportunity (SDG 10). The Universal Declaration of Human Rights (UDHR) also focuses on equality at least 13 times.

However, more recently, there is increasing focus on equity as well. While the principle of equality in the context of gender and human rights is critical, so is the concept of equity which requires a recognition and acknowledgement of the inherent differences between the genders and the systemic disadvantage experienced by one gender. Only the responses based on the principles of equity will be effective in achieving equality. Equitable system solutions aim to focus on promoting health, access to services, and economic stability among marginalized communities and systems. Supporting those that are underserved ensures equality of all people, including all genders. Women and girls around the world experience inequality, discrimination, exploitation, marginalization, and powerlessness. Addressing these multiple forms of oppression and closing the gender gaps between men and women would entail re-evaluating the aforementioned practices and choosing to redistribute resources, responsibilities, and opportunities, while purposefully reducing discriminatory practices (ILO, 2016).

Universality of Human Rights and the Public–Private Divide

Human rights and freedoms are inalienable and recognize the dignity and worth of every human, everywhere. The UDHR is written under these universal terms, affirming that all humans are entitled to freedom and equal rights to health, food, education, and housing. Regardless of countries' and states' beliefs, religious practices, culture, and demographics, human rights are entitled to all and must be adhered to. All rights, including civil, political, social, cultural, are intrinsically interrelated, and must be treated with equal importance. For example, the right to health and related objectives can be directly impacted by the right to education and access to knowledge.

> Every moment spent debating the universality of human rights is one more opportunity lost to achieve effective implementation of all human rights. Universality is, in fact, the essence of human rights: all people are entitled to them, all governments are bound to observe them, all state and civil actors should defend them. The goal is nothing less than all human rights for all.
>
> (Robinson, 2000)

Women's rights are heavily impacted by the distinct divide between the public and private sectors, such as the state and family systems, and work versus family life and labor (Boyd, 1997). This divide between public and private is critical for gender and human rights because historically violation of women's human rights within the private domain and by private entities, which typically consisted of families, and community was considered as an exception and not bound by international human rights. It is only more recently accepted that international human rights must address public and private divides in order to address women's lack of rights in various ways (Radačić, 2007). The lack of attention to women's rights in the private sphere is an abuse to the equalization of human rights. Private rights infringements, such as domestic violence, child marriage, and female genital mutilation, are no longer considered outside the purview of human rights. Infringements of women's rights not only on a national level, but in familial, religious, and cultural domains, as well, for the protection of their women and girls must be recognized and addressed.

Theories

FEMINIST THEORY

Feminist theory has many of the same basic concepts as empowerment and oppression theories as it focuses on the power of the social, political, and economic structures that shape human societies and puts the focus on gender as the most important consideration of the effects of domination, oppression, power, and powerlessness in our society (Turner & Maschi, 2015). There have been at least three "waves" in the development of feminist theory as it has evolved from being primarily a focus on the oppression of individual white middle-class women as they struggled to win the right to vote, to a broader focus on domination and oppression in our patriarchal society. Most recently, feminists of color have discarded the "wave" theory of feminism due to its exclusive focus on white women and shift to move diverse narratives of history that analyze the intersections of race, class, gender, and sexual orientation. Post-1990 feminism focuses on intersectionality, which is articulated by biracial, bicultural identities. The focus is on capitalism and the history of slavery in the United States and the limits in social justice put on all women (Greer, 2021; McCann & Kim, 2016).

Women of color and other progressive people point to the how the US capitalist economy was built on the free labor provided by slavery and point out the extent to which white people will go to hold on to power (Greer, 2021) and will seek racial justice only when there is something in it for them. Walker (1983) connects "womanism," a term she feels is more capacious than feminism for women of color, to environmentalism and sees the contemporary environmental destruction as being connected to the destruction of her female ancestors. Womanism represents an escape from slavery and seeks justice and freedom.

More recently, transnational feminism (Chevez-Duenas & Adames, 2021) looks at the complex multidimensional and interactive oppression experienced by women of color. The focus is on creating equalitarian collaborations that support critical consciousness and social change. Intersectionality is a cornerstone of multicultural feminist and social justice approaches (Crenshaw, 1991). Postcolonial feminism rejects Euro-American feminism that universalizes women's oppression and suggests taking stock of one's assumptions, values, and social locations to understand how we might consciously or unconsciously be supporting oppressive patriarchal systems.

Oppression Theory

Oppression theory addresses the power imbalance in any organizational structure and the larger society that fosters and sustains an unjust use of power of one individual or group over another. There are generally considered to be four levels of oppression: personal, structural, cultural, and internalized.

Internalized oppression refers to the way an individual has incorporated discrimination, poverty, racism, and powerlessness into one's psyche (Mullaly, 2017). Personal oppression is often reflected in microaggressions, and violence toward others, usually subordinate groups. Cultural oppression is transmitted by societal judgments often portrayed by the media. Structural level oppression is transmitted via institutions, organizations, governments, laws, and policies. Inequalities are imposed on subordinate groups often with impunity (Mullaly, 2017; Dominelli, 2003).

The concept of intersectionality shows how important it is to look at discrimination and oppression using many lenses. The #Me Too movement often overlooks the fact that minority cisgender and transgender women are discriminated against differently when a straightforward narrative of men being the abusers and women the victims is promoted. This approach does not recognize the harassment of transgender women by cisgender women as well as the oppression of cisgender minority women (Brodsky, 2019). In fact, the invisibility of race in the #MeToo movement means that often the experiences of women of color are overlooked. For example, Native American women have the highest rate of sexual assault in the United States (one in three Indigenous women are raped). If people of color, queer, disabled, and poor aren't centered in our anti-oppression movements, they tend to become no more than a footnote (Garza, 2020). However, the #MeToo movement, started in 2006 by Tarana Burke, has helped to empower and embolden women to speak out, protest, and bring charges when they are sexually, verbally, and physically abused. Women have seen the advantage of joining together and supporting each other (Brodsky, 2019).

Empowerment Theory

Empowerment will be discussed as both a theory and a practice. Empowerment was first conceptualized by Paulo Freire (1973) in the 1970s as he was working with oppressed people in Brazil. When social work shifted from a focus on deficits and problems to the strengths perspective, empowerment practice followed as an outgrowth of this human rights and social justice approach. Freire developed the concept of "conscientization" or critical consciousness, which involved using skills of reflection, action, and joining with others. He worked with poor children in schools, first joining with them to understand their oppression and disempowerment, and then to help them increase their strength and sense of interpersonal power. The belief that you must enter into the lives of oppressed people to work with them toward achieving strength and well-functioning is also the foundation of feminist practice based on the concept of mutuality, which is establishing reciprocal relationships with those you are working with (Jordan, 2017).

Social workers and educators who work from an empowerment perspective believe that oppressions have to be recognized and acknowledged which then leads to what Friere called "conscientization," which can lead to the first step in becoming empowered (Friere, 1973; Carr, 2003).

There are generally considered to be four levels of empowerment: intrapersonal, interpersonal, collective (community), and political. Personal empowerment is gaining the ability to develop self-efficacy or competence. Individual empowerment is generally not sufficient to overcome powerlessness (Miley et al., 2011). Interpersonal empowerment involves developing capacity to work in groups and organizations successfully to achieve change. Political and/or community empowerment achieves the redistribution of power and resources to foster the empowerment of oppressed people (Gutierrez et al., 1998; Christens et al., 2011).

The Caring Justice Framework

The Caring Justice Partnership Perspective (CJPP) utilizes a care-centered conceptualization to approach simple and complex problems of care and justice that affect multiple systems, such as local and global social, economic, political, and health systems (Maschi et al., 2020). Problems in these domains may include health, crime, justice disparities, and violence. Areas of oppression that are externalized (e.g., victimization, marginalization) and internalized (e.g., sexism, classism) are dismantled or transformed through the CJPP process (Maschi & Kaye, 2019). In alignment with feminist and human rights perspectives, the CJPP seeks to promote awareness, empowerment, and liberation to all (Maschi et al., 2020). It recognizes the healing powers of masculine and feminine principles innate in all individuals, regardless of their gender identification, which occur by taking responsibility and finding inner peace to return to a state of balance and unconditional love for the self and for others. Individual healing can precipitate mutual love and co-creation of world peace and care and justice enhancement. It is imperative to recognize the inherent rights of ALL humans regardless of gender identification. This includes the dignity, value, and worth of each person.

The CJPP includes developing present-oriented, creative ways to promote care, justice, ethics, and principles that enhance the capacity of people and groups to survive life adversities and gain the strength to flourish (Maschi & Morgen, 2020). The CJPP replaces fear-based, negative thinking with solution-focused, positive thinking to assess diversity, inclusivity, peace, equity, safety, and health. Problem-focused thinking favors binary, hierarchical, dualistic, and negative viewpoints; solution-focused thinking avoids these negative foci and prevents competition, conflict, and repetitions of tragedies (Maschi et al., 2020; Maschi et al., 2021). According to the CJPP, "caring" is defined as emotional and behavioral aspects, which encompass empathy, compassion, authenticity, unconditional love, dignity, and respect for all, optimism, intrapersonal, and interpersonal unity, "I/We" statements, wellness of the self and others, worthiness of all humans, and being of service to others. CJPP sees "justice" as balance, rationality, harmony, orderliness, truth ideals, mortality, equity, and equality. The unconditional love found through these channels of care and justice surpasses that which is found in sympathy or even empathy.

Protection of the Human Rights of Women and Girls Under International Law

The Commission on the Status of Women (CSW) first met in 1947, soon after the founding of the United Nations, is the principal global intergovernmental body exclusively dedicated to the promotion of gender equality and the empowerment of women. From 1947 to 1962, the Commission focused on setting standards and formulating international conventions to change discriminatory legislation and foster global awareness of women's issues. It contributed to the drafting of the Universal Declaration of Human Rights, and also drafted the early international conventions on women's rights, such as the 1953 Convention on the Political Rights of Women; the 1957 Convention on the Nationality of Married Women; the 1962 Convention on Consent to Marriage, Minimum Age for Marriage and Registration of Marriages; the International Labor Organization's 1951 Convention concerning Equal Remuneration for Men and Women Workers for Work of Equal Value; and in 1979, the Commission drafted the Convention on the Elimination of All Forms of Discrimination against Women (CEDAW), and also worked on the Beijing Declaration and Platform for Action.

Convention on the Elimination of All Forms of Discrimination Against Women (CEDAW, 1979)

The Convention on the Elimination of All Forms of Discrimination against Women (CEDAW) is an international treaty adopted by the UN General Assembly in 1979. It is considered an international bill of women's rights and has been ratified by 189 countries except for the United States and Palau. In its preamble and a total of 30 articles, it defines what constitutes discrimination against women and provides an action agenda to end that discrimination. The CEDAW Committee consists of 23 global experts on women's rights, and its primary goal is to work toward achieving equality between men and women and end discrimination against women.

Vienna Declaration, 1993

When the agenda for the 1993 World Conference on Human Rights in Vienna, Austria did not originally mention women or any gender aspects of human rights, the women's rights movement brought attention to the issue of violence against women. As a result, the Vienna Declaration addressed the elimination of violence against women in public and private life as a human rights obligation. When the UN General Assembly adopted the

Declaration on the Elimination of Violence against Women in December 1993, it was the first international instrument to specifically address the issue that violence against women constitutes a violation of the rights and fundamental freedoms of women.

Beijing Declaration, 1995

The Beijing Declaration focused on 12 areas concerning the implementation of women's human rights and an agenda for women's empowerment. It was at the Beijing Conference that Hilary Clinton famously stated, "Women's rights are human rights." Participating governments agreed on a comprehensive plan to achieve global legal equality called the Beijing Platform for Action, which covered areas of concern such as women in power and decision-making, girl children, women and poverty, women in the economy, violence against women, human rights of women, the environment, women in power, education and training of women, institutional mechanisms for the advancement of women, women and health, women and the media, and women and armed conflict.

Sustainable Development Goals (SDGs)

The SDGs are 17 global goals designed to be a "blueprint to achieve a better and more sustainable future for all" and were set up in 2015 by the United Nations General Assembly and are intended to be achieved by the year 2030. The 2030 Agenda for Sustainable Development (2030 Agenda) is a landmark agreement negotiated and approved by the 193 Member States of the United Nations. The 17 SDGs include 169 targets and 232 indicators of sustainable development (Boudet et al., 2018) and provide a framework for action for member states. SDG #5, that is, Gender Equality is a dedicated goal that aims to end discrimination between women and men. The focus of SDG 5 Gender Equality is to achieve gender equality and empower all women and girls. There are 9 targets and 14 indicators defined for this SDG.

1. 5.1. End all forms of discrimination against all women and girls everywhere
2. 5.2. Eliminate all forms of violence against all women and girls in the public and private spheres, including trafficking and sexual and other types of exploitation
3. 5.3 Eliminate all harmful practices, such as child, early and forced marriage and female genital mutilation
4. 5.4. Recognize and value unpaid care and domestic work through the provision of public services, infrastructure and social protection policies and the promotion of shared responsibility within the household and the family as nationally appropriate

5 5.5. Ensure women's full and effective participation and equal opportunities for leadership at all levels of decision-making in political, economic and public life
6 5.6. Ensure universal access to sexual and reproductive health and reproductive rights as agreed in accordance with the Program of Action of the International Conference on Population and Development and the Beijing Platform for Action and the outcome documents of their review conferences
7 5.a. Undertake reforms to give women equal rights to economic resources, as well as access to ownership and control over land and other forms of property, financial services, inheritance and natural resources, in accordance with national laws
8 5.b. Enhance the use of enabling technology, in particular information and communications technology, to promote the empowerment of women
9 5.c. Adopt and strengthen sound policies and enforceable legislation for the promotion of gender equality and the empowerment of all women and girls at all levels

These goals recognize the multiple forms of disadvantages experienced by women and girls especially as it relates to access to quality education, health and well-being, and protections against inequalities and gender discrimination. These SDGs also acknowledge that many of the deprivations experienced by women and girls are intensified for women and girls who are living at the intersection of inequalities and discrimination. Gender equality is also central to the achievement of all 17 SDGs even if gender might not be the focus of a particular SDG. The 2030 Agenda reflects the indivisibility and interdependence of rights, the interlinkages between gender equality, and the three dimensions of sustainable development, that is, social, economic, and environmental. For women and girls, different dimensions of their well-being and deprivations are deeply intertwined. For example, a girl who is born into a poor household (Target 1.2) and forced into early marriage (Target 5.3), for example, is more likely to drop out of school (Target 4.1), give birth at an early age (Target 3.7), suffer complications during childbirth (Target 3.1) and experience violence (Target 5.2) than a girl from a higher-income household who marries at a later age (Boudet et al., 2018).

Despite the global agreement and commitment to the cause of women and children, in an analysis of the SDGs related to gender, it was found that of the 129 countries studied, no country has fully achieved the promise of gender equality envisioned in the 2030 Agenda. Nearly 40% of the world's girls and women—1.4 billion—live in countries that are failing on gender equality (scores of 59 or less out of 100) and another 1.4 billion live in countries that "barely pass" (scores of 60–69 out of 100; Boudet et al., 2018).

The Human Rights Framework in Practice

Women and Poverty—Standard of Living and Implications Throughout the Lifespan

Table 13.1 lists the UDHR Articles and SDGs that address issues related to women living in poverty.

Gender inequalities make women and girls more vulnerable than men and boys to poverty (Boudet et al., 2018). Other gender based differences in families and communities related to gender norms, division of assets, work and responsibility, and relations of power further widen these disparities (Grown, 2014). Gender inequalities in labor markets also contribute to women's greater vulnerability to poverty. Women are more likely to participate in the informal economy, which lacks non-wage protective benefits such as health insurance, pensions, paid sick leave, and maternity leave (ILO, 2016). Women and girls are also more likely to be providers of unpaid care within the household. For women and girls, certain life events at specific age groups correlate with higher poverty rates. For women and girls who are married, widowhood, divorce, or separation affect them more negatively than men (Boudet et al., 2018). Poverty experienced by women and girls is also a result of accumulated deprivation of quality education, decent work, health, and well-being. These disadvantages are further intensified for those living at the intersection of inequalities and discrimination. Gendered social norms influence institutional policies and laws that define women's and men's access to productive resources. Persistent gender inequality maintained and sustained by many social policies further make it impossible for women to emerge out of poverty.

While there is substantial research to support the claim of gendered poverty, emerging theories have challenged the indicators used to measure female poverty. Poverty measured through income alone does not capture the entirety of the experience of women or girls who work. Chant (2011) has posited the concepts of time poverty, asset poverty, and power poverty

Table 13.1 Poverty

Universal Declaration of Human Rights	*Sustainable Development Goals*
Article 25: Right to adequate standard of living	SDG 1: End Poverty in all forms
Article 22: Right to social security	SDG 2: End hunger, achieve food security and promote sustainable agriculture
Article 2: Right to equality and non-discrimination	SDG 5: Gender Equality Achieve gender equality and empower all women and girls
Article 3: Right to life, liberty and security of person	SDG 10: Reduce inequalities

which are all interrelated to some extent. Time poverty, for example, refers to the type of poverty that emerges because of the loss of time engaged in earnings due to childbirth, child rearing, or other familial-care providing duties. In this instance, while the women are engaging in income-generating activities while potentially reducing their income poverty, the fact that they exit and reenter the income-generating activity because of their care-providing responsibilities lead them to be "time poor." Other contributing factors to time poverty are also poorer indicators for health, which is a direct result of neglect due to their already subservient position in the family and community. Asset poverty is reflected in the lack of ownership of assets that could be in the form of savings, land, or property ownership. Power poverty refers to circumstances in gendered cultural and/or social norms that result in women and girls having limited control over their lives and decision-making processes that impact them. These three types of poverty are direct outcomes of human rights laid out in the UDHR.

Time poverty: right to rest and leisure, work conditions
Asset poverty: right to own property
Power poverty: right to decision making

Strategies to address poverty experienced by women and girls must address the gender dimensions of health, education, employment, climate change, environmental degradation, urbanization, migration, and conflict and peace.

As a result of the current pandemic, studies suggest that up to 400 million people will be forced below the poverty line of $1.90 a day when the immediate impact of the pandemic is combined with the effects of the profound global economic slowdown that many economists are forecasting (Chadwick, 2021). Continuing with the pre-pandemic global trends, the majority of these people will be women.

Right to Education for Women and Girls

Table 13.2 lists the UDHR Articles and SDGs that address issues related to education for women and girls.

Table 13.2 Education

Universal Declaration of Human Rights	*Sustainable Development Goals*
Article 26: Right to education.	SDG 4: Inclusive and equitable quality education and life-long learning opportunities
Article 2: Right to equality and non-discrimination	SDG 5: Gender Equality and empowerment of all women and girls
Article 3: Right to life, liberty and security of person	SDG 10: Reduce inequalities

Another issue of women's and girl's rights is the imbalance in a lack of access to education and information. The lack of access to quality education for girls has lifelong implications for women. The Global Citizen organization lists seven main causes of a lack of access to education faced by young girls (Rodriguez, 2019). First, oftentimes when families around the world are lacking in funds necessary for education, they choose to send their sons, rather than daughters, for a formal education. Parents may choose to have their daughters marry as teens so the financial responsibilities for them are no longer incumbent upon them, which leads into the second cause. Child marriage around the world perpetuates teenage pregnancy, pregnancy issues, and domestic violence rates. It also prevents women from getting proper, uninterrupted education. Next, in many countries, school attendance drops for girls as they reach puberty when families are unable to buy sanitary products or due to the stigma of the "impurity" of menstruation. Household chores and gender-based violence are other issues that preclude women and girls from becoming educated and literate. Yet another cause is women and girls on the move due to displacement or migration or a combination of both. The ensuing instability directly impacts their access to quality education. Lastly, in countries with political or civil unrest due to wars or conflicts, schools are often targeted. Children, especially girls, already have less access to education but during conflicts and attacks on schools have long-lasting impacts when girls lose access to education.

The lack of education of girls affects their life trajectory into womanhood and beyond. For example, mothers' levels of health literacy and education directly impact their children's health outcomes (Robinson, 2000). This poses the danger of intergenerational inequity. Women's lack of education in childhood can lead to them becoming unpaid laborers. Another issue in adulthood after a lack of education during childhood is that of unpaid laborers in the world, of which women make up three quarters (Right to Education, 2018a). Contrarily, when girls' education is fairly equalized, according to UNICEF (n.d.), the following domains in women's lives begin to improve. These include the decline of child marriage rates, the decrease of child mortality, lower rates of maternal mortality, less child stunting and growth rate declines, and an increase in the lifetime earnings of girls and women.

Some rights infringements when it comes to women's rights are included in various human rights conventions and covenants over the years (Right to Education, 2018b). These include the Convention on the Elimination of All Forms of Discrimination against Women of 1979. In Article 10, section a, stages of education throughout the lifespan are addressed. The demanded equality in education includes that of preschool education, general and technical education, vocational training, and higher education. Section C of this article calls for the elimination of stereotyping of female roles in education, which includes coeducation and equalizing texts and education materials.

The Right to Education (2018b) also lists the UNESCO Convention against Discrimination in Education of 1960 as another stand against education imbalance. Article 1 defines education access as equality and acceptable standards of learning conditions, levels, and overall access.

Women's and Girl's Right to Health

Table 13.3 lists the UDHR Articles and SDGs that address issues related to health of women and girls.

Women's right to health includes their rights to sexual and reproductive health. A wide range of human rights conventions and policy instruments developed since the 1960s address the issue of women's sexual and reproductive health rights. These include the rights of women to control matters related to their sexuality; to decide on whether, when and how many children to have; to be informed about and have access to family planning; to be able to access reproductive and maternal healthcare; and to access safe abortion under some circumstances (Boudet et al., 2018). International human rights frameworks set important normative standards around women's reproductive rights because women's reproductive agency has a critical bearing on the broader conditions of their lives, including their physical and emotional well-being, their economic opportunities, and their participation in political processes. In general, discriminatory social norms and inadequate reproductive healthcare services pose major barriers to women's ability to negotiate their rights within families, communities, and even in the larger economy and polity.

Some examples human rights laws related to sexual and reproductive health are as follows:

1. Article 12 of the International Covenant on Economic, Social and Cultural Rights (ICESCR, 1966).
2. Article 16 of CEDAW (1979) guarantees women equal rights in deciding "freely and responsibly on the number and spacing of their children and to have access to the information, education and means to enable them to exercise these rights."

Table 13.3 Health

Universal Declaration of Human Rights	*Sustainable Development Goals*
Article 3: Right to life, liberty and security of person	SDG 3: Good Health and Well-being.
Article 2: Right to equality and non-discrimination	SDG 5: Gender Equality and empowerment of all women and girls
Article 27: Right to enjoy the benefits of scientific progress and its application	SDG 10 Reduce inequalities

3 The 1994 International Conference on Population and Development (ICPD) which provided a first comprehensive definition of reproductive rights, which rests on "the recognition of the basic right of all couples and individuals to decide freely and responsibly the number, spacing and timing of their children and to have the information and means to do so, and the right to attain the highest standards of sexual and reproductive health."
4 The Beijing Platform for Action (1995) reinforced these commitments, stating that "the human rights of women include their right to have control over and decide freely and responsibly on matters related to their sexuality, including sexual and reproductive health, free of coercion, discrimination and violence." (Cornwall et al., 2008)
5 In 2016, the Committee on the Rights of the Child urged States "to adopt comprehensive gender and sexuality-sensitive sexual and reproductive health policies for adolescents, emphasizing that unequal access by adolescents to such information, commodities and services amounts to discrimination."
6 The CEDAW Committee and the Committee on the Rights of Persons with Disabilities have emphasized the need to guarantee the sexual and reproductive health and rights of women with disabilities.
7 In 2018, the Human Rights Committee stated in General Comment 36: "States parties must provide safe, legal and effective access to abortion where the life and health of the pregnant woman or girl is at risk, or where carrying a pregnancy to term would cause the pregnant woman or girl substantial pain or suffering, most notably where the pregnancy is the result of rape or incest or is not viable."

Those who identify outside of gender norms, whether in terms of gender identity, gender expression, or otherwise, often experience discrimination, violence, and stigma, as well as mental health struggles and suicidality (WHO, 2019). These issues are perpetuated by strict gender norms. One form of discrimination experienced by those outside of gender norms or the dominating gender(s) is less access to proper health care service, health information, support, and positive medical outcomes. Healthcare should be equitable, affordable, and accessible to all. Additionally, it should be acceptable and provided with quality and dignity. However, women and girls have consistently received poorer health services and information than men and boys, contributing to a greater risk to their wellbeing and overall health. This inequality extends to areas of adverse community and provider attitudes, lower decision-making power, poorer literacy rates, mobility restrictions, and less-than-desirable training and awareness for healthcare providers, all of which negatively impact health outcomes in women and girls. Statistically, women and girls are disadvantaged when it comes to health challenges such as sexually transmitted diseases (STDs), including human immunodeficiency virus (HIV), unintended pregnancies, cervical cancer, poorer vision, and respiratory infections. Women also face greater levels of malnutrition, gender-based violence, and elder abuse.

Violence Against Women and Girls

Table 13.4 lists the UDHR Articles and SDGs that address issues related to violence experienced by women and girls.

Violence against women and girls (VAWG) is one of the most prevalent and systemic human rights violations in the world, often described as a public health crisis or a pandemic. The following forms of violence include:

- Sexual violence: Any conduct or behavior that by threat, intimidation, coercion or use of force—results in a woman or girl witnessing or participating in non-consensual sexual contact or behavior that violates her bodily integrity and sexual autonomy.
- Physical violence: Any conduct or behavior that inflicts physical harm and offends the bodily integrity or health of women and girls.
- Psychological violence: A range of behaviors that encompass any act of emotional abuse and controlling behavior that causes "emotional damage, reduces self-worth or self-esteem, or aims at degrading or controlling a woman's actions, behaviors, beliefs and decisions."
- Economic violence: Any conduct or behavior whereby an individual denies their intimate partner access to financial resources, typically as a form of abuse or control or in order to isolate them or to impose other adverse consequences on their well-being.

Women and girls throughout the world experience physical, sexual, psychological, and economic violence with long-term effects to their physical, mental, and emotional wellbeing. Around one-third of women worldwide have experienced physical and/or sexual violence by an intimate partner and 18% have experienced such violence in the past 12 months. Regardless of where the women live, that is, developed countries or developing countries,

Table 13.4 Violence

Universal Declaration of Human Rights	*Sustainable Development Goals*
Article 3: Right to life, liberty and security of person	SDG 5: Gender Equality and empowerment of all women and girls
Article 4: No one shall be held in slavery or servitude	SDG 3: Good Health and Well-being.
Article 5: No one shall be subjected to torture or to cruel, inhuman or degrading treatment or punishment.	SDG 16: Peace, Justice and Strong Institutions for inclusive societies.
Article 2: Right to equality and non-discrimination	SDG 10 Reduce inequalities

violence experienced by women often peaks during their reproductive years and although it declines somewhat with age, it persists among older women. While intimate partner violence is the most common form of violence, women and girls are subject to a range of other forms of violence within the family and community. Violence is also perpetuated at local, national, and global levels due to political, economic, and social factors.

Experiencing violence has serious and enduring impacts on the lives of women and girls detrimentally affecting their psychological and physical health, well-being, educational outcomes, political participation, economic security, and their ability to engage in socio-cultural aspects of their lives. For example, women and girls who have been physically or sexually abused are almost twice as likely to experience depression and, in some regions, are 1.5 times more likely to contract HIV, compared to women who have not experienced partner violence. VAWG in the family also has significant intergenerational impacts, increasing the risk of violence for future generations.

Decades of relentless efforts by advocates of women's rights, feminists, and other activists to protect the human rights of women against violence has resulted in some progress. UN data from 2012 or 2019 shows significant attitude changes—women's acceptance of violence by their partners decreased in almost 75% countries; a few countries have recorded a decrease in intimate partner violence and female genital mutilation is becoming less common. There is also a growing global recognition of violence against women and girls as a priority for sustainable development, which has led to the introduction of laws, action plans, protection and support services, and prevention measures.

Despite these positive developments, many of these initiatives remain poorly implemented in countries all over the world. A reaction against this culture of impunity and state-sanctioned violence against women and girls, especially sexual violence and harassment, can be seen in recent global and national movements such as #MeToo, #TimesUp, #BalanceTonPorc, #NiUnaMenos, and HollaBack! These movements have demanded and led to an increased focus on the accountability of perpetrators and the systems and institutions that were created to protect women against violence. These movements have also drawn attention to the common systemic and structural causes that underpin all forms of violence. Persisting violence against women and girls reflects the existence of underlying social norms and attitudes that normalize, justify, and excuse violence. In many cultures, violence is a tool to reinforce male dominance and as a means of discipline and subordination when patriarchal authority and power are being threatened. Violence is also more likely to be perpetrated when support for its use is normalized. And extreme evidence of this can be commonly found in regions where armed conflict takes place. Conflict-related sexual violence—including rape, forced sterilization, and sexual slavery—is widespread but grossly underreported. In many cases, there is a lack of support from the state, whether in the form of investigation and prosecution or support for the survivors.

Even before being born, girls are susceptible to violence when women are forced to abort female fetuses. For example, in India, despite laws that ban gender identification of fetuses, infanticide is very common. Girls are at risk of child marriage, female genital mutilation, honor killings, kidnappings, forced sex work, forced servitude, and human trafficking. While there is lack of global data, many research studies have highlighted that being a woman or girl who is Indigenous, identifies as queer, living with a disability, or an insecure migration status increases their risk of violence.

Violence against women and girls is recognized as a gross violation of human rights and several human rights instruments, including the Universal Declaration of Human Rights (UDHR), emphasize that the right to live a life free of violence is an unalienable human right. Elimination of violence against women is also imperative to meeting SDG 5, gender equality, and the empowerment of all women and girls. Other SDGs such as SDG 3 (ensure healthy lives and promote well-being for all) and SDG 8 (Promote sustained, inclusive and sustainable economic growth, full and productive employment and decent work for all) also require that there are structures and policies in place to prevent violence and protect women and girls who are vulnerable to violence. In addition to the SDGs, General Recommendation No. 35 of UN CEDAW (issued in 2017), set out state obligations to punish perpetrators, prevent violence, and empower and support affected women.

Despite many national and international legal instruments, many women fall through the cracks and are still severely vulnerable to violence. They include Indigenous women, women with disabilities, older women, and queer women. Women also experience violence in the workplace, especially in countries where labor laws are very weak or, sometimes, non-existent. In order to protect women and girls from violence, states not only have a negative obligation to not discriminate but also have a positive duty to recognize differences and inherent inequalities and take measures to achieve and promote equality.

Human Rights of Women and Girls Who Work

Table 13.5 lists the UDHR Articles and SDGs that address work related issues for women and girls.

The labor of women and girls are broadly used in two distinct forms—paid work and unpaid work. In the past few decades, more and more women are entering the paid labor workforce. Much of the global economy consists of a service sector that far outweighs manufacturing in terms of output and the number of people employed. While professional/managerial and service positions have opened up for women in wealthier countries, women in many developing countries have been restricted to low-paying or rapidly disappearing agricultural and industrial work (Boudet et al., 2018). In most developing countries, however, even maternity leave is often unavailable except for a small group of formal sector employees. Globally,

Table 13.5 Work

Universal Declaration of Human Rights	*Sustainable Development Goals*
Article 23: Right to work in just and favorable conditions	SDG 8: Decent Work and Economic Growth
Article 4: Prohibition of slavery or forced labor	
Article 2: Right to equality and non-discrimination	SDG 5: Gender Equality and empowerment of all women and girls
Article 3: Right to life, liberty and security of person	SDG 10: Reduce inequalities

only 28% of working women are effectively covered by cash benefits in the event of maternity (Boudet et al., 2018). Women around the world experience work-related discrimination, exploitation, and poor labor conditions. The International Labour Organization (2016) cites various targets within the Sustainable Development Goals (SDGs) that relate to gender inequality, such as equal access to education (SDG 4), overall gender equality (SDG 5), decent work for all (SDG 8), equal pay (SDG 8), and equal opportunity (SDG 10). Those who identify as a sexual, gender, racial, ethnic, ability, or migrant minority are at further risk, as seen from an intersectionality lens. Women's discrimination faced at work includes voicelessness, lack of opportunity, social exclusion, and indecent work conditions and hours, all of which perpetuate poverty among women.

The disproportionate responsibility for unpaid care falls on women and girls and is further responsible for creating many constraints to their income-earning capacity. The reduced earning capacity increases their financial dependence on husbands and partners while weakening their families' ability to escape poverty (Boudet et al., 2018). As a result of globalization and a highly internationalized economy, many women, regardless of their educational levels and professional training, are becoming more mobile in seeking economic opportunities, often moving to a closer urban setting or even across countries. As migrant women workers, they are already disadvantaged by their migrant status and racial identity and are more susceptible to the poor conditions and a lack of labor protections that characterize the low-wage economy of care and domestic work. Not having access to income-generating work to escape poverty and to be financially independent directly influences their ability to accumulate savings, invest in assets, and plan for their retirement. The disproportionately high time spent on providing unpaid care renders them to be "time poor" and "income poor" and can have intergenerational ramifications.

A number of international human rights treaties such as the Beijing declaration, the International Covenant on Economic, Social and Cultural Rights, the Convention on the Elimination of All Forms of Discrimination against Women, and the Convention on the Rights of the Child recognize this and highlight the importance of addressing the unequal distribution of paid and unpaid work between women and men as critical toward achieving gender equality. These treaties contain specific provisions guaranteeing the right to work, just and favorable conditions of work, freedom to form trade unions, and the prohibition of discrimination based on sex. Most recently, the ILO has also passed a convention on eliminating violence and harassment at work. This is much needed considering the trends related to technological changes, demographic changes, accelerated globalization, and environmental degradation. Improving and protecting the human rights of women to work will involve the redistribution of power and resources. The COVID-19 pandemic further exacerbates many of the negative outcomes for women who engage in paid and unpaid work. Globally, women make up 70% of frontline workers in the health and social sector across a range of occupations and also already bear a disproportionate responsibility for the care of children, the elderly, and people with disabilities (United Nations [UN], 2020). The pandemic is further intensifying and increasing the risk and vulnerability toward economic insecurity. To protect the rights of women and girls at work, it is imperative that structural and systemic discrimination is specially addressed.

Women in Power and Decision-Making

Table 13.6 lists the UDHR Articles and SDGs that address issues related to power and decision making for women and girls.

A recent video that has been widely circulated in the United States shows images of women heads of state from 23 countries plus the United States with Vice President Kamala Harris, as well as women's and girl's inspirational leaders such as Greta Thunberg and Amanda Gorman. The introduction

Table 13.6 Power and decision-making

Universal Declaration of Human Rights	*Sustainable Development Goals*
Article 6: Right to recognition everywhere as a person before the law.	SDG 5: Gender Equality and empowerment of all women and girls
Article 7: All are equal before the law without any discrimination	SDG 16: Peace, Justice and Strong Institutions for inclusive societies.
Article 20: Right to freedom of peaceful assembly and association.	SDG 10: Reduce inequalities
Article 21: Right to take part in the government directly or through representatives and right to equal access to public service.	
Article 2: Right to equality and non-discrimination	
Article 3: Right to life, liberty and security of person	

is "While the world has been distracted by all those resistant to change, change has been happening." This portrayal of the strength and compassion of women leaders is consistent with the data retrieved from the most recent report of the 17 SDGs that showed the countries that showed achievement on SDG 3 (insuring healthy lives and promotion of well-being for all at all ages), SDG 5 (achieve gender equality and empower all women and girls), SDG 10 (reduced inequality within and among countries), and SDG 16 (achievement of peace and justice) were more likely to be headed by a woman. The five countries that showed achievement on SDG 16 (peace and justice) are Finland, Austria, Slovenia, Ireland, and Iceland (De Neve & Sachs, 2020). Of these five countries, Finland and Iceland are headed by women, and Ireland was headed by a woman up until several years ago. Although Norway has not yet shown achievement on SDG 16, it does show achievement on all of the other three SDGs we analyzed, and the prime minister is a woman (Erna Solberg), and 40% of the parliamentarians are women. It is the only country that reached achievement on all of the three SDGs that were compared, as well as affordable and clean energy (7); decent work and economic growth (8); sustainable cities and communities (11); life on land (15); and partnerships for the goals (17). Norway also has free or low-cost access to health care, education, and welfare, and it is a gender-egalitarian society with parental benefits and full access to day-care for all.

We note that the United States is ranked 31 overall and has not reached achievement on any of the 4 SDGs we analyzed. However, with the election of Kamala Harris as Vice-President and great numbers of women in the Biden administration, there is some reason to be hopeful for change.

Environment and the Human Rights of Women and Girls

Table 13.7 lists the UDHR Articles and SDGs that address issues related to the environment and women and girls.

The state of the environment has a direct relationship with the human rights of women and girls. In every humanitarian crisis that follows a natural disaster or an environmental adversity, women and girls face significant vulnerability to their health, safety, and their economic, social, and political well-being. For example, research studies have underscored the heightened risk of violence that women and girls face, loss of livelihood, and displacement (Boudet et al., 2018). This also triggers off complex trajectories of combined and accumulated vulnerabilities that spill over to all domains of human rights for women and girls. While many developing countries grapple with the dilemma of development at the cost of environmental sustainability, women who are already marginalized in those communities are worse off due to underlying structural discrimination, unequal access to land and natural resources, and lack of access to sustainable infrastructure. Declining access to natural resources in the context of climate change also

Table 13.7 Environment

Universal Declaration of Human Rights	*Sustainable Development Goals*
Article 25: Right to a standard of living and the right to security	SDG 5: Gender Equality and empowerment of all women and girls
Article 27: right to enjoy the benefits of scientific progress and its application.	SDG 11: Sustainable Cities and Communities which are inclusive, safe, resilient and sustainable
Article 2: Right to equality and non-discrimination	SDG 6: Ensure availability and sustainable management of water and sanitation for all
Article 3: Right to life, liberty and security of person	SDG 7: Affordable and Clean Energy Ensure access to affordable, reliable, sustainable and modern energy for all
	SDG 10: Reduce inequalities
	SDG 15: Protect, restore and promote sustainable use of ecosystems
	SDG 13: Climate Action-combat climate change and its impacts

increases the burden of heavy unpaid care and domestic workloads for the poorest women and girls.

At the same time, women often play an important role, particularly in developing countries, in the conservation of the natural environment and ensuring that the efforts toward climate interventions are more effective. Women also play a key role in agriculture by promoting natural resources management, which is critical to adaptation to climate change (UN, 2020). However, the secondary social status due to gender and other means of social exclusion renders their expertise in local and traditional knowledge to not being recognized.

Eco-feminists have long propounded that when principles of feminist theory are combined with ecological restoration and preservation, there will be positive outcomes for the human rights of women because eco-feminism challenges the oppressive forces of economic exploitation, patriarchy, racism, and sexism.

Migration and the Human Rights of Women and Girls

Table 13.8 lists the UDHR Articles and SDGs that address issues related to migration and women and girls.

A gender perspective is essential to understanding both the causes and consequences of international migration. Gender inequality can be a powerful factor in precipitating migration for women and girls when they lack economic, political, and social opportunities in their home countries. While migration can be an empowering experience for women and girls as they

Table 13.8 Migration

Universal Declaration of Human Rights	*Sustainable Development Goals*
Article 22: Right to Social Security	SDG 1: End Poverty in all forms SDG 3: Good Health and Well-being.
Article 2: Freedom from Discrimination	SDG 5: Gender Equality and empowerment of all women and girls SDG 10: Reduced inequality
Article 23: Right to Work Article 24: Right to Rest and Leisure Article 9: Freedom from Arbitrary Detention Article 13: Freedom of Movement Article 14: Right to Asylum Article 15: Right to Nationality	SDG 8: Decent Work and Economic Growth GOAL 16: Peace and Justice Strong Institutions

move away from traditional patriarchal societies, it also exposes them to many vulnerabilities during their migratory journey as well as post migration.

Various international human rights instruments specifically or generally enumerate the rights of migrants such as the International Covenant on Civil and Political Rights; the International Covenant on Economic, Social and Cultural Rights; International Convention on the Protection Rights of All Migrant Workers and Members of Their Families; the Protocol to Prevent, Suppress and Punish Trafficking in Persons, Especially Women and Children, supplementing the United Nations Convention against Transnational Organized Crime; and the Protocol against the Smuggling of Migrants by Land, Sea, and Air, supplementing the United Nations Convention against Transnational Organized Crime.

However, there are many national laws on emigration and immigration of voluntary migrants that include discriminatory provisions that affect the protection of migrant women. For example, policies exist that make it harder for female migrants to bring their husbands and children to join them, require pregnancy tests, bar emigration of women without their guardian's permission, and impose age limits on immigration or emigration of women and girls.

Women and girls who are refugees or asylum seekers face additional threats to their physical safety in addition to legal problems. Many factors contribute to the vulnerability of refugee and displaced women and girls to sexual violence and exploitation as they navigate new laws and policies far from home while lacking the traditional communal support systems. Power relations in situations where women and children are dependent on aid may increase vulnerability to sexual exploitation. Equal access to food and other essential items is a key issue for refugee and displaced women and children, as is their participation in decisions regarding their future and that of their families.

Another sub-group of migrant women are those that are trafficked for prostitution and forced labor and often find themselves trapped into forced prostitution, marriage, domestic work, sweatshops, and types of exploitation that constitute a contemporary form of slavery. While this is a very common occurrence within any country in the world, it has severe ramifications when women experience it as migrants as the migrant status adds to their vulnerability. International migration affects gender roles and opportunities for women in destination countries and in transit countries. In general, labor participation by female immigrants is lower than among the native population, and unemployment rates among women immigrants in the labor force are generally higher. Migrant women workers are also less likely to be protected by labor laws, especially when they are engaged in the informal sector of the economy.

Migration can profoundly affect the health and well-being of both migrating women and their families, as well as women and families that stay behind when spouses migrate. The impact on women's mental health and well-being along with their physical health and wellbeing is complex and involves many factors including access to healthcare, language and cultural barriers, and lack of resources. The mental and physical health and wellbeing is further compromised when women are a part of irregular migration. For example, women and girls who are victims of trafficking are at high risk of injuries and sexually transmitted diseases along with mental health problems resulting from the trauma. Similarly, refugee women and girls may suffer from post-traumatic stress disorder with little or no recourse to adequate care, treatment, or support owing to the lack of a social support network.

Conclusion

We have provided an overview of the human rights and the lack thereof of women and girls globally, using a theoretical and conceptual framework. While our focus is on the inequalities and violations of their human rights that women and girls worldwide have experienced and continue to suffer, we offer some positive signs of change such as the increase in numbers of women leaders globally and the relationship between women leaders and an increase in equality and well-being in the countries they head. The #MeToo and Black Lives Matter Movement have a positive impact on women and girl's access to equity and equality and freedom from poverty, abuse, oppression, and discrimination.

Although the human rights of women and girls have been enshrined in the UDHR and then later in CEDAW, 1979, and the Beijing World Conference, 1995, the gender gaps in "traditional" data (women's activities, women's needs, interests, threats, achievements) have been largely invisible. The UN SDGs offer some real-time monitoring of gender progress and highlight a few countries where women and girls experience gains in well-being, equality, and social justice. It is our hope that social work practice can have a more positive political and personal influence on supporting and realizing the human rights of women and girls.

References

Boudet, M., Maria, A., Buitrago, P., De La Briere, L., Newhouse, B., Locke, D., Matulevich, R., Carolina, E., Kinnon, S., Becerra, S., & Pablo. (2018). *Gender differences in poverty and household composition through the life-cycle: A global perspective (English)* (Policy Research working paper; no. WPS 8360). Washington, DC: World Bank Group.

Boyd, S. B. (1997). *Challenging the public/private divide: Feminism, law, and public policy* (Revised ed.). University of Toronto Press, Scholarly Publishing Division. Retrieved from https://books.google.com/books?id=g4LEkytI0RwC&printsec=frontcover#v=onepage&q&f=false

Brodsky, J. (2019, June 12). Law and the #MeToo movement. *Fordham Law*. Retrieved from https://news.law.fordham.edu/blog/2019/06/12/law-and-the-metoo-movement/

Carr, E. S. (2003). Rethinking empowerment theory using a feminist lens: The importance of process. *Affilia*, (18), 1.

Chadwick, A. (2021). Afterword: Poverty and human rights. In *Poverty and Human Rights*. Edward Elgar Publishing.

Chant, S. H. (Ed.). (2011). *The international handbook of gender and poverty: concepts, research, policy*. Edward Elgar Publishing.

Chevez-Duenas, Y., & Adames, Y. (2021). Intersectionality awakening model of womanista: A transnational treatment approach for Latinx women. *Women & Therapy, 44*(1–2), 83–100.

Christens, B., Peterson, N. A., & Speer, P.W. (2011). Community participation and psychological empowerment: Testing reciprocal causality using a cross-lagged panel design and latent constructs. *Health Education & Behavior, 38*(4), 589–598.

Convention on the Elimination of All Forms of Discrimination against Women. (1979). Retrieved from https://www.ohchr.org/sites/default/files/cedaw.pdf

Cornwall, A., Correa, S., & Jolly, S. (2008). *Development with a body: Sexuality, human rights and development*. London: Zed Books.

Crenshaw, K. (1991). Mapping the margins: Intersectionality, identity, politics and violence against women of color. *Stanford Law Review, 43*, 1241–1299.

De Neve, J. E., & Sachs, J. D. (2020). The SDGs and human well-being: A global analysis of synergies, trade-offs, and regional differences. *Scientific Reports, 10*(1), 1–12.

Dominelli, L. (2003). *Anti-oppressive social work theory and practice*. New York, NY: Red Grove Press.

Freire, P. (1973). *Education for critical consciousness*. Seabury, NY: Crossroad Publishing Company.

Garza, A. (2020). *The purpose of power: How we come together when we fall apart*. New York, NY: Random House.

Greer, C. (2021, March 18). *Interlocking pandemics* (Webinar). New York, NY: Black History Month Webinar.

Grown, C. (2014). Missing women: Gender and the extreme poverty debate. *A Paper Prepared for USAID under Award# AID-OAA-0-13-00103 Mod, 1.*

Gutierrez, L. M., Parsons, R. J., & Cox, E. O. (1998). *Empowerment in Social Work Practice. A Sourcebook*. Brooks/Cole Publishing Co.

Hamilton, L., Hunt, V., Murphy, Y., Norris, A. N., & Zajicek, A. M. (2009). *Incorporating intersectionality in social work practice, research, policy, and education*. Baltimore, MD: Port City Press.

International Covenant on Economic, Social and Cultural Rights. (1966). Retrieved from https://www.ohchr.org/sites/default/files/cescr.pdf

International Labour Organization. (2016). *10. Gender equality and non-discrimination*. Retrieved from www.ilo.org/global/topics/dw4sd/themes/gender-equality/lang--en/index.htm

Jordan, J. (2017). *Relational-cultural psychotherapy*. Washington, DC: American Psychological Association.

Maschi, T., & Kaye, A. (2019). *Unconditionally LGBTQIA+: Moving from victimization and criminalization to liberation* (PowerPoint slides). New York: Fordham University

Maschi, T., Kaye, A., & Rios, J. (2020, Fall/Winter). Co-constructing community with 2020 vision of care and justice. In *National association of social work specialty practice. Sections: Mental health newsletter*, pp. 5–9.

Maschi, T., & Morgen, K. (2020). *Aging behind prison walls: Trauma and resilience*. New York, NY: Columbia University Press.

Maschi, T., Morgen, K., Bullock, K., Kaye, A., & Hintenach, A. M. (2021). Aging in prison and the social mirror: Reflections and insights on care and justice. *Journal of Elder Policy, 1*(2), https://doi.org/10.18278/jep.1.2.6

McCann C, & Kim S. (2016). *Feminist theory reader: Local and global perspectives*. New York, NY: Routledge.

Miley, K., O'Melia, M., & DuBois, B. (2011). Assessing resource capabilities. *Generalist social work practice: An Empowering Approach*, 235–271.

Mullaly, B. (2017). *Challenging oppression and confronting privilege*. New York: Oxford.

Radačić, Ivana. (2007). Human rights of women and the public/private divide in international human rights law. *Croatian Yearbook of European Law and Policy, 3*(3). https://doi.org/10.3935/cyelp.03.2007.42

Right to Education. (2018a). *Early childhood care and education*. Retrieved from www.right-to-education.org/issue-page/early-childhood-care-and-education

Right to Education. (2018b). *International instruments: Girls' and women's right to education*. Retrieved from www.right-to-education.org/sites/right-to-education.org/files/resource-attachments/RTE_International_Instruments_Girls_Women_Right_to_Education.pdf

Robinson, M. (2000). *Universality and priorities*. United Nations Development Programme: Human Developments Reports. Retrieved from www.hdr.undp.org/en/content/universality-and-priorities#:%7E:text=Simply%20stated%2C%20universality%20of%20human,to%20inalienable%20rights%20and%20freedoms.&text=%E2%80%9CEveryone%E2%80%9D%20is%20entitled%20to%20rights,race%2C%20sex%20or%20other%20status.

Rodriguez, L. (2019, September 24). *7 Obstacles to girls' education and how to overcome them*. Global Citizen. Retrieved from www.globalcitizen.org/en/content/barriers-to-girls-education-around-the-world/

Turner, S., & Maschi, T. (2015). Feminist and empowerment theory and social work practice. *Journal of Social Work Practice, 29*(2), 151–162.

UNICEF. (n.d.). *Girls' education*. Retrieved from www.unicef.org/education/girls-education

United Nations. (2020, April). *Women's human rights in the changing world of work* (A/HRC/44/51). United Nations General Assembly. Retrieved from https://documents-dds-ny.un.org/doc/UNDOC/GEN/G20/094/80/PDF/G2009480.pdf?OpenElement

Walker, A. (1983). *In search of our mother's gardens*. New York, NY: Random House.

World Health Organization. (2019, June 19). *Gender and health*. Retrieved from www.who.int/health-topics/gender#tab=tab

14 Refugees and Migrants

Stacey A. Shaw

Introduction

> *Rana was born in Afghanistan. She and her family reside temporarily in a country in Southeast Asia. During a mental health program, Rana shared her concerns about her mother, who mourned the deaths of family members and feared for those still in Afghanistan. Rana then talked about her future: she wanted to be an engineer, to build tall buildings in the devastated cities back home. What does the future hold for a young person like Rana? Her life is shaped not only by her goals, personality, intelligence, close-knit family, and religious beliefs, but by entrenched warfare, national priorities, and anti-Muslim prejudice.*

The migration of people across borders is a major feature of contemporary life. Over 3.5% of the global population reside in a nation different from that of their birth (International Organization for Migration [IOM], 2020) and over 1% have been forcibly displaced (United Nations High Commissioner for Refugees [UNHCR], 2020; terminology defined in Table 14.1). Mobility is driven by many factors, including desires for safety, livelihood, health, family, education, and survival. Opportunities to migrate and experience post-migration are shaped by global inequities of wealth and power. Among migrants, the 80 million forcibly displaced persons worldwide (UNHCR, 2020) experience barriers to social and economic justice most acutely.

This chapter examines migration in light of social justice and social work practice. Historical and current contexts of migration are explored first, with attention to forced displacement and international agreements governing refugee policy. Social work values and competencies are then discussed as a foundation for rights-based social work with migrant communities. With attention to the lived experiences of people like Rana and her family, we also examine macro, mezzo, and micro social work approaches that promote social justice. Throughout the chapter, examples are drawn primarily from U.S. refugee resettlement but also attend to international contexts of protracted displacement. Research on migrant experiences and services is incorporated throughout the chapter, including qualitative, historical, longitudinal, systematic review, and intervention methods utilized in the

DOI: 10.4324/9781003111269-17

Table 14.1 Migrant Definitions

Term	*Definition*
International migrant[a]	Someone who has changed his or her country of usual residence (IOM, 2020)
Forcibly displaced person	Refugees, asylum-seekers, internally displaced people, and Venezuelans displaced abroad (UNHCR, 2019)
Asylum seeker	Someone whose request for sanctuary has yet to be processed (UNHCR, 2021b)
Internally displaced person	Someone who has been forced to flee their home but never crossed an international border (UNHCR, 2021a)
Refugee	Someone who has been forced to flee his or her country because of persecution, war, or violence. A refugee has a well-founded fear of persecution for reasons of race, religion, nationality, political opinion, or membership in a particular social group (UNHCR, 2021a)
Stateless person	Someone who is not a citizen of any country (UNHCR, 2021a)

a Terms such as "migrant" and "forced migrant" do not have universally agreed-upon definitions (IOM, 2020; UNHCR, 2018a)

United States and internationally by the author.4 Each section begins with a scenario and ends with bullet points that summarize action-oriented strategies for social workers.

Historical Context

> *In the late 1930s, social worker Cecilia Razovsky was inundated with requests from people seeking to help their loved ones flee Europe. Working primarily with Jewish communities in the U.S., Cecilia sought to raise awareness among policy makers, community leaders, and the general public. She worked strategically within prejudiced systems to assist the few individuals who qualified for quota spots to meet strict policy guidelines. While the role of such advocates was significant, the lack of asylum opportunities for so many was devastating. After World War II, Cecilia continued to advocate for resettlement globally and improvement in refugee camp conditions.*
>
> ***(Shaw, 2018; Zucker, 2008)***

Throughout history, people have migrated with varying levels of agency. Some chose to flee when facing limited options for survival. Others moved against their will, as in the brutal displacement of enslaved peoples from the African continent during the transatlantic slave trade, and in the destruction and displacement of Indigenous peoples during European colonization of the Americas. Migration is physical: bodies in new environments adjust to new sounds, landscapes, and food sources. Migration is also social: people encounter new cultures, ideas, practices, and relationships. Over time, countries choose how to govern migration, with public opinion surrounding migrant desirability shaping national policies. In many countries, only certain types of people, and certain amounts of people, are welcomed. In the United States, policies have long restricted migration from particular regions. Examples include the Chinese Exclusion Act of 1882, prohibitions on immigration from the "Asiatic barred zone" in 1917, and national origin quotas of the 1924 Immigration Act (Gyory, 1998; Munshi, 2015; Ngai, 1999). Due to racialized notions of desirability, U.S. immigration policy through the mid-20th century favored White, Protestant immigrants from Northern European countries and the British Isles (Reimers, 1998; Smith, 1995).

Witnessing the horrors of the Holocaust during World War II, many recognized the failure of nations to respond to people facing persecution and death at the hands of the Nazi regime. In response, 149 countries agreed to global protocols, including the 1951 Refugee Convention and its 1967 Protocol, which defined refugee rights and country responsibilities. The principal of non-refoulement stipulated that people legally designated as refugees should not be returned to a country where they face threats to life or freedom (UNHCR, 2021c). These agreements guide policies regarding forcibly displaced persons and include both promises and limitations. While recognizing refugee rights, they also protect countries' interests. For example, though refugees should not be returned to an environment of persecution, there is no parallel commitment that nations accept people into a new country. This gap in commitments to civil, political, and social rights and protections has led to the proliferation of refugee camps and statelessness, where people live perpetually at borders without permanent legal status (Besteman, 2016; Chimni, 2004).

National responses to forced displacement in the decades since World War II have been influenced by both humanitarian and political motives (Darrow, 2018; Haines, 2012). Throughout the 1960s and 1970s, the United States only admitted refugees who were fleeing communism (Hamlin & Wolgin, 2012). When the United States withdrew military troops from Southeast Asia in the aftermath of the war in Vietnam, thousands fled incoming communist governments. Those with close ties to the U.S. military were prioritized for resettlement, with approximately 130,000 people from Vietnam, Cambodia, and Laos authorized for resettlement in 1975 (Bankston & Zhou, 2020). Following this conflict, the U.S. Refugee Act of 1980 formalized resettlement processes (Office of Refugee Resettlement, 2012). Founded on market-based priorities including privatization and workfare (Benson, 2016), this legislation formed the resettlement program as it exists through the present. However, after the terrorist attacks in New York on September 11, 2001, immigration and resettlement policy increasingly prioritized security and border control (Kerwin, 2005). This shift away from humanitarian aims continues to evolve.

Social Work Strategies

- *Recognition*: Social workers see limits to social justice, human rights, and human capabilities that are embedded in global and national policy frameworks.
- *Persistence*: Social workers like Cecilia Razovsky serve individuals within limited systems, while also trying to improve those systems.

Current Context

> *Uyen, who resettled to the U.S. from Vietnam, talked about recent political and social changes during an interview conducted in 2018. She described shifting meanings of symbols and a sense that prejudice had increased in the U.S., saying, "I felt a bit unsafe when I went running. If I saw . . . a truck with the American flag, then I got really nervous because I really don't know what they are going to do."*
>
> ***(Funk & Shaw, 2021)***

In the 21st century, national discontent and division have led to a re-examination of the post-World War II political order (IOM, 2020). Globally, people are increasingly connected due to the accessibility of air travel and availability of information through the Internet. The past five decades witnessed higher rates of migration, with people moving for opportunities shaped by economic growth, trade liberalization, and globalization (IOM, 2020). Forced displacement also increased due to ongoing conflicts, crises, violence, statelessness, and climate change, alongside persecution of those with minority ethnic and religious identities and lesbian, gay, bisexual, transgender, and intersex individuals (UNHCR, 2015; UNHCR, 2019). From 2010 to 2019, over 100 million people were forcibly displaced, few of whom accessed permanent, durable solutions. Half of those forcibly displaced were children, nearly half were female, and many had disabilities (UNHCR, 2019). Countries responded both with hostility and with support (Hangartner et al., 2019; Koos & Seibel, 2019). Turkey hosts the largest number of displaced people, with over 3 million refugees from Syria. The largest numbers of internally displaced people reside in Colombia (8 million), Syria (6 million), and the Democratic Republic of Congo (5 million) (UNHCR, 2019).

Growing nationalism and right-wing movements led to political realignments such as Brexit in the European Union and the election of Donald Trump in the United States. (Hogan & Haltinner, 2015; Inglehart & Norris, 2016). In addition to labeling refugees and migrants as deviant and undesirable (Khan et al., 2019), recent U.S. policies barred migrants from predominantly Muslim countries and reduced opportunities for refugee resettlement (Pierce & Bolter, 2020). Policing and profiling within migrant communities increased and gross injustices were perpetuated toward migrants and asylum seekers at the southern U.S. border (Garrett, 2020). When U.S. refugee resettlement services were reduced post-2016, many agencies closed (Darrow & Scholl, 2020), though others were able to shift to alternative sources of funding and other aspects of service provision.

In 2020, the global COVID-19 pandemic illustrated global connectivity and vulnerabilities. During the pandemic, prejudices led to increased harassment and violence toward Asian communities and migrants (Cai et al., 2021; Ruiz et al., 2020). Many refugees and migrants faced heightened risk for infection due to living and workplace conditions, as well as a lack of healthcare and protective resources (Kluge et al., 2020). Economic vulnerabilities were also heightened among refugee communities during the pandemic, with widespread loss of employment and difficulties accessing remote resources and education (Morrissey, 2021). Organizations adapted services to provide testing, address pandemic-related education and work challenges, and serve communities by phone, Internet, and socially distant visits (International Rescue Committee, 2020; National Resource Center for Refugees, Immigrants, and Migrants, 2021).

Social Work Strategies

- *Awareness:* Social workers see how structural and cultural oppression targets the most vulnerable due to gender, race, migrant status, and other intersecting identities.
- *Flexibility and creativity:* As conditions change, including policy restrictions and pandemic conditions, social workers' roles adapt, with continued attention to community rights and capabilities.

Social Work Values, Competence, and Theory

> *Devon was passionate about migrant rights and excited to begin an internship in an agency that served refugees. Soon he faced questions around how to manage cultural expectations, program and policy limitations, and professional standards. For example, should he share a meal with clients? Share his cell phone number? Develop friendships with particular clients? He also recognized that staff did not have time to fully engage with a large caseload of diverse clients. What else could he do to ensure basic needs were being met? How could he deal with the stress, frustrations, and biases he encountered in this new role?*

Professional values and theoretical paradigms guide social work responses to migration. Values of service, social justice, dignity and worth of the person, the importance of human relationships, integrity, and competence ground social work practice (NASW, 2021). In applying these values, social workers recognize that each individual who migrates has dignity and worth, meaningful relationships, and a right to be treated justly. Social workers see how conflict and oppression drive refugees and asylum seekers to migrate, and how structural and cultural oppression limit people's rights, opportunities, and capabilities post-migration (Ostrander et al., 2017).

Competencies gained through social work education guide the operationalization of values in practice, where social workers learn to effectively engage, assess, intervene, and evaluate with migrant individuals, families, groups, communities, and organizations. Social workers also learn to engage in policy practice and advance migrant rights (CSWE, 2015). Recognizing how power and oppression influence all levels of practice with migrants, social workers engage in anti-racist and anti-oppressive practices. In policy work, social workers understand social determinants of health and see how racist and anti-immigrant policies affect people's lives. Engagement with migrant communities in policy advocacy, community development, and direct practice requires the ability to work effectively across differences (Potocky-Tripodi, 2002). Social workers learn to competently engage diversity and difference related to race, ethnicity, language, legal status, national origin, sexual orientation, gender identity, and other identities, through ongoing reflection, learning, and advocacy.

The development of competency also involves application of the theories that guide social work practice. These include theories regarding social justice and human development, conflict, trauma, the strength's perspective, empowerment, systems theory, the ecological framework, and other health and behavioral models. Utilization of social work theories enables social workers to be effective in serving people while addressing systems of oppression. Both attention to unjust systems and the promotion of migrant rights and capabilities within existing systems are essential. Social workers have key roles to play in developing equitable migration polices, building responsive services, and empowering individuals and communities, including those who migrate and those who become their neighbors.

Social Work Strategies

- *Competence*: Work with migrant communities requires awareness of social work values, skills, and theory. Social workers value differences, respect client autonomy, and understand legal and service systems. In the scenario discussed, Devon learned to follow agency guidelines regarding roles and boundaries, respect client choices, and support access to other resources when needed.
- *Vision*: Social workers prioritize social justice and human rights in implementing anti-oppressive practice.

Macro: Policy Change

> *Selena, a social worker leading a resettlement agency, listened to feedback from clients and staff that the brief resettlement services provided to refugees were insufficient for many. To address this, she first secured a grant to provide extended service for clients identified as most vulnerable. State support was then received to provide extended case management services to all new arrivals in the state, utilizing federal funds. Advocates elsewhere implemented similar programs through state legislation, hoping that in time, comprehensive service models will become policy nationwide.*

Policies at the global, national, state, and local levels affect migration possibilities and conditions. Global policies point to sustainable solutions for forced displacement but have limited power to implement these solutions. In 2018, the United Nations Global Compact on Refugees re-affirmed a global framework for responding to forced displacement, with an aim to expand solutions for refugees as well as to "ease the pressures on host countries" (UN, 2018, p. 2). Durable solutions identified include voluntary repatriation or return to one's country of origin and support for those countries, permanent resettlement to a third country, and local integration within the country of first asylum (UN, 2018). These durable solutions highlight the range of pathways through which refugees can achieve permanence. Despite these solutions, the majority of the world's forcibly displaced persons remain in limbo, unable to safely repatriate, integrate locally, or resettle. Of 79.5 million forcibly displaced persons in 2020, the majority live in neighboring areas or countries with limited resources, including acute food insecurity (UNHCR, 2020). Some people are able to return to their homes, including 5.3 million internally displaced persons and 317,200 refugees in 2019 (UNHCR, 2019). But only 22,800 accessed third-country resettlement in 2020 and few accessed naturalization within their country of asylum (UNHCR, 2019; UNHCR, 2021d).

National policies form the possibilities for and conditions of migration. In the United States, federal law determines how and when people can visit or immigrate and the pathways available for accessing permanent residence (U.S. Citizenship and Immigration Services, 2021a; U.S. Department of State, 2021a). Those seeking asylum in the United States must meet the legal definition of a refugee (see Table 14.1) and can apply for asylum while in the United States or at a U.S. border (U.S. Citizenship and Immigration Services, 2021b). In 2019, 96,952 people applied for asylum at a U.S. port of entry and 210,752 applied for asylum after being placed in removal proceedings (Baugh, 2020). However, asylum proceedings generally take years within backlogged court systems. In 2019, 46,508 people were granted asylum, representing approximately 15% of the number who filed claims in the same year (Baugh, 2020).

Recent restrictive policies such as the Migrant Protection Protocols and Asylum Cooperative Agreements banned asylum for those who passed through another country prior to reaching the United States and forced people to wait in Mexico for court proceedings (American Immigration Council, 2020). Additional policies implemented to deter asylum seekers separated children from their parents and detained asylum seekers in inhumane conditions (Garrett, 2020). Structurally oppressive policies and practices such as these have devastating effects on children and families and violate basic human rights as well as international agreements regarding migrant protection (Monico et al., 2019; Wood, 2018).

Refugee resettlement involves a legal migration pathway for a limited number of people each year. Since the establishment of the U.S. Refugee Resettlement Act in 1980, a presidential determination is submitted to and approved annually by Congress. This includes the number of refugees that can be admitted as well as characteristics (such as regional origin) of those to be admitted. In 2021, a revised determination after the election of President Joe Biden indicated 62,500 refugees can be admitted to the United States during fiscal year 2021, superseding the initial allocation of 15,000 by President Trump (U.S. Department of State, 2021b). While advocates for resettlement celebrate this increase, the allocation's tie to an annual presidential designation leads to unpredictability in arrival numbers, where shifting political priorities dominate national response. Opportunities for third-country resettlement and asylum remain a solution available to only a small fraction of the world's forcibly displaced persons, and many advocates call for increased opportunities for resettlement and asylum.

Policies also govern people's post-migration experiences. Post-resettlement to the U.S., refugees can apply for permanent residence after one year and citizenship after five years. Asylum seekers access a similar pathway to permanent residence after receiving asylum but do not receive targeted resettlement services. While economic self-sufficiency remains the aim of U.S. resettlement services and policy (Halpern, 2008), longer-term assistance navigating systems is often needed. As discussed in the scenario earlier, extended case management services support refugee adjustment over time (Shaw & Poulin, 2015). Advocacy efforts to expand resettlement services in multiple states indicate the power of practitioners to influence resettlement policy and programming, though federal legislation is ultimately needed to standardize service provision nationally.

Advocacy strategies include voting for elected officials who support migrant rights, educating elected officials on problematic effects of restrictive policies, and collaborating with organizations and communities to develop and promote solutions. Campaigns that raise public awareness of migrant experiences and unite communities around specific policy goals are needed. For example, widespread, bipartisan condemnation of family separation policies at the southern U.S. border led to political backlash and policy re-evaluation (Associated Press, 2018; Pramuk, 2018). Protests, demonstrations, and messaging campaigns (Slawson, 2016) are useful tools in raising awareness and shifting discourse regarding needed policy changes.

Social Work Strategies

- *Partner in seeking solutions*: Social workers collaborate to identify and advocate for durable solutions and improve services. Strengths-based framing prioritizes migrant rights, contributions, and opportunities.
- *Advocate through civic engagement*: Social workers press for an end to inhumane policies; protection for children and families; and access to legal, humane pathways for asylum and resettlement.

Macro: Public Perceptions and Attitudes

> *Jared's community was divided. Recent experiences of bullying towards refugee Muslim youth in local public schools led to expressions of anger and fear from the targeted community and from those who felt threatened by "outsiders." Jared worked with other social work students to promote messages of solidarity. They invited families to visit a local mosque, where the Imam conducted weekly meetings with those from any religious background to learn more about Islam. Interested neighbors sought opportunities to develop friendships, celebrate events and holidays, share food, and collaborate in building understanding and solidarity.*

Global responses to migrants are influenced by a range of views. In the pre-World War II era, Jewish refugees were feared due to notions of economic competition, cultural and religious difference, and infiltration of spies or deviants (Friedman, 2017; Shaw, 2018). In recent years, similar fears are evident in discourse portraying migrants as invaders, floods, waves, and parasites (Hogan & Haltinner, 2015; Stearns, 2020). Muslim refugees in particular have been targeted, with fears reminiscent of those targeting Jewish refugees in the 1930s surrounding competition for jobs, cultural differences, and terrorist threats. In the United States, candidate and later President Donald Trump portrayed Muslims as different from Americans within an us versus them dichotomy, describing a large and diverse group of people as anti-democratic, terrorists, and religious extremists (Khan et al., 2019). Such language dehumanizes, demeans, and posits groups of people as "other," exemplifying cultural oppression. Terms such as "illegal" or "alien" also dehumanize when applied to people. Description of a person's "undocumented," "unauthorized," or "irregular" status is preferable, though this terminology also has limits (Hiltner, 2017; UNHCR, 2018b).

Othering perspectives view people as a faceless danger and may lead to conclusions that policy restrictions or unfair treatment are justified. Negative perceptions toward people who migrate center on the most vulnerable: those who have been forcibly displaced. Conversely, demeaning language is rare toward people who migrate for employment, expatriates, students, or people who cross borders temporarily as tourists. Recognizing this targeting of the most vulnerable, advocacy efforts must incorporate attention to migrant representation and public understanding.

In contrast, migrants may also be viewed as helpless victims in need of savings. When this occurs, migrants are placed on a pedestal, forced into a position of dependency, or expected to abase themselves in performative gratitude (Nayeri, 2019). Migrants deserve protection, rights, and access because of their humanity, not because they are helpless or saintly. While it is critical that the global community is aware of conflict and persecution, care is needed in the portrayal of people's experiences. Media and organizations often reduce complex lives and situations to desperate victimization and images of suffering (also termed "disaster-porn"). In response, culpable consumers often develop compassion fatigue and tune out. Phrases such as "first world problems" suggest a sense that lived experiences globally are inherently different and suffering outside high-income countries is prevalent. Such notions, including that of a "third world" or "developed country" divide and over-simplify.

Social workers can avoid these and other attitudinal pitfalls by expanding awareness of their own positionality, biases, and privileges. In addition to the learning that occurs through practice and professional training, educational resources that explore migration experiences are valuable means of improving cultural competency. Many texts, films, podcasts, and events can be used to deepen understanding (for examples, see RefugeeOne, 2019). Further, research and academic literature inform and guide evidence-based practice. Such resources can help social workers expand their understanding of migrant lived experiences as well as recognize how migrant identities intersect with gender, race, social class, and other identities in particular contexts.

Education, interaction, and advocacy are also useful in enhancing community awareness. Migrant stereotyping must be faced directly, with attention to dehumanizing language within media, community settings, and by elected leaders. Individuals with a migrant or refugee background often address these biases through sharing their experiences and vision. Prominent examples include poet Emi Mahmoud and author Kao Kalia Yang, who inspire and educate through their personal stories (Mahmoud, 2016; Yang, 2019). An elected representative to the U.S. Congress from the state of Minnesota, Ilhan Omar, originally from Somalia, advocates at the federal level for a range of policy priorities, including increased admittance of refugees and investigation of human rights abuses perpetrated against migrants and asylum seekers (Omar, 2021). Allied citizens and organizations also raise public awareness through pro-refugee campaigns, affirming media portrayals, educative events, celebratory cultural performances, sports and youth activities, volunteer and mentor opportunities, and partnership with diverse groups.

Social Work Strategies

- *Self-awareness and a holistic perspective*: Social workers see migrants as people with complex histories, desires, and strengths. They seek opportunities to learn about diverse migrant perspectives and experiences, and foster self-reflection.

- *Address community perspectives*: Social workers recognize and respond to dehumanizing stereotypes regarding migrants. They work collaboratively with migrant communities to build awareness and empathy within organizations, media, and political leadership.

Mezzo-Level Engagement With Organizations and Communities

> *Suya and her family resettled to the U.S. when she was a child. Though she recently graduated from college, she sees many friends and family members who struggle to develop literacy, find meaningful employment, and feel they belong. Suya runs a coalition with others promoting refugee access to higher education. Based on community feedback, they started a mentoring program for young adults seeking to go to college. They are also raising awareness across college campuses, creating environments where refugee students feel welcomed and included. In these efforts, she partners with national and local organizations, many of whom are represented on the coalition.*

Migrant adaptation is influenced by environmental factors and service access within the country of asylum or resettlement. Post-migration adjustment is often described as *integration*; a process influenced by migrant characteristics and dynamics in the receiving community (Strang & Ager, 2010). Efforts to achieve integration guide service provision for migrants and refugees, generally prioritizing a list of migrant outcomes or economic indicators (Taccolini & Gonzalez-Benson, 2019). The emphasis in these framings on refugee outcomes fails to adequately attend to structures and opportunities available within receiving societies (Phillimore, 2020). Possibilities for migrant integration, acceptance, and belonging are shaped not only by migrant characteristics and achievements but also by biases, fears, and socioeconomic conditions within the surrounding communities. In the United States, migrants are often viewed in light of racialized tropes. For example, model-minority myths toward Asian communities create problematic stereotypes, while also being used as a weapon to pathologize inner-city Black communities (Ong, 2003; Tang, 2015).

Newcomers may be categorized based on racial or other characteristics that take on new meanings after migrating. For example, individuals from diverse ethnic and cultural backgrounds, where race was not a salient marker of identity may resist being identified as Black post-arrival in the United States (Benson, 2006). While navigating assumptions, in-group, and out-group dynamics, migrants use agency and creativity to establish community (Besteman, 2016; Ong, 2003). In a study examining integration experiences post-resettlement, refugees emphasized the importance of social engagement and expressions of welcome (Shaw & Wachter, under review). Participants valued choosing to belong in their new home in addition to maintaining distinct cultural identities. They also described demands to "fit in" and efforts to navigate and fight assimilation. Research among Muslim American immigrants identified efforts both to aspire to and to reject dominant Whiteness (Yazdiha, 2021). This illustrates both the importance of receiving community dynamics and the social-relational components of adjustment post-arrival.

To support adaptation, government and non-profit organizations provide services to migrants and refugees based on policy, eligibility requirements, and local community resources. Agency scope is further shaped by leadership and staff capacity. Post-arrival, refugees in the U.S. access services from designated resettlement agencies, many of which are religiously affiliated (Bureau of Population, Refugees, and Migration, 2020; U.S. Department of State, 2020). Resettlement agencies' reception and placement services focus on the first 30-days post-arrival, with a check in at 90-days and 180-days. Federal government benefits are provided through state Workforce Service offices and include food stamps, Medicaid, and workfare-based cash assistance for eight months after arrival, with an aim of rapid employment and self-sufficiency (Halpern 2008; U.S. Department of State, 2020). Additional programs are available based on state and local priorities (Shaw & Funk, 2019).

People resettling in the United States as refugees prioritize safety, education, financial stability, and social connections (Shaw et al., 2021). Effective and empowering services respond to these aims rather than the limited focus on economic self-sufficiency that drives current U.S. resettlement policy. For staff members working in resettlement, balancing paperwork and reporting requirements with attention to client needs can be challenging (Fee, 2019). Effective leadership is needed within agency settings to ensure staff and clients are adequately supported. In addition, attention to client feedback through ongoing assessment, evaluation, and research can help identify organizational successes and service gaps. Such efforts to improve programs prioritize client wellbeing, allowing organizations to adjust and expand services when needed. Furthermore, migrant leadership is fostered through listening to and supporting the aims of community leaders, as well as hiring and promoting migrants in professional roles. Partnership between organizations is essential to ensure mainstream services available to migrants are linguistically and logistically accessible.

Community organizations and diaspora networks also shape refugee and migrant experiences. Mutual assistance associations include people with a shared ethnic, linguistic, or regional background, providing opportunities to promote identity and solidarity, address community issues, and raise awareness (Gonzales Benson, 2020). Religious institutions, as well as meeting places including mosques, churches, and temples, can also be important sources of identity, meaning, and social support (Allen, 2010). Neighborhood locations such as stores with foods from one's region of origin, parks, libraries, and community centers provide spaces for networking and belonging. Creative forms of community building and exchange, including gardening, farming, sports, theater, music, and food, can strengthen relationships and promote understanding. For example, mural paintings among Rohingya refugees residing in the Balukhali camp in Bangladesh inspired and educated camp residents (Brown, 2021). Gardening among Bhutanese-Nepali refugees in the United States provided opportunities for socialization, education, enhanced wellbeing, and access to traditional foods (Zavon, 2020). Social service organizations can promote creative and culturally accessible forms of community building.

Social Work Strategies

- *Evaluate experiences and services*: Practitioners invite and respond to client feedback regarding post-migration experiences and service limitations. Agency leaders prioritize client wellbeing while recognizing the influence of receiving community dynamics.
- *Promote community development*: Social workers support refugee-led organizations and foster refugee and migrant leadership. In partnership with community leaders, social workers help build responsive programs and services.

Micro-Level Casework and Mental Health Service Provision

> *Rahim valued his role as a facilitator providing mental health services to other refugees. Though he and his family faced similar challenges living in the large refugee camp, he was able to set those aside while listening to community members describe ways they coped with stress, uncertainty, and anger. He saw how mindfulness exercises and creative activities helped people relax, open up, and laugh. While such approaches would not solve people's ultimate needs for permanence and security, he felt a renewed sense of hope when seeing the way group members supported one another.*

Micro-level social work practice involves direct engagement with individuals and families. Though refugees and asylum seekers experience common challenges, each client's background and context is unique. Social workers engage with an individualized approach based on cultural humility and an awareness of structural inequalities (Ostrander et al., 2017). Empathy for client concerns is key, alongside an ability to adapt skills and practices in culturally and spiritually responsive ways (George & Ellison, 2014). Respectful engagement occurs through listening and creating a safe environment (Lau & Rodgers, 2021). Effective social workers are aware of provider-client power dynamics and openly discuss confidentiality and service limitations. Practitioners are mindful of past and present traumas and ask for permission before addressing sensitive topics. Additionally, social workers value the whole person, including social and spiritual needs (Lau & Rodgers, 2021). Successful engagement occurs when social workers value people as diverse individuals and approach practice with skills, including empathy and cultural humility.

When social workers and migrant clients do not speak a shared language, partnership with interpreters is often necessary. In many service settings, interpretation provision is legally required. In cases when interpretation is not available, families may rely on a child who has higher language proficiency than other family members. Social workers are aware of the strains this creates within families, value language skills, and develop relationships with professional interpreters. In addition to translating, interpreters can provide important guidance, understanding, and feedback as cultural brokers (Lau & Rodgers, 2021). Attention to interpreter training, supervision, and roles can ensure interpreter involvement supports beneficial client outcomes (Fenning & Denov, 2021).

Social workers who speak the same language and share a cultural background with migrant clients have valuable experiences and skills that enable connection and enhance understanding among colleagues and agency partners. While prior experience navigating asylum and resettlement is useful, it is important to remain mindful of differing circumstances for each client. Social service professionals with a refugee background often face heightened expectations from clients and communities to exceed professional roles and boundaries (Shaw, 2014). Regardless of background, social workers benefit from organizational environments that provide ongoing training, feedback, and support.

For social workers in direct practice, knowledge of local resources and an ability to support client access is essential. Due to language and cultural differences as well as the complexity of systems such as healthcare (Fadiman, 2012), some migrants need assistance learning how to ensure they and their families access adequate services. Social workers support client capacity to navigate systems and advocate for client rights, for example, through ensuring competent interpretation is provided when discussing choices regarding medical procedures or educational plans. Further, when working with migrant families, social workers attend to each family member's needs and capacities, not only to the primary applicant within the resettlement case or the individual initially presenting for services.

Mental health services comprise another component of micro-level practice and include assessment, clinical services with individuals and families, and group modalities. Some individuals benefit from individual counseling and psycho-tropic medications. Treatment approaches that have demonstrated effectiveness in reducing depression, anxiety, and post-traumatic stress disorder symptoms among refugee samples include Cognitive Behavioral Therapy, Narrative Exposure Therapy, and Eye Movement Desensitization and Reprocessing (Lambert & Alhassoon, 2015; Murray et al., 2010; Nosè et al., 2017; Robjant & Fazel, 2010). Group models are also effective in reducing mental health symptoms among refugees and asylum seekers (Badali et al., 2017; Shaw et al., 2019a; Williams & Thompson, 2011).

Barriers to formal mental health service access include stigma, language, insufficient interpretation, unstable housing, financial strain, cultural and religious beliefs, and a lack of knowledge regarding how to access services (Byrow et al., 2020). Recognizing these barriers, community engagement or spiritual and religious approaches to increasing mental wellbeing may be preferable for many. Additionally, peer outreach and peer support models in camp settings or post-resettlement are useful in overcoming barriers to mental health service access (Badali et al., 2017; Block et al., 2018; Wilber, 2009).

As much of the research examining mental health treatment among forcibly displaced persons has been conducted in high-income countries, additional resources for service provision in lower-income settings where most refugees reside is needed. When developing relevant mental health services, community partners and potential participants can guide the selection of content and process. For example, feedback on participant priorities, challenges, cultural and religious perspectives, availability, time preferences, and barriers to participation in direct intervention selection and adaptation (Shaw et al., 2019b). Providing group services in an accessible location with transportation, food, and childcare promotes participation. As service provision in camps, detention centers, and other transitory locations vary from those conducted post-resettlement settings, attention to particular contexts and capacities is needed. For example, an intervention addressing stress within camps for internally displaced persons in Northern Iraq was implemented by paraprofessionals, building resiliency through religiousness, thankfulness, kindness, courage, and hope (Lancaster & Gaede, 2020). When people reside in a state of uncertainty, with limited legal rights and opportunities, services must address migrant priorities. These may involve family reunification; support in applying for asylum, refugee status, and resettlement; advocacy for those detained or subjected to abuses; and basic needs including food, adequate housing, and health care. Psycho-social and mental health services are also valuable in these settings, but stability and emotional wellbeing may remain out of reach due to the stressors associated with displacement.

Social Work Strategies

- *Cultural humility*: Social workers in case management and clinical roles intervene with empathy and openness regarding possible solutions. They chart pathways to healing with attention to client values, strengths, and priorities. Social workers are aware of resources and ensure clients have access to needed information and professional interpretation.
- *Responsive programming*: Services are adapted to environmental contexts, with incorporation of peer support and group approaches.

Conclusion

> *Mara described mixed feelings about resettling as a child. She laughed reflecting on how shocked her family was after arriving to see homeless people living in the U.S. She appreciated her education and the pride it brought her family, but often experienced conflict with her Mother and Grandmother regarding priorities and ways of living. Mara worried about graduate school plans and dating relationships as well as the struggles facing relatives still in refugee camps in Kenya.*

Social work practice and policy enhance social justice through promoting freedom of movement, resource access, social acceptance, and opportunities for thriving. In practice, micro, mezzo, and macro efforts to support migrant wellbeing intersect. Whether working in camp settings, with migrant communities near borders, or post-resettlement, social workers engage with individuals and advocate for needed organizational, community, and political change. Key to these efforts is an ability to listen and respond with empathy. The stories, desires, and lived realities of people who migrate drive social work understanding and action. Social workers build responsive programs that treat people with respect and dignity. They advocate for migrant rights, just policies, and access to resources that enable survival as well as wellbeing and belonging.

Forced displacement due to persecution and oppression affects millions of individuals and families. While global responses indicate a level of concern through commitments not to force people to return to dangerous environments, efforts to achieve safety and permanence reach only a small fraction of people. The vast majority of forcibly displaced people survive in oppressive conditions with limited rights and few opportunities for permanence. In large part, efforts to promote human rights have failed to reach refugees and stateless persons. For the few refugees who access resettlement or asylum, services are limited. Racism and anti-immigrant perspectives within receiving communities restrict opportunities for acceptance and belonging. The traumas of displacement and integration shape people's lives and the lives of their children.

Efforts to achieve justice and honor the capabilities of refugees and asylum seekers invite social workers to engage with empathy, vision, and humility. Individuals are more than their immigration or legal status, and no one should be viewed solely by ethnicity, religion, class, sexual orientation, or any other characteristic. No child should be detained or separated from their family for seeking asylum. No family should wait decades for a chance at asylum without opportunities to learn, work, and heal. Global systems of power and governance have the potential to prioritize human life and wellbeing, but existing frameworks, including those that incorporate human rights, have not brought solutions to the vast majority of forcibly displaced persons. Going forward, realistic and creative solutions are needed to build a world that literally and figuratively makes space to welcome and value people without a country and without a home. In addition to micro-, mezzo-, and macro-level efforts, social workers can follow refugees and migrants in rethinking notions of shared responsibility, belonging, and global community.

Note

1 Recognizing limits in my experience as someone who has not experienced forced displacement, I value opportunities to learn from and work with clients and colleagues of diverse refugee backgrounds. This chapter is informed by my experiences working as a social worker in resettlement services, researching services and refugee experiences, teaching, and engaging with refugee communities in the United States and abroad. All scenarios presented draw from real experiences, though names and details have been modified (for all but Cecilia Razovsky) to maintain confidentiality.

References

Allen, R. (2010). The bonding and bridging roles of religious institutions for refugees in a non-gateway context. *Ethnic and Racial Studies*, *33*(6), 1049–1068.

American Immigration Council (2020, June 11). Fact sheet: Asylum in the United States. Retrieved from https://www.americanimmigrationcouncil.org/research/asylum-united-states

Associated Press (2018, June 18). *What's happening: Border policy fuels backlash against Trump.* Retrieved from https://apnews.com/article/1e6fbcde65664a348e3720c76e23089c

Badali, J. J., Grande, S., & Mardikian, K. (2017). From passive recipient to community advocate: Reflections on peer-based resettlement programs for Arabic-speaking refugees in Canada. *Global Journal of Community Psychology Practice*, *8*(2), 1–31.

Bankston III, C. L., & Zhou, M. (2020). Involuntary migration, context of reception, and social mobility: The case of Vietnamese refugee resettlement in the United States. *Journal of Ethnic and Migration Studies*, 1–20.

Baugh, R. (2020). *Refugees and asylees: 2019. U.S. Department of Homeland Security*. Office of Immigration Statistics. Retrieved from https://www.dhs.gov/sites/default/files/publications/immigration-statistics/yearbook/2019/refugee_and_asylee_2019.pdf

Bazant, M. (n.d.). *Micah Bazant. Refugees are welcome here*. Retrieved from https://www.micahbazant.com/welcome-here

Benson, J. E. (2006). Exploring the racial identities of Black immigrants in the United States. *Sociological Forum*, *21*(2), 219–247.

Benson, O. G. (2016). Refugee resettlement policy in an era of neoliberalization: A policy discourse analysis of the Refugee Act of 1980. *Social Service Review*, *90*(3), 515–549.

Besteman, C. (2016). *Making refuge: Somali Bantu refugees and Lewiston*. Maine, NC: Duke University Press.

Block, A. M., Aizenman, L., Saad, A., Harrison, S., Sloan, A., Vecchio, S., & Wilson, V. (2018). Peer support groups: Evaluating a culturally grounded, strengths-based approach for work with refugees. *Advances in Social Work*, *18*(3), 930–948.

Brown, P. L. (2021, Mar 19). For Rohingya survivors, art bears witness. *New York Times*. Retrieved from https://www.nytimes.com/2021/03/19/arts/design/rohingya-survivors-art-bangladesh.html

Bureau of Population, Refugees, and Migration. (2020). *Reception and placement. U.S. Department of State*. Retrieved from https://www.state.gov/refugee-admissions/reception-and-placement/

Byrow, Y., Pajak, R., Specker, P., & Nickerson, A. (2020). Perceptions of mental health and perceived barriers to mental health help-seeking amongst refugees: A systematic review. *Clinical psychology review*, *75*, 101812.

Cai, W., Burch, A. D. S., & Patel, J. K. (2021, April 3). Swelling anti-Asian violence: Who is being attacked where. *New York Times*. Retrieved from https://www.nytimes.com/interactive/2021/04/03/us/anti-asian-attacks.html

Chimni, B. S. (2004). From resettlement to involuntary repatriation: Towards a critical history of durable solutions to refugee problems. *Refugee Survey Quarterly*, *23*(3), 55–73.

CSWE. (2015). *2015 educational policy and accreditation standards for baccalaureate and master's social work programs*. Retrieved from https://www.cswe.org/getattachment/Accreditation/Accreditation-Process/2015EPAS_Web_FINAL-(1).pdf.aspx

Darrow, J. H. (2018). *Working it out in practice: Tensions embedded in the US refugee resettlement program resolved through implementation. Refugee resettlement: Power, politics and Humanitarian governance*. New York: Berghahn Books.

Darrow, J. H., & Scholl, J. H. (2020). Chaos and confusion: Impacts of the Trump administration executive orders on the U.S. refugee resettlement system. *Human Service Organizations: Management, Leadership & Governance*: 1–19.

Fadiman, A. (2012). *The spirit catches you and you fall down: A Hmong child, her American doctors, and the collision of two cultures*. Macmillan.

Fee, M. (2019). Paper integration: The structural constraints and consequences of the US refugee resettlement program. *Migration Studies*, 7(4): 477–495.

Fennig, M., & Denov, M. (2021). Interpreters working in mental health settings with refugees: An interdisciplinary scoping review. *American Journal of Orthopsychiatry*, *91*(1), 50–65.

Friedman, S. S. (2017). *No haven for the oppressed: United States policy toward Jewish refugees, 1938–1945*. Detroit, MI: Wayne State University Press.

Funk, M., & Shaw, S. A. (2021). "I remember when Donald Trump was elected. It broke a lot of refugees' hearts": Refugee perspectives on the post-2016 US political climate. *Advances in Social Work*, *21*(4), 1100–1123.

Garrett, T. M. (2020). COVID-19, wall building, and the effects on Migrant Protection Protocols by the Trump administration: The spectacle of the worsening human rights disaster on the Mexico-US border. *Administrative Theory & Praxis*, *42*(2), 240–248.

George, M., & Ellison, V. (2014). Incorporating spirituality into social work practice with migrants. *British Journal of Social Work*, *45*(6), 1717–1733.

Gonzalez Benson, O. (2020). Welfare support activities of grassroots refugee-run community organizations: a reframing. *Journal of Community Practice*, *28*(1), 1–17.

Gyory, A. (1998). *Closing the gate: Race, politics, and the Chinese Exclusion Act*. Chapel Hill, NC: Univ of North Carolina Press.

Haines, D. (2012). *Safe haven? A history of refugees in America*. Sterling, VA: Kumarian.

Halpern, P. (2008). Refugee economic self-sufficiency: An exploratory study of approaches used in office of refugee resettlement programs. *U.S. Department of Health and Human Services*. Retrieved from http://citeseerx.ist.psu.edu/viewdoc/download?doi=10.1.1.473.1584&rep=rep1&type=pdf

Hamlin, R., & Wolgin, P. E. (2012). Symbolic politics and policy feedback: The United Nations Protocol relating to the status of refugees and American refugee policy in the Cold War. *International Migration Review*, *46*(3), 586–624.

Hangartner, D., Dinas, E., Marbach, M., Matakos, K., & Xefteris, D. (2019). Does exposure to the refugee crisis make natives more hostile? *American Political Science Review*, *113*(2), 442–455.

Hiltner, S. (2017, March 10). Illegal, undocumented, unauthorized: The terms of immigration reporting. *The New York Times*. Retrieved from https://www.nytimes.com/2017/03/10/insider/illegal-undocumented-unauthorized-the-terms-of-immigration-reporting.html

Hogan, J., & Haltinner, K. (2015). 'Floods, invaders, and parasites: Immigration threat narratives and right-wing populism in the USA, UK and Australia'. *Journal of Intercultural Studies* 36(5): 520–543.

Inglehart, R. F., & Norris, P. (2016). Trump, Brexit, and the rise of populism: Economic have-nots and cultural backlash (HKS Working Paper No. RWP16–026). Retrieved from SSRN: https://ssrn.com/abstract=2818659

International Rescue Committee. (2020). *IRC in Salt Lake City responds to COVID-19*. Retrieved from www.rescue.org/announcement/irc-salt-lake-city-responds-covid-19

International Organization for Migration [IOM]. (2020). *World Migration Report 2020*. Retrieved from https://publications.iom.int/system/files/pdf/wmr_2020.pdf

Kerwin, D. (2005). The use and misuse of 'national security' rationale in crafting US refugee and immigration policies. *International Journal of Refugee Law, 17*(4), 749–763.

Khan, M. H., Adnan, H. M., Kaur, S., Khuhro, R. A., Asghar, R., & Jabeen, S. (2019). Muslims' representation in Donald Trump's anti-Muslim-Islam statement: A critical discourse analysis. *Religions, 10*(2), 115.

Kluge, H. H. P., Jakab, Z., Bartovic, J., d'Anna, V., & Severoni, S. (2020). Refugee and migrant health in the COVID-19 response. *The Lancet, 395*(10232), 1237–1239.

Koos, S., & Seibel, V. (2019). Solidarity with refugees across Europe. A comparative analysis of public support for helping forced migrants. *European Societies, 21*(5), 704–728.

Lambert, J. E., & Alhassoon, O. M. (2015). Trauma-focused therapy for refugees: Meta-analytic findings. *Journal of Counseling Psychology, 62*(1), 28–37.

Lancaster, S. L., & Gaede, C. (2020). A test of a resilience based intervention for mental health problems in Iraqi internally displaced person camps. *Anxiety, Stress, & Coping, 33*(6), 698–705.

Lau, L. S., & Rodgers, G. (2021). Cultural competence in refugee service settings: A scoping review. *Health Equity, 5*(1), 124–134.

Mahmoud, E. (2016). A young poet tells the story of Darfur. Retrieved from www.ted.com/talks/emtithal_mahmoud_a_young_poet_tells_the_story_of_darfur/transcri pt

Monico, C., Rotabi, K. S., & Lee, J. (2019). Forced child—family separations in the Southwestern US border under the "Zero-Tolerance" Policy: Preventing human rights violations and child abduction into adoption (Part 1). *Journal of Human Rights and Social Work, 4*(3), 164–179.

Morrissey, K. (2021, April 4). *Life as a refugee in San Diego was challenging enough: Then the pandemic hit*. San Diego Union Tribune. Retrieved from www.latimes.com/california/story/2021-04-04/pandemic-challenges-san-diego-refugees

Munshi, S. (2015). Race, geography, and mobility. *Georgetown Immigration Law Journal, 30*, 245.

Murray, K. E., Davidson, G. R., & Schweitzer, R. D. (2010). Review of refugee mental health interventions following resettlement: Best practices and recommendations. *American Journal of Orthopsychiatry, 80*(4), 576–585.

NASW. (2021). *Read the code of ethics*. Retrieved from www.socialworkers.org/About/Ethics/Code-of-Ethics/Code-of-Ethics-English

National Resource Center for Refugees, Immigrants, and Migrants (2021). *Bringing Covid-19 testing services directly to communities*. University of Minnesota. Retrieved from https://nrcrim.org/bringing-covid-19-testing-services-directly-communities

Nayeri, D. (2019). *The ungrateful refugee: What immigrants never tell you*. Catapult.

Ngai, M. M. (1999). The architecture of race in American immigration law: A reexamination of the Immigration Act of 1924. *The Journal of American History, 86*(1), 67–92.

Nosè, M., Ballette, F., Bighelli, I., Turrini, G., Purgato, M., Tol, W., Priebe, S., & Barbui, C. (2017). Psychosocial interventions for post-traumatic stress disorder in refugees and asylum seekers resettled in high-income countries: Systematic review and meta-analysis. *Plos One, 12*(2).

Office of Refugee Resettlement. (2012). *The refugee act*. Retrieved from www.acf.hhs.gov/orr/policy-guidance/refugee-act

Omar, I. (2021). Immigration. Retrieved from https://omar.house.gov/issues/immigration

Ong, A. (2003). *Buddha is hiding: Refugees, citizenship, the new America, vol. 5*. Univ of California Press.

Ostrander, J., Melville, A., & Berthold, S. M. (2017). Working with refugees in the US: Trauma-informed and structurally competent social work approaches. *Advances in Social Work, 18*(1), 66–79.

Phillimore, J. (2020). Refugee-integration-opportunity structures: Shifting the focus from refugees to context. *Journal of Refugee Studies, 34*(2), 1946–1966.

Pierce, S., & Bolter, J. (2020). *Dismantling and reconstructing the U.S. immigration system: A catalog of changes under the Trump presidency*. Retrieved from www.migrationpolicy.org/research/us-immigration-system-changes-trump-presidency

Potocky-Tripodi, M. (2002). *Best practices for social work with refugees and immigrants*. New York, NY: Columbia University Press.

Pramuk, J. (2018, June 18). *Trump risks political damage as he barrels forward with separating migrant families*. Retrieved from www.cnbc.com/2018/06/18/trump-risks-midterm-backlash-with-immigration-family-separation-policy.html.

Reimers, D. M. (1998). *Unwelcome strangers: American identity and the turn against immigration*. New York, NY: Columbia University Press.

RefugeeOne. (2019). *Resources for adults about the refugee and immigrant experience*. Retrieved from www.refugeeone.org/uploads/1/2/8/1/12814267/book_list_for_adults_final_version_may_2019.pdf

Robjant, K., & Fazel, M. (2010). The emerging evidence for narrative exposure therapy: A review. *Clinical Psychology Review, 30*(8), 1030–1039.

Ruiz, N. G., Horowitz, J. M., & Tamir, C. (2020). Many Black and Asian Americans say they have experienced discrimination amid the COVID-19 outbreak. *Pew Research Center*.

Shaw, S. A. (2014). Bridge builders: A qualitative study exploring the experiences of former refugees working as caseworkers in the United States. *Journal of Social Service Research, 40*(3), 284–296.

Shaw, S. A. (2018). Implications of the World War II U.S. refugee resettlement efforts of Cecilia Razovsky and Varian Fry. *Journal of Migration History, 4*, 111–133.

Shaw, S. A., & Funk, M. (2019). A systematic review of social service programs serving refugees. *Research on Social Work Practice, 29*(8), 847–862.

Shaw, S. A., Funk, M., Garlock, E. S., & Arok, A. (2021). Understanding successful refugee resettlement in the United States. *Journal of Refugee Studies, 34*(4), 4034–4052.

Shaw, S. A., Pillai, V., & Ward, K. P. (2019b). Assessing mental health and service needs among refugees in Malaysia. *International Journal of Social Welfare, 28*(1), 44–52.

Shaw, S. A., & Poulin, P. (2015). Findings from an extended case management U.S. refugee resettlement program. *Journal of International Migration and Integration, 16*(4), 1099–1120.

Shaw, S. A., & Wachter, K. (under review). "Integration is accepting refugees as equals:" Refugee perspectives on integration post-resettlement.

Shaw, S. A., Ward, K. P., Pillai, V., Hinton, D. E. (2019a). A group mental health randomized controlled trial for female refugees in Malaysia. *American Journal of Orthopsychiatry, 89*(6), 665–674.

Slawson, N. (2016, September 20). *Thousands march in London during pro-refugee demonstration*. Retrieved from www.theguardian.com/world/2016/sep/17/thousands-march-in-refugees-welcome-rally-in-london.

Smith, J. F. (1995). A nation that welcomes immigrants-An historical examination of United States immigration policy. *UC Davis J. Int'l l. & Pol'y*, 1, 227.

Stearns, J. (2020, February 28). Quick take: *Europe's Refugees*. Bloomberg. Retrieved from www.bloomberg.com/quicktake/europe-refugees

Strang, A., & Ager, A. (2010). Refugee integration: Emerging trends and remaining agendas. *Journal of Refugee Studies, 23*(4), 589–607.

Taccolini, A., & Gonzalez-Benson, O. (2019). "And slowly, the integration and the growing and the learning": Nuancing integration of Bhutanese refugees in U.S. cities. *Social Sciences, 8*(6), 1–11.

Tang, E. (2015). *Unsettled: Cambodian Refugees in the New York City Hyperghetto, Vol. 222.* Philadelphia, PA: Temple University Press.

UN. (2018). *Report of the United Nations High Commissioner for Refugees. Part II: Global compact for refugees.* New York, NY: United Nations. Retrieved from www.unhcr.org/gcr/GCR_English.pdf

UNHCR. (2018a). *'Refugees' and 'Migrants'—Frequently asked questions.* Retrieved from www.unhcr.org/en-us/news/latest/2016/3/56e95c676/refugees-migrants-frequently-asked-questions-faqs.html

UNHCR. (2018b). *Why 'undocumented' or 'irregular'?* Retrieved from www.unhcr.org/cy/wp-content/uploads/sites/41/2018/09/TerminologyLeaflet_EN_PICUM.pdf

UNHCR. (2019). *Global trends: Forced displacement in 2019.* Retrieved from www.unhcr.org/globaltrends2019/

UNHCR. (2020). *Figures at a glance.* Retrieved from www.unhcr.org/en-us/figures-at-a-glance.html

UNHCR. (2021a). *Refugee facts: What is a refugee?* Retrieved from www.unrefugees.org/refugee-facts/what-is-a-refugee/

UNHCR. (2021b). *Asylum-seekers.* Retrieved from www.unhcr.org/en-us/asylum-seekers.html/

UNHCR. (2021c). *The 1951 Refugee Convention.* Retrieved from www.unhcr.org/en-us/1951-refugee-convention.html

UNHCR. (2021d). *Resettlement data.* Retrieved from www.unhcr.org/en-us/resettlement-data.html

United Nations High Commissioner for Refugees. (2015). *Protecting persons with diverse sexual orientation and gender identities.* Retrieved from www.unhcr.org/en-us/publications/brochures/5ebe6b8d4/protecting-persons-diverse-sexual-orientation-gender-identities.html

U.S. Citizenship and Immigration Services. (2021a). *Green card eligibility categories.* Retrieved from www.uscis.gov/green-card/green-card-eligibility-categories

U.S. Citizenship and Immigration Services. (2021b). *Obtaining asylum in the United States.* Retrieved from www.uscis.gov/humanitarian/refugees-and-asylum/asylum/obtaining-asylum-in-the-united-states

U.S. Department of State. (2020). *Report to Congress on proposed refugee admissions for FY2021*. Retrieved from www.state.gov/reports/report-to-congress-on-proposed-refugee-admissions-for-fy-2020/

U.S. Department of State. (2021a). *Directory of visa categories*. Retrieved from https://travel.state.gov/content/travel/en/us-visas/visa-information-resources/all-visa-categories.html

U.S. Department of State. (2021b). *Report to Congress on the proposed emergency presidential determination on refugee admissions for fiscal year 2021*. Retrieved from www.state.gov/proposed-emergency-presidential-determination-on-refugee-admissions-for-fy21/

Wilber, R. (2009). Leveraging women's community Leadership: A model for outreach in urban refugee populations. *Policy, 30*.

Williams, M. E., & Thompson, S. C. (2011). The use of community-based interventions in reducing morbidity from the psychological impact of conflict-related trauma among refugee populations: A systematic review of the literature. *Journal of Immigrant and Minority Health, 13*(4), 780–794.

Wood, L. C. (2018). Impact of punitive immigration policies, parent-child separation and child detention on the mental health and development of children. *BMJ Paediatrics Open, 2*(1).

Yang, K. K. (2019). *About Kao Kalia*. Retrieved from https://kaokaliayang.com/

Yazdiha, H. (2021). Toward a Du Boisian framework of immigrant incorporation: Racialized contexts, relational identities, and Muslim American collective action. *Social Problems, 68*(2), 300–320.

Zavon, J. (2020). *Cultivating community and identity: Urban gardening in the Bhutanese-Nepali refugee community of Columbus, Ohio* [Doctoral dissertation]. The Ohio State University).

Zucker, B. A. (2008). *Cecilia Razovsky and the American Jewish women's rescue operations in the Second World War*. Vallentine Mitchell.

15 Conclusions

Carole Cox and Tina Maschi

The many chapters in this book underscore the critical role of human rights in a socially just society. Indeed, they emphasize how human rights and social justice are indivisible and interconnected and their crucial roles in laying the foundation for a supportive and peaceful world in which all people can thrive with dignity. At the same time, while human rights are unalterable, social justice has varying interpretations as it encompasses social, economic, and cultural meanings. The COVID-19 pandemic, which has decimated entire populations, is a vivid reminder of how human rights are still imperiled and social justice not yet a reality. The immense toll on vulnerable groups, those in poverty, older adults, and those without adequate health care has exposed how countries, even those we may consider the most developed, are still challenged to create societies where human rights and social justice are recognized and dominate.

Social justice and human rights cannot coexist with oppression, discrimination, and marginalization or in a world where the environment itself is threatened. Many of the chapters have discussed how specific populations have suffered due to oppressive attitudes and policies that deny their basic human rights and contribute to their inequality in society. Social work, among all professions, as it focuses on the individual in society and the factors that impact the individual, including dignity, autonomy, and well-being, has the responsibility to assure that all are treated in a just manner with equal access to opportunities, resources, and well-being. Understanding the barriers that obstruct groups from accessing these rights is the foundation for social work involvement.

As social workers, we are witnesses to the impact of inequalities and disparities impacting individuals and communities and the ways that human rights are violated. To be a witness and not take action for change is tantamount to ignoring our professional responsibility. Such actions can be as small as assisting a client to advocate for their children with regard to improving school services and recognizing special educational needs or as large as organizing a protest around gun violence or voter suppression. Although issues vary, social workers can play prominent roles as change agents in the pursuit of new legislation that promotes social justice.

DOI: 10.4324/9781003111269-18

As we write this book, examples of social injustice and human rights violations are occurring across the globe. Among other issues, unemployment, poverty, women's rights, reproductive rights, and the absence of appropriate medical care are impacting many countries with drastic impacts on the most vulnerable groups. Human rights violations against specific groups, noticeably migrants, have become common. All of these situations present challenges for social work involvement while also offering opportunities for social work advocacy and leadership.

The National Association of Social Workers (NASW) lists five social justice priorities for the United States (NASW, 2021).

- Voting Rights
- Criminal Justice/Juvenile Justice
- Environmental Justice
- Immigration
- Economic Justice

Each of the aforementioned priorities responds to the national concerns and disparities that continue to affect large populations within the country. Moreover, state and local chapters are encouraged to become active in one of the priority areas. This call for action is important as it sets the stage for and encourages advocacy for social change that can lead to a more just society.

The International Federation of Social Work (IFSW, 2020) asserts that the principles of social justice, human rights, collective responsibility, and respect for diversities are central to social work as they reflect its core values and principles. Building upon this foundation, IFSW has developed a new Global Agenda that stresses the future of social work as a profession that shifts from providing to people in crisis to becoming "agencies of social transformation that prevent social crisis" (IFSW, 2020). Accordingly, social work skills must be involved in co-building and co-designing communities, building relationships and networks, strengthening protections that underscore human dignity and rights, promoting the strengths of people and their roles in social development. Consequently, it calls upon social workers to advocate for policies and systems that challenge oppression, support diversity, and give voices to all of the people.

The Sustainable Development Goals (UN, 2018) discussed earlier in this book further underscore the crucial role that social work can have in creating a socially just society. The underlying pledge that no one be left behind in a world that ensures and promotes security and dignity for all. Unfortunately, the COVID-19 pandemic highlighted the extent of disparities throughout the world and the impact that they have on the most vulnerable. As countries continue to recover and strive to create stronger and more equitable systems, social work involvement can help to assure that disparities are rectified in societies that are inclusive and the rights of all are recognized.

Throughout the chapters, the roles that social workers play at the micro, meso, and macro levels have been discussed. Interventions at each level are essential to assure human rights and establish social justice. However, effectiveness necessitates self-awareness of one's own beliefs, stereotypes, and biases as these are the lenses through which one perceives and experiences the world. Concomitantly, understanding the lenses of others and how their experiences and histories have shaped their lens is equally important for the establishment of relationships and trust that are the base of all successful interventions.

Each of the chapters dealing with a special population has vividly described the specific human rights violations encountered and the accompanying social justice abuses that impinge on well-being. Micro interventions frequently involve assessments, counseling, education, and information coupled with empowerment strategies that strengthen and enable persons to advocate for their own rights. Meso interventions focus on organizations, systems, and communities that have the power to support and provide services and resources that can strengthen individuals and groups necessary for assuring their inclusion in society. Macro interventions must include advocacy and actions that seek policy changes that promote human rights while removing barriers that impede and exclude social justice.

The quest for environmental justice offers a vivid example of the linkages between these approaches. Micro interventions may involve educating persons about the dangers of pollutants and the impact they can have on health and well-being. Meso interventions can focus on businesses and governments, which permit hazardous materials to infiltrate communities while macro interventions work toward policy changes that support the environment and the people depending on it. Involving stakeholders in all phases of the interventions is important for obtaining the overarching goal of a sustainable and just environment that is inclusive of all people.

The issue of systemic racism that plagues the United States and is reflected in a myriad of policies impacting individuals and communities is another example of where social work involvement can be an important force for change. Working with individuals in the affected groups to deal with the many effects that the oppression has on them is a needed intervention. Working with Black and Brown youth who are often targeted by the police or Asian older adults who may be targeted by community persons and are liable to become fearful and isolated are important areas for micro interventions.

Dealing with systemic racism must also involve working with organizations and systems that contribute to oppression, even if unintentional. Assuring that schools have the resources to support the educational goals of students is an example of a meso intervention that can help children to succeed. At the macro level, engaging with community residents and leaders and collaborating with alliances and others concerned about the same issue can be critical for achieving sustainable change and supportive policies.

Through all change efforts, social workers should focus on working with those who will benefit from the changes. Empowering groups that have been disenfranchised and ignored by the political process to become actively involved by as participants and stakeholders. The Black Lives Matters Movement is a striking example of how a mass movement of those who had been victimized can become a strong catalyst for change. Involving all stakeholders as participants in change efforts is integral to strengthening and developing just societies.

Research Agenda

Social work scholars have asserted that applying a human rights approach to research and evaluation with vulnerable populations must move beyond deductive and quantitative ways of knowing (e.g., Maschi, 2015; Wronka, 2007). For example, in a *'Rights' Research Manifesto*, Maschi (2015) introduced a "rights research approach" that infuses a human rights lens with the practice of social work research and evaluation to address issues of individual to social structural factors that influence the life course experiences of diverse populations in diverse locations. Given that individuals who experience abuse and injustices, social workers are encouraged to emancipate themselves from mental slavery and "manifest" instead their own free minds to recognize and respond to oppression and promote equality. We suggest that adopting a rights research approach to practice research and evaluation is a pathway to personal and professional freedom and empowerment. As helpers of others, it also is a prerequisite to work most effectively to guide others through a similar liberating and empowerment process (Maschi, 2015). That is, any collective efforts of social work profession must first start with each individual social worker in which the research question lies within the self-regarding one's life purpose and passion to serve others.

Adopting a rights research approach is in fact initial step in one's ability to integrate the thinking, feeling, and doing of human rights research for the purposes of individual, group, and societal transformation. It calls for each social worker to engage in their own personal liberation in order to achieve the *mass liberation* of the profession to achieve its historical vision of the liberation of the historical and emerging underrepresented and underserved populations that the profession is charged to serve. Historical examples of how a rights research approach in theory and practice, such as the settlement house movement or friendly visitors programs, have formed the underpinnings of the art and science of contemporary human rights informed intersectional social work practice. To incorporate six theme-based strategies of a rights research approach: (1) understanding and applying a human rights lens, (2) research and evaluation that makes a difference, (3) informed decision-making, multiple perspectives, approaches, and methods, (4) social contexts, meaningful participation, relational communication, (4) holistic analysis, discerning meaning from narrative and numeric data, and (5) thoughtful sharing (dissemination) and action. These strategies can be infused in the design and implementation of research projects that are most consistent with promoting human rights and individual, family, and community well-being (Maschi, 2015; Maschi & Leibowitz, 2018).

Part of every social worker's journey ideally involves cultivating critical consciousness as the mental picture of the connection between the personal and political. For example, a clinical social work must be able to recognize the psychological and emotional impact of anti-gay legislation when working with an LGBT person and/or their family members. Social workers also refine their sixth sense to recognize power dynamics at all levels. As Reeser (2009) refers to the sociopolitical level: social workers should be aware of strategies used by the status quo (e.g., those that hold power) to maintain power and control and strategies that advance equity and fairness. Social workers also should be aware of how grassroots or the rank and file has the power to change unjust structures. And just as importantly, their social work literature on human rights and social justice underscores that social workers should engage in thoughtful reflection to guide their actions. This involves engaging in critical self-reflection and assessment of one's position (e.g., race, class, sex, and class) and how it is linked to the larger environmental context (Reeser, 2009). A social worker who has inner awareness of the self in context of the sociopolitical environment can apply this understanding to a rights-based approach to research.

Finally, as we conclude, we hope that this book offers a foundation for social work involvement in many different areas and at many different levels, from the micro practitioner to the social researcher. The problems facing societies will undoubtedly shift in the coming years, but the ethics and principles of the profession are clear. Social work is a profession of change that aims to improve lives, reduce disparities, and promote dignity and well-being. The profession recognizes that the promotion of human rights and social justice are core concepts that are critical for both individual and social development. Realizing these concepts remains a challenge, but by attempting to do so, social work can have a far-reaching impact on the world and those who inhabit it. We truly hope you enjoy the journey.

References

IFSW. (2018). *Global social work statement of ethical principles*. Retrieved from www.ifsw.org/global-social-work-statement-of-ethical-principles/

IFSW. (2020). *The Global Agenda*. Retrieved from www.ifsw.org/social-work-action/the-global-agenda/

Maschi, T. (2015). *Applying a Human Rights Approach to Social Work Research and Evaluation: A Rights Research Manifesto*. New York, NY: Springer Publishing.

Maschi, T., & Leibowitz, G. (2017). *Forensic social work: Psychosocial and legal issues across diverse populations and settings* (2nd ed.). NY, NY: Springer.

NASW (2021). Social Justice Priorities. Retrieved from https://www.socialworkers.org/Advocacy/Social-Justice/Social-Justice-Priorities

Reeser, L.C. (2009). Educating for social change in the human service profession. In E. Aldarando (Ed.), *Advancing social justice through clinical practice* (pp. 459–476). Mahwah, NJ: Lawrence Erlbaum Associates.

United Nations (2015). *The sustainable development goals*. Retrieved from https://www.undp.org/sustainable-development-goals

Wronka, J. (2007). *Human rights and social justice: Social action and service for the helping and health professions*. Thousand Oaks, CA: Sage Publications.

Index

Note: Page numbers in *italics* indicate a figure and page numbers in **bold** indicate a table on the corresponding page. Page numbers followed by "n" indicate a note.

Printed in Great Britain
by Amazon

11867701R00190